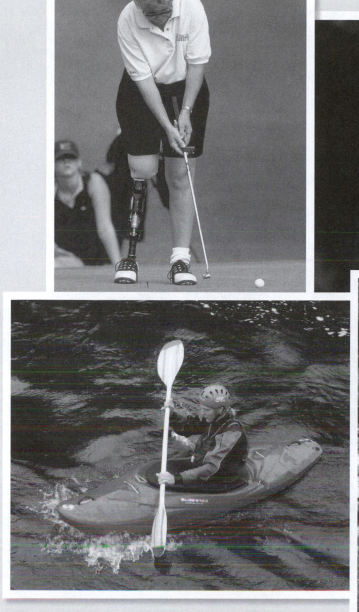
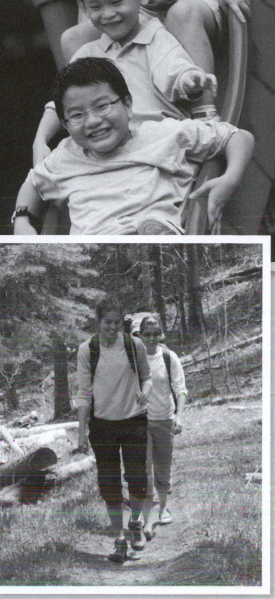
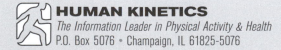

ABOUT THE AUTHOR

Diane C. Blankenship, EdD, is an associate professor at Frostburg State University in Frostburg, Maryland, where she teaches courses in research methods in the recreation and parks management program. She also serves on the program's graduate thesis and project committee.

Blankenship has extensive and varied experience, having worked as a professional Boy Scout and a recreation therapist; in residential camps, aquatic facilities, recreation centers, and outdoor recreation facilities; and for the Department of the Army in Germany.

Blankenship has used her skills in recreation and leisure research methods to assist local and state organizations in the evaluation of their programs and facilities and in strategic planning. She is a member of the Maryland Recreation and Parks Association (MRPA) and has served numerous times on the conference committee and as the coordinator of data analysis for all conference evaluations. In addition, she serves as a site visitor for the Commission for Accreditation of Park and Recreation Agencies (CAPRA) and as a recreation commissioner for the City of Frostburg.

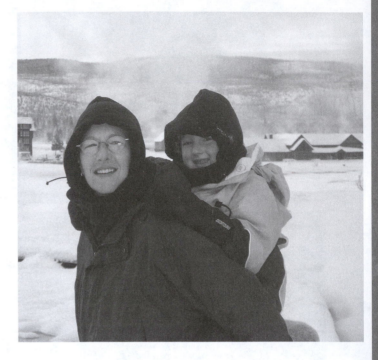

In her free time, Blankenship enjoys walking rail-trails, knitting, and traveling with her daughter to Native American reservations. She and her husband, Calvin, and their daughter reside in Frostburg.

Atlas of Vascular and Endovascular Surgical Techniques

System requirements:

- **Operating System—Windows Vista or above**
- **Web Browser—Google Chrome, Mozilla Firefox, Internet Explorer 9 and above**
- **Essential plugins—Java & Flash Player**
  - If you are experiencing problems viewing content, please check that your system has Java enabled.
  - If the video clips do not appear, your system may require Flash Player or require an update to Flash Player settings. To learn more about Flash Player settings, please click on the link in the "Help" section of the DVD.
  - You can test Java and Flash Player by using the associated links available in the "Help" section of the DVD.

Please note that this CD/DVD will only play in a computer or laptop and will not work properly in a DVD player.

This CD/DVD come with an "Autorun" function; it may take a few seconds to load on your computer. If the content does not load, please follow the steps listed below to access the contents manually:

- Click on "My Computer".
- Select the CD/DVD drive and Click "Open/Explore". A list of available files will appear.
- Find and double click the file "launch.html".

For more information about troubleshooting, please click on http://support.microsoft.com/kb/330135.

Atlas of Vascular and Endovascular Surgical Techniques

Editor-in-Chief

M Ashraf Mansour MD RPVI FACS
Professor and Chairman
Department of Surgery and
Director of Cardiovascular Medicine
Michigan State University
College of Human Medicine
Academic Chair of Surgical Specialties
Spectrum Health Medical Group
Grand Rapids, Michigan, USA

Editors

Erica Mitchell MD MEd SE FACS
Associate Professor of Surgery
Division of Vascular Surgery
Oregon Health and Science University
Portland, Oregon, USA

Murray Shames MD RPVI FACS
Professor of Surgery and Radiology
Program Director for Vascular Surgery
University of South Florida
Health Division of Vascular and
Endovascular Surgery
Tampa, Florida, USA

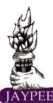

JAYPEE

The Health Sciences Publisher

New Delhi | London | Philadelphia | Panama

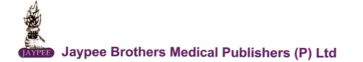
 Jaypee Brothers Medical Publishers (P) Ltd

Headquarters
Jaypee Brothers Medical Publishers (P) Ltd.
4838/24, Ansari Road, Daryaganj
New Delhi 110 002, India
Phone: +91-11-43574357
Fax: +91-11-43574314
E-mail: jaypee@jaypeebrothers.com

Overseas Offices

J.P. Medical Ltd.
83, Victoria Street, London
SW1H 0HW (UK)
Phone: +44-20 3170 8910
Fax: +44(0)20 3008 6180
E-mail: info@jpmedpub.com

Jaypee Medical Inc.
The Bourse
111 South Independence Mall East
Suite 835
Philadelphia, PA 19106, USA
Phone: +1 267-519-9789
E-mail: jpmed.us@gmail.com

Jaypee Brothers Medical Publishers (P) Ltd.
Bhotahity, Kathmandu, Nepal
Phone: +977-9741283608
E-mail: kathmandu@jaypeebrothers.com

Jaypee-Highlights Medical Publishers Inc.
City of Knowledge, Bld. 237, Clayton
Panama City, Panama
Phone: +1 507-301-0496
Fax: +1 507-301-0499
E-mail: cservice@jphmedical.com

Jaypee Brothers Medical Publishers (P) Ltd.
17/1-B, Babar Road, Block-B, Shaymali
Mohammadpur, Dhaka-1207
Bangladesh
Mobile: +08801912003485
E-mail: jaypeedhaka@gmail.com

Website: www.jaypeebrothers.com
Website: www.jaypeedigital.com

Inquiries for bulk sales may be solicited at: jaypee@jaypeebrothers.com

Atlas of Vascular and Endovascular Surgical Techniques

First Edition: **2016**

ISBN: 978-93-5152-527-1

Printed at: Ajanta Offset & Packagings Ltd., New Delhi

Dedicated to

Students, residents, and fellows
who are learning the tricks of the trade.

Contributors

S Sadie Ahanchi MD RPVI
Surgeon
Sentara Heart Hospital
Norfolk, Virginia, USA

Mark P Androes MD
Division Chief of Vascular Surgery
Department of Surgery
Greenville Hospital System
University Medical Center
Greenville, South Carolina, USA

Paul Armstrong DO
Associate Professor of Surgery
Division of Vascular and
Endovascular Surgery
University of South Florida
Tampa, Florida, USA

Amir Azarbal MD
Assistant Professor
Department of Surgery
Oregon Health and Science University
Portland, Oregon, USA

Ali Azizzadeh MD
Professor and Chief Program
Director in Vascular Surgery
Department of Cardiothoracic
and Vascular Surgery
The University of Texas
Medical School at Houston
Houston, Texas, USA

Charles Bailey MD
Vascular Surgeon
Brandon Regional Hospital
Brandon, Florida, USA

James R Ballard MD
Vascular Surgeon
Intermountain Health Care
Provo, Utah, USA

Shonda Banegas DO
Vascular Surgeon
Carondelet Heart and
Vascular Institute
Tucson, Arizona, USA

Adam W Beck MD
Assistant Professor
Vascular Surgery and
Endovascular Therapy
University of Florida
Gainesville, Florida, USA

Michael Brewer MD
Vascular Surgery Fellow
Department of Surgery
University of Southern California
Los Angeles, California, USA

Luke P Brewster MD PhD MA
Assistant Professor
Department of Surgery
Emory Clinic
Atlanta VA Medical Center
Atlanta, Georgia, USA

John G Carson MD
Assistant Professor of Surgery
University of California Davis
Sacramento, California, USA

Christopher M Chambers MD PhD
Division Chief, Surgical
Vascular Department
Spectrum Health Medical Group
Grand Rapids, Michigan, USA

Kristofer M Charlton-Ouw MD
Assistant Professor
Department of Cardiothoracic
and Vascular Surgery
The University of Texas
Medical School at Houston
Houston, Texas, USA

LeAnn A Chavez MD
Vascular Fellow
University of California Davis
Sacramento, California, USA

Tina Chen MD
Department of Dermatology
Sharp Rees-Stealy, Medical Group
Sharp Memorial Hospital
La Mesa, California, USA

Giye Choe MD
Resident
Department of General Surgery
Oregon Health and Science
University
Portland, Oregon, USA

Robert F Cuff MD RVT RPVI FACS
Assistant Professor of Surgery
Department of Vascular Surgery
Spectrum Health Medical Group/
Michigan State University
Grand Rapids, Michigan, USA

Rachel C Danczyk MD
Resident
Division of Vascular Surgery
Oregon Health and Science University
Portland, Oregon, USA

Sapan S Desai MD PhD
Vascular Surgery Fellow
Department of Cardiothoracic and
Vascular Surgery
The University of Texas
Medical School at Houston
Houston, Texas, USA

John Eidt MD
Professor
Department of Surgery—
Vascular Division
University of South Carolina
School of Medicine, Greenville
Greenville, South Carolina, USA

Mark K Eskandari MD
Chief, Division of Vascular Surgery
Northwestern University
Chicago, Illinois, USA

Anthony L Estrera MD
Professor and Chief of
Cardiac Surgery
Department of Cardiothoracic and
Vascular Surgery
The University of Texas Medical
School at Houston
Houston, Texas, USA

Lindsay Gates MD
Vascular Surgeon
Yale-New Haven Hospital
New Haven, Connecticut, USA

Patrick J Geraghty MD
Associate Professor of
Surgery and Radiology
Department of Surgery
Washington University
Medical School
St Louis, Missouri, USA

Bruce Gray DO
Department of Surgery/
Vascular Medicine
University of South Carolina
School of Medicine, Greenville
Greenville, South Carolina, USA

Tod M Hanover MD
Vascular Surgery
Greenville Health System
Greenville, South Carolina, USA

Peter Henke MD
Professor
Department of Surgery
University of Michigan
Ann Arbor, Michigan, USA

Jonathan A Higgins MBBS
Vascular and Endovascular
Surgery Fellow, Eastern Virginia
Medical School
Norfolk, Virginia, USA

Justin Hurie MD
Assistant Professor
Wake Forest University
Winston-Salem, North Carolina, USA

Jeffrey Indes MD FACS
Assistant Professor
Vascular Surgery, Yale University
New Haven, Connecticut, USA

Jason Jundt MD
Staff Vascular Surgeon
Department of Vascular Surgery
St. Charles Health System
Bend, Oregon, USA

Sharon Kiang MD
Vascular Surgeon
Ronald Reagan University
of California, Los Angeles
Medical Center
Los Angeles, California, USA

Lindsey M Korepta MD
Resident Physician
Department of Vascular Surgery
Michigan State University/
Grand Rapids Medical
Education Partners
Grand Rapids, Michigan, USA

Michelle C Kosovec MD
Clinical Instructor
Department of Vascular Surgery
Michigan State University
Spectrum Health
Grand Rapids, Michigan, USA

Marcus R Kret MD
Fellow—Vascular Surgery
Division of Vascular and
Endovascular Surgery
Stanford University
Medical Center
Stanford, California, USA

M Ashraf Mansour MD RPVI FACS
Professor and Chairman
Department of Surgery and
Director of Cardiovascular Medicine
Michigan State University
College of Human Medicine
Academic Chair of Surgical Specialties
Spectrum Health Medical Group
Grand Rapids, Michigan, USA

Kamal Massis MD
Assistant Professor
Department of Radiology
University of South Florida
Tampa, Florida, USA

Michael M McNally MD
Vascular Fellow
Department of Vascular Surgery
University of Florida
Gainesville, Florida, USA

Barend ME Mees MD PhD FEBVS
Department of Vascular Surgery
Maastricht University
Medical Center
Maastricht, The Netherlands
Royal Melbourne Hospital
Parkville, Victoria, Australia

Ross Milner MD
Associate Professor
Department of Vascular
Surgery
University of Chicago
Chicago, Illinois, USA

Erica Mitchell MD MEd SE
Associate Professor of Surgery
Division of Vascular Surgery
Oregon Health and
Science University
Portland, Oregon, USA

Maria Molnar
BSN Candidate
St. Mary's College
Notre Dame, Indiana, USA

Robert Molnar MD
Assistant Program Director
Vascular Surgery Fellowship
Michigan Vascular Center
Assistant Program Director
General Surgery Residency
Michigan State University
Director of Surgical Education
McLaren Regional Medical Center
Flint, Michigan, USA

Greg Moneta MD
Professor of Surgery,
Chief Vascular Surgery
Department of Surgery and
Knight Cardiovascular Institute
Oregon Health and
Science University
Portland, Oregon, USA

Mark D Morasch MD
Vascular Surgeon
Cardiac—Vascular Surgery
St Vincent Healthcare
Billings, Montana, USA

Neil Moudgill MD
Associate Professor
Division of Vascular and
Endovascular Surgery
University of South Florida
Tampa, Florida, USA

J Westley Ohman MD
Vascular Surgery Resident
Department of Surgery
Washington University in St. Louis
St. Louis, Missouri, USA

Jean M Panneton MD FRCSC FACS
Professor of Surgery
Chief and Program Director
Division of Vascular Surgery
Eastern Virginia Medical School
Norfolk, Virginia, USA

F Ezequiel Parodi MD
Staff
Department of Vascular Surgery
Cleveland Clinic Foundation
Cleveland, Ohio, USA

Scott Perrin MD
IR Fellow
International Radiology
University of South Florida
Tampa, Florida, USA

Alexis Powell MD
Vascular Surgeon
Assistant Professor
Case Western Reserve
University School of Medicine
Cleveland, Ohio, USA

Basel Ramlawi MD
Associate Professor of Surgery
Department of Cardiovascular Surgery
Methodist DeBakey
Heart Center
Houston, Texas, USA

Michael J Reardon MD
Professor, Cardiothoracic Surgery
Department of
Cardiovascular Surgery
Houston Methodist Hospital
Houston, Texas, USA

David Rigberg MD
Associate Professor
Department of Surgery
University of California Los Angeles
Los Angeles, California, USA

Domenic R Robinson MBBS FRACS
Department of Vascular Surgery
St. Vincent's Hospital
Melbourne, Victoria, Australia

Jean Marie Ruddy MD
Fellow
Vascular Surgery
Emory University
Atlanta, Georgia, USA

Hazim J Safi MD
Professor and Chair
Department of Cardiothoracic
and Vascular Surgery
The University of Texas
Medical School at Houston
Houston, Texas, USA

Steven Satterly BS MD
Resident
Vascular Department
Madigan Army Medical Center
Tacoma, Washington, USA

Susan M Shafii MD
Assistant Professor of Surgery
Department of Surgery
Division of Vascular Surgery and
Endovascular Therapy
Emory University, School of Medicine
Atlanta, Georgia, USA

Murray Shames MD RPVI FACS
Professor of Surgery and Radiology
Program Director for Vascular Surgery
University of South Florida
Health Division of Vascular and
Endovascular Surgery
Tampa, Florida, USA

Alexander D Shepard MD
Head
Division of Vascular Surgery
Henry Ford Hospital
Detroit, Michigan, USA

Niten Singh MD
Associate Professor of Surgery
Department of Surgery USUHS
Madigan Army Medical Center
Tacoma, Washington, USA

Jason D Slaikeu MD
Vascular Surgeon
Spectrum Health
Grand Rapids, Michigan, USA

Christopher Smolock MD
Assistant Professor
Department of Vascular Surgery
The Cleveland Clinic
Cleveland, Ohio, USA

Elliot Stephenson MD
Vascular Surgeon
Department of Vascular and
Endovascular Surgery
Minneapolis Heart Institute at
Abbott Northwestern
Minneapolis Heart Institute
Minneapolis, Minnesota, USA

Jordan R Stern MD
Resident, Department of Surgery
The University of Chicago Medicine
Chicago, Illinois, USA

Allan W Tulloch MD
Vascular Surgery Fellow
Division of Vascular Surgery
University of California Los Angeles
Los Angeles, California, USA

Ramon L Varcoe MD MBBS MS FRACS
Department of Surgery
Prince of Wales Hospital
Randwick, New South Wales, Australia

Ashley K Vavra MD
Assistant Professor of Vascular Surgery
Department of Surgery
University of Colorado
School of Medicine
Aurora, Colorado, USA

Ravi K Veeraswamy MD
Department of Surgery
Emory University School of Medicine
Atlanta, Georgia, USA

Jennifer J Watson MD
Vascular Surgeon
Spectrum Health Medical Group
The Vein Center
Grand Rapids, Michigan, USA

Mitchell R Weaver MD
Clinical Assistant Professor
Wayne State School of Medicine
Department of Vascular Surgery
Henry Ford Hospital
Detroit, Michigan, USA

Karen Woo MD MS
Assistant Professor of Surgery
Department of Surgery
University of Southern California
Los Angeles, California, USA

Bruce Zwiebel MD
Associate Professor of Radiology
Department of Radiology
University of South Florida
Tampa, Florida, USA

Preface

Our aim in writing this book is to provide a reference for learners trying to get organized before they observe, assist, or perform a vascular procedure. Many textbooks and articles are exhaustive about the indications for a procedure and the expected outcomes, but lack operational details such as positioning the patient or having the right instruments to perform the procedure. The authors and co-authors endeavor to describe how they approach some of the most commonly performed vascular procedures, whether open or endovascular. Whenever pictures or drawings are illustrative, we include them. The main references have been cited but the lists included in the chapters in this book are not meant to be comprehensive.

The chapters in this Atlas are intended to capture the little details that are often left out from the main textbook references. A lot of this information gets passed down from attending to senior fellow to junior fellow and so forth. All surgeons can attest that a difficult operation can be even more difficult if the right instruments are not there or if the patient is not positioned or prepared optimally. Most chapters include pearls and pitfalls that should help the reader stay out of trouble.

In the conceptual stages, we strive to be comprehensive in scope, covering bypass to balloon angioplasty to toe amputation. In the end, we had to compromise and leave out some procedures adequately described in other text-books. If the inclusion of additional chapters is deemed helpful to readers, we would certainly want to hear about it and to consider it for a future edition.

As technology and medicine advance, we anticipate that revisions and updates will be necessary. We hope this work will be helpful to neophytes and even young surgeons starting out their career in vascular surgery. We welcome your feedback so that future editions may fill a particular gap on your library shelf.

M Ashraf Mansour MD RPVI FACS

Acknowledgments

The writing of a medical textbook takes the effort of many individuals. I am very grateful to my associate editors who have been a tremendous help in organizing this work and executing their assignments.

I would like to thank all the authors and co-authors who have contributed time and effort to finish this Atlas. The editors would also like to thank the Senior Management Team and Production staff of Jaypee Brothers Medical Publishers in New Delhi, India, and Philadelphia, USA.

Contents

Section 6: Venous

Video Legends

Video 34.1: Initial aortogram with the flush catheter positioned in the infrarenal aorta showing lumbar arteries from the aorta, the aortoiliac bifurcation, and a stenosis in the left common iliac artery

Video 34.2: Pelvic angiogram showing a stenosis within the left common iliac artery, with patency of bilateral hypogastric and common femoral arteries as well as the proximal bilateral superficial femoral and profunda arteries

Video 34.3: Completion angiogram after deployment of a 8 × 37 mm express stent showing improved flow in the left common iliac artery

Video 44.1: Infusion catheter

Video 44.2: AngioJet

Video 44.3: Trellis

SECTION

1

Cerebrovascular

Carotid Endarterectomy

M Ashraf Mansour

1 PREOPERATIVE

1.1 Indications

- Symptomatic carotid stenosis including amaurosis fugax, transient ischemic attack, or mild stroke.
- Asymptomatic severe carotid stenosis. A risk—benefit analysis should be individualized for each patient, taking into account factors such as age, functional capacity, life expectancy, comorbidities, proven outcomes in the hospital, and operating surgeon.

1.2 Evidence

- For symptomatic carotid stenosis ECST, NASCET, and VA trial
- For asymptomatic carotid stenosis ACAS
- Comparison with carotid stenting option: CREST trial

1.3 Instruments Needed

- Picture of back table (Fig. 1.1)
- Vascular instruments and clamps
- Suture material 6.0 or 7.0 monofilament
- Back pressure line, shunt (these include: Pruitt-Inahara, Javid, and Sundt shunts)
- Patch (PTFE, Dacron, bovine pericardium)
- Cw-Doppler unit or portable duplex machine for completion study (Fig. 1.2)

1.4 Preoperative Planning and Risk Assessment

Planning:

- *Diagnostic studies*: Carotid duplex from an accredited vascular laboratory, CT angiogram, magenetic resonance angiography (MRA) or digital subtraction angiogram showing the carotid bifurcation and must include

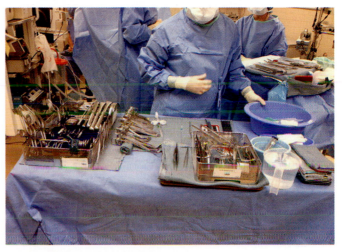

Fig. 1.1: Picture of back table.

the common and internal carotid, proximal and distal to the lesion, respectively.

- Is the patient for general or regional anesthesia?
- *Is the patient fit for surgery*: Good cardiopulmonary reserve?
- Previous operations or radiation to the neck make dissection more difficult.
- Osteoarthritis of the cervical spine and morbid obesity make positioning the neck in surgery difficult.
- High carotid bifurcation and high lesion (at C2 or higher) are best approached with nasotracheal intubation and temporary subluxation of the mandible.

Risk assessment:

- *Low risk*: No cardiopulmonary disease, no anatomical risks, e.g. previous radiation or neck surgery, degenerative disease of the spine precluding rotation, and extension (Flowchart 1.1).
- *Intermediate risk*: Low cardiac or pulmonary risk, comorbid disease such as obesity, poorly controlled hypertension and hyperlipidemia, tobacco use, and mild chronic obstructive pulmonary disease (COPD).

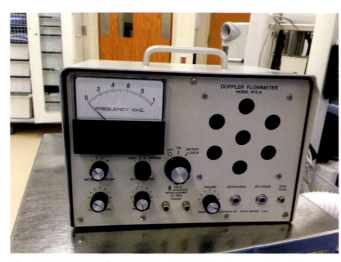

Fig. 1.2: CW-Doppler unit or portable duplex machine for completion study.

- *High risk*: Poor ejection fraction (<20%), angina or recent myocardial infarction (MI), oxygen-dependent COPD, previous radical neck dissection or neck radiation, tracheostomy, frozen neck (consider carotid stenting).

1.5 Preoperative Checklist

- Preoperative β-blockers, statins, and aspirin should be started preoperatively.
- There is no contraindication for maintaining Plavix preoperatively; however, there is an increased risk of bleeding.

Special considerations for diabetic patients:

Sign in	Time out	Sign out
Patient confirms: Identity Site Procedure Appropriate consent form	Team members introduction	Procedure performed Instrument and needle final count Labeling specimen Equipment problems to address
Site marked	Verbal confirmation from surgeon, anesthesiologist and nurse	Anesthesia and surgeon report key concerns to PACU
Anesthesia safety checklist	Anticipated critical events	
Allergy, special considerations	Antibiotic prophylaxis Preoperative imaging	

Flowchart 1.1: Decision-making algorithm.

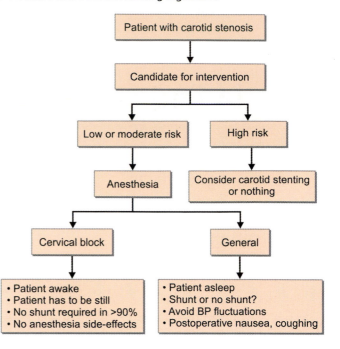

1.6 Decision-Making Algorithm

- *See* Flowchart 1.1.

1.7 Pearls and Pitfalls

Pearls:

- The length of the incision can be shortened if the carotid bifurcation is located preoperatively by duplex scan. An experienced operator with an ultrasound machine in the operating room can do this in less than a minute [(Figs. 1.3A and B). Note small oblique incision, and the angle of the mandible is marked in blue ink, note eversion endarterectomy suture line].
- An oblique incision in a skin crease is cosmetically more acceptable to patients.
- Regional cervical block is tolerated quite well and obviates the need for a shunt in over 90% of patients.
- If you plan to use a vein, don not forget to prepare a groin for vein harvest.
- The ideal position to access the neck fully is having the patient semisitting (30–45° Fowler) with the arms tucked in at the sides after insertion of arterial lines and proper intravenous access.
- In a large neck, the mini Omni retractor can be very helpful.
- Dividing the digastric muscle and ligating the small tethering vessel posterior to the hypoglossal nerve can help expose the distal internal carotid artery.

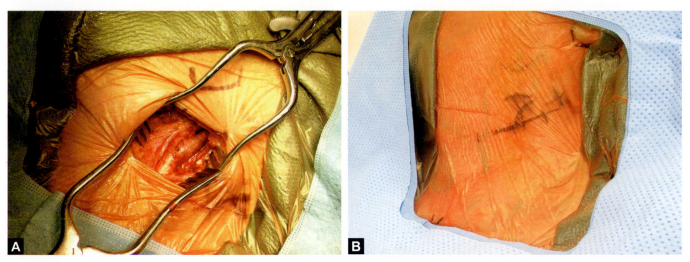

Figs. 1.3A and B: The precise location of the incision can be determined by a quick carotid duplex to show the bifurcation and mark it before prepping.

Pitfalls:
- Do not be surprised by a high bifurcation and plaque, it is better to plan for a difficult exposure with nasotracheal intubation and mandibular subluxation.
- The carotid bifurcation can be quite tortuous with the internal carotid in a posterior position.
- Be careful with dividing the facial vein, the hypoglossal can be adherent to it [(Fig. 1.4). Note hypoglossal nerve crossing the external carotid].
- Vigorous retraction can cause marginal mandibular nerve injury.

1.8 Surgical Anatomy

See Figures 1.3A and B.
- The best exposure to the carotid bifurcation is from the anterior approach.
- Beware of nerves, vagus, hypoglossal, descendens hypoglossi.
- Ligation of common facial vein to provide exposure.
- Occasionally, ligation of a tethering vessel posterior to the hypoglossal is required for high exposure.
- Injection of lidocaine in the bifurcation is necessary to treat bradycardia that occurs with carotid manipulation.

1.9 Positioning

See Figures 1.5A and B.
- I prefer a modified Fowler position, which is semisitting, with knees resting on a pillow and a small shoulder role behind the shoulders and have the neck turned to the opposite side.

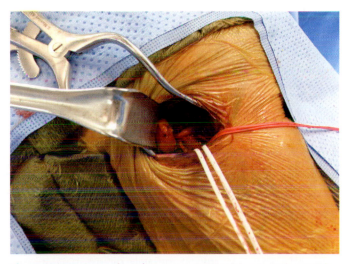

Fig. 1.4: Note hypoglossal nerve crossing the external carotid.

1.10 Anesthesia

- Most surgeons and anesthesiologists prefer general endotracheal anesthesia. There are many benefits to regional cervical block, providing the patient is able to be still, the anesthesiologist able to use minimal sedation, and the surgeon confident and relaxed.
- Supplemental local anesthesia is sometimes required after a regional cervical block, some patients experience pain with arterial manipulation.
- If bradycardia occurs during manipulation of the carotid bifurcation during dissection, Lidocaine 1% may be injected in the bifurcation with a 25G or 27G needle, or placed topically.

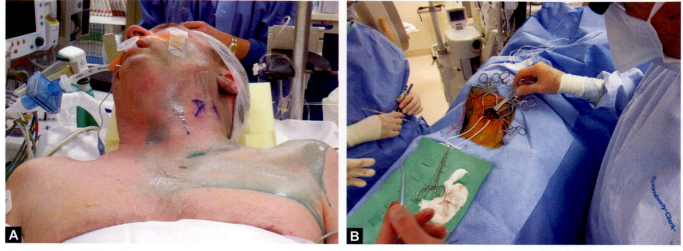

Figs. 1.5A and B: Positioning.

- A radial arterial line helps with close hemodynamic monitoring and guiding the use of pressors or antihypertensives as needed.
- Avoiding wild fluctuation in the blood pressure is important throughout the case, but especially with induction and emergence from anesthesia.

2 PERIOPERATIVE

2.1 Incision

See Figures 1.3A and B.
- The most common type of incision is a longitudinal one, along the anterior border of the sternocleidomastoid.
- Some surgeons prefer an oblique incision or an incision placed in a skin crease, it has a better patient acceptance. The precise location of the incision can be determined by a quick carotid duplex to show the bifurcation and mark it before prepping (*See* Figs. 1.3A and B).
- The disadvantage of oblique or transverse incisions is the inability to extend caudad for common carotid exposure or cephalad for a high lesion in the internal carotid artery.

2.2 Steps

- Exposure of the carotid bifurcation.
- Avoid manipulation of the vessels because a plaque may be dislodged causing a neurological complications.
- Clamp the distal internal carotid artery first.

- Decision to shunt or not, based on back pressure, or if the patient is awake and can tolerate the clamp.
- Arteriotomy on the common carotid opposite the take-off of the external carotid to allow endarterectomy and placement of a patch.
- For eversion, I prefer an oblique incision on the common carotid artery extending to the bifurcation and complete detachment of the internal carotid artery.
- The most important step of the procedure is to ensure an adequate removal of the distal plaque, and proper visualization of the end point. In rare cases, tacking sutures are necessary to avoid "lifting" of the distal shelf.
- Removal of the plaque from the common and external carotid also has to be very meticulous and avoid leaving any residual loose atheroma (Fig. 1.6).
- Copious flushing of the endarterectomy site with heparinized saline is very helpful.

2.3 Closure

- The endarterectomy site is closed primarily with 6.0 or 7.0 Prolene in eversion endarterectomy.
- A patch with Dacron, ePTFE, bovine pericardium, or vein is recommended in all other cases. Vein is preferred if infection is suspected.
- A subcuticular closure is preferred. Most patients can be discharged on postoperative day 1 and do not need to be seen for 1–2 weeks.

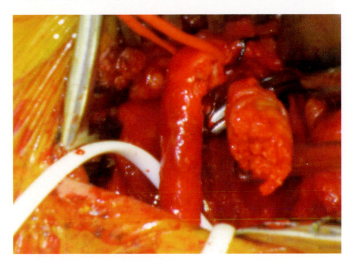

Fig. 1.6: Eversion endarterectomy.

- Some surgeons use closed suction drains, either routinely or selectively; however, there is no evidence this decreases the incidence of wound hematoma.

3 POSTOPERATIVE

3.1 Complications

- The most serious and feared complication is stroke.
- Stroke rate is higher for symptomatic lesions and redo operations.
- *Cranial nerve injury*: Vagus, hypoglossal, marginal mandibular, rarely glossopharyngeal.
- Wound hematoma requiring re-exploration.
- *Patch blowout*: More common with vein patches.
- *Wound infection or synthetic patch infection*: Quite rare in carotids.

3.2 Outcomes

- The ideal stroke rate is 1–2% in centers of excellence.
- Perioperative stroke rate is higher for symptomatic patients, and redo endarterectomy.
- The incidence of myocardial infarction should be <5%.
- Patients with cardiac risk factors had a higher MI rate in the Sapphire trial.

3.3 Postoperative Hospitalization

- After a period of 2–4 hours of close monitoring in a postanesthesia care unit, most patients may go to a vascular ward for neurological checks and vital signs every 4 hours.
- Patients with blood pressure lability require monitoring in an ICU with vasopressors if hypotensive and antihypertensive drips if hypertensive.

3.4 Discharge Instruction

- Patients should monitor their blood pressure postoperatively, and continue to take their medications (especially statins, antihypertensives, and antiplatelet agents).
- We counsel patients not to drive for a week, avoid strenuous activity, and heavy lifting.
- Wound infection is rare, but routine wound care, keeping the wound clean, and avoiding contamination is good advice.

3.5 Follow-Up

- A follow-up visit in the office 2–4 weeks postoperative is recommended for wound and neuro check.

3.6 E-mail an Expert

- *E-mail address*: ashraf.mansour@spectrumhealth.org

SUGGESTED READING

Hobson RW, Weiss DG, Fields WS, et al. Efficacy of carotid endarterectomy for asymptomatic carotid stenosis. N Engl J Med. 1993;328:221-7.

Moore WS, Barnett HJM, Beebe HG, et al. Guidelines for carotid endarterectomy: a multi-disciplinary consensus statement form the Ad Hoc Committee, American Heart Association. Stroke. 1995;26:188-201.

North American Symptomatic Carotid Endarterectomy Trial Collaborators. Beneficial effect of carotid endarterectomy in symptomatic patients with high-grade carotid stenosis. N Engl J Med. 1991;325:445-53.

Walker MD, Marler JR, Goldstein M, et al. Executive Committee for the Asymptomatic Carotid Atherosclerosis Study. Endarterectomy for asymptomatic carotid artery stenosis. JAMA. 1995;273:1421-8.

Warlow, C. European Carotid Surgery Trial: Interim results for symptomatic patients with severe (70–99%) or with mild (0–29%) carotid stenosis. Lancet. 1991;337:1235-43.

QUIZ

Question 1: Carotid endarterectomy has been proven to be superior to best medical therapy:

a. In the European Carotid Trial only (ECST)
b. In the North American Trial only (NASCET)
c. In the VA asymptomatic carotid trial only
d. In the Asymptomatic Carotid Atherosclerosis Study only (ACAS)
e. All the above.

Question 2: The benefit of carotid endarterectomy hinges on the track record of the surgeon performing the operation and keeping stroke rates at a minimum. The guidelines suggest that stroke rates after carotid endarterectomy should be:

a. Less than 3% for asymptomatic patients
b. Less than 5% for symptomatic patients
c. Less than 10% for redo surgery
d. A and B are correct
e. A, B and C are correct.

Question 3: Carotid eversion endarterectomy:

a. Cannot be performed if the patient needs an indwelling shunt
b. Has a higher rate of restenosis compared to endarterectomy with patch closure
c. Cannot be performed in awake patients
d. Its main advantage is that it is faster and does not require a patch
e. Cannot be performed if the internal carotid is redundant.

Aortic Arch and Four-Vessel Cerebral Angiography

Lindsey M Korepta, Jason D Slaikeu

1 PREOPERATIVE

1.1 Indications

- Diagnosis of acquired or congenital vascular disease of the aortic arch, carotid arteries, vertebral arteries, or intracranial arteries
- Preparation and planning for arterial interventions and procedures
- Evaluation after an arterial intervention

Contraindications:

- Severe obesity
- Inability of patient to lay still and supine during the procedure
- Severe peripheral artery disease that limits access

Relative contraindications:

- Iodinated contrast allergy
- Metformin
- Anticoagulation (e.g. warfarin with elevated INR)
- Severe coagulopathy, thrombocytopenia
- Pregnancy (require shielding of the fetus)
- Acute or chronic renal failure
- Active bleeding (e.g. gastrointestinal)
- Uncontrolled hypertension
- Renal insufficiency

1.2 Evidence

- Cerebral angiography is safe, cost-effective, and yields an accurate estimate of stenosis and plaque composition in cerebrovascular disease.
- Cerebral angiography is the gold standard for diagnosis of four-vessel cerebrovascular disease.[1-3]
- Approximately 74–85% of the general population have a "classical" arch configuration (Fig. 2.1).[4]
- Anatomical variants have important implications in the planning of future endovascular interventions.

- The most common anatomical variants include a bovine arch (20%) and an aberrant takeoff of the left common carotid artery (36%), as demonstrated in Figure 2.2.[5-7]
  - Aortic arch aberrancies are depicted in Figures 2.3A to F.
- The remaining arch anomalies are rare and include an aberrant left vertebral artery, an aberrant right subclavian, a right-sided aortic arch, a double aortic arch, and an aberrant left subclavian.
- In addition to congenital abnormalities, the aortic arch changes shape with age and hypertension. Different classifications schemes have been proposed for classifying types of arches.
- The classification scheme that we employ divides aortic arches into three types (Fig. 2.4).

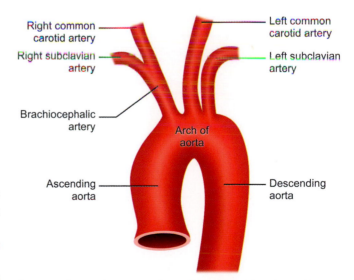

Fig. 2.1: Classical aortic arch configuration. The classical aortic arch consists of a left-sided aortic arch with three branches in the order of first the brachiocephalic trunk, second the right common carotid artery, and third the right subclavian artery.

- The aortic arch type has implications for future endovascular interventions.

1.3 Materials Needed

Imaging equipment:
- Standard imaging equipment is necessary. This includes a fixed-mounted imaging unit or portable fluoroscopy unit with video screens (Figs. 2.5A and B and 2.6).
- Floating-table carbon fiber bed

- Power injector
- Iodinated or nonionic contrast agents

Personal protective equipment:
- Leaded apron
- Thyroid shield
- Leaded eye shields

Arterial access:
- Clamp (e.g. hemostat), local anesthetic, 22-gauge arterial puncture needle, starting guidewire (0.035 in.), scalpel blade, 4-Fr or 5-Fr sheath (Fig. 2.7).

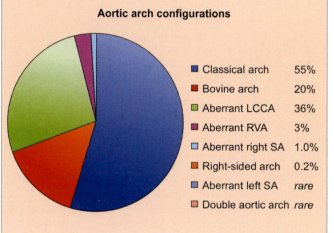

Aortic arch configurations

Classical arch	55%
Bovine arch	20%
Aberrant LCCA	36%
Aberrant RVA	3%
Aberrant right SA	1.0%
Right-sided arch	0.2%
Aberrant left SA	*rare*
Double aortic arch	*rare*

Fig. 2.2: Percentages of aortic arch configurations. While the majority of persons have a classical aortic arch configuration, the most common variants include a bovine arch, an aberrant left common carotid artery (LCCA) with the remainder of rare anatomical configurations include an aberrant right vertebral artery (RVA), an aberrant right subclavian artery, a right-sided arch, an aberrant left subclavian artery (SA), or a double aortic arch.

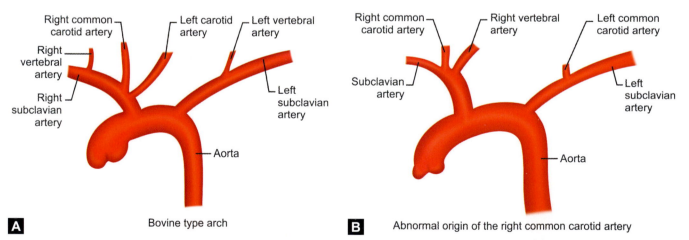

A Bovine type arch

B Abnormal origin of the right common carotid artery

Figs. 2.3A and B: Diagrams of aortic arch variants. A bovine arch has a common origin of the BCT and right CCA. The left CCA can have a common origin with the BCT or arise off of the BCT. The left VA can arise from the arch between the LCCA and the LSA. An aberrant right SA can arise posterior to the left subclavian artery. A right-sided aortic arch crosses the right mainstem bronchus and then descends along the spine. A double aortic arch occurs when the ascending aorta bifurcates anteriorly to the trachea and esophagus, with one coursing to the left of the trachea and esophagus and the other to the right. (A) Bovine type arch. (B) Aberrant right common carotid artery.

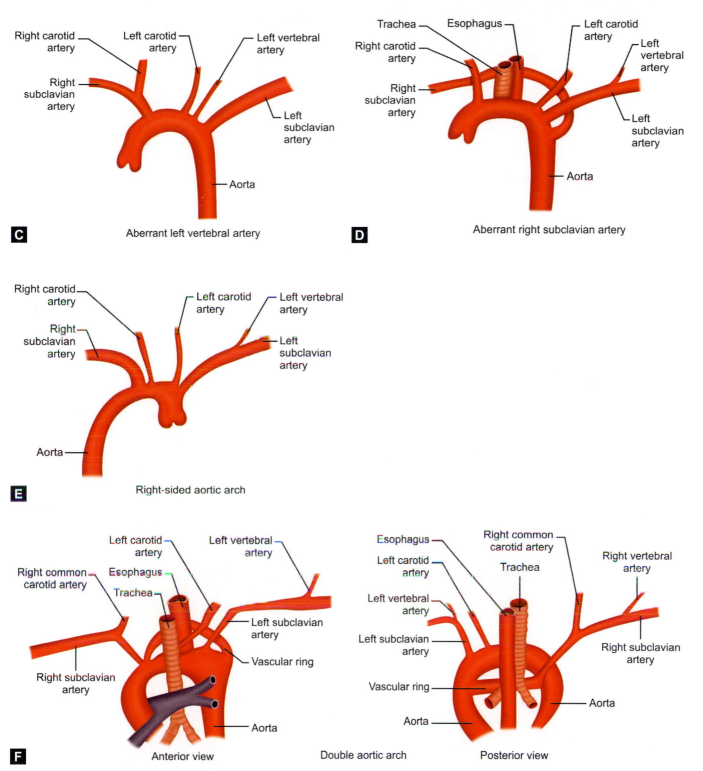

Figs. 2.3C to F: (C) Aberrant left vertebral artery. (D) Aberrant right subclavian artery. (E) Right-sided aortic arch. (F) Double aortic arch. (BCT: Brachiocephalic trunk; CCA: Common carotid artery; LCCA: Left common carotid artery; LSA: Left subclavian artery; SA: Subclavian artery).[7]

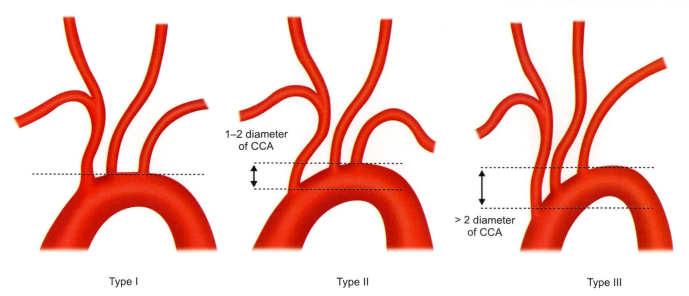

Fig. 2.4: How to classify aortic arch types. The vertical distance from the origin of the BCT to the top of the arch determines the arch type. This distance is <1 diameter of the CCA in a type 1 arch, between 1 and 2 CCA diameters in a type 2 arch, and >2 CCA diameters in a type 3 arch. (BCT: Brachiocephalic trunk; CCA: Common carotid artery)
Source: Uchino et al.[6]

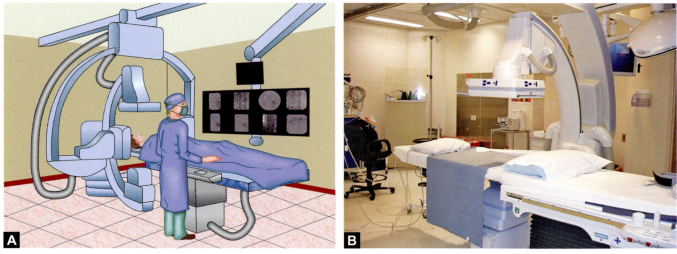

Figs. 2.5A and B: Artist rendering (A) illustrating positioning and screens. Actual hybrid operating room photograph (B).

Wires:
- Exchange length Newton or Bentson wire (0.035 in.)
- Selective glidewire 260 cm (angled tip 0.035 in.)

Catheters:
- 100-cm pigtail flush catheter
- Inventory of 4-Fr or 5-Fr catheters with lengths ≥100 cm (Fig. 2.8)
- Selection of the appropriate catheter is dependent on arch anatomy

Closure devices (optional):
- An inventory of closure devices based on surgeon preference should be available, if desired

Tips:
- H1 Headhunter catheter can be used to enter the branches of the aortic arch.
- Simmons catheter is used to cannulate the carotid and brachiocephalic arteries.[8,9]
- Shepherd hook catheter is used to cross the aortic bifurcation.

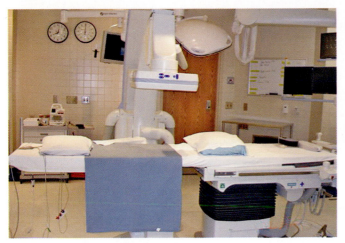

Fig. 2.6: Endovascular suite. Another image of our hybrid endovascular suite.

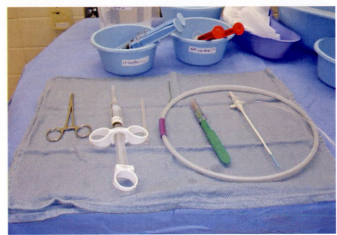

Fig. 2.7: Sterile access devices. The proper setup for arterial access includes a syringe for local anesthetics, a scalpel, a clamp, a 22-gauge arterial puncture needle, No. 11 scalpel blade, gauze pads, and a starting guidewire.

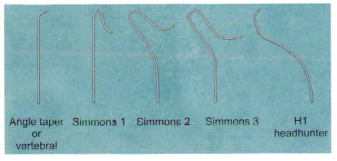

Angle taper or vertebral   Simmons 1   Simmons 2   Simmons 3   H1 headhunter

Fig. 2.8: Choosing a catheter for selective arteriography. 4-Fr or 5-Fr, 100 cm or greater selective cerebral catheters with either a simple curve (angled Glidecath, angled Glidecath, Vert, or H1 Headhunter), or complex curve (Simmons 1, Simmons 2, Simmons 3).

- Simmons catheters are especially useful in type 3 aortic arches.

1.4 Preoperative Risk Assessment

- *Low risk*:
  - Patients without hypertension, diabetes, or significant comorbidities
- *Medium/high risk*:
  - Significant atherosclerosis of access vessels and aortic arch
  - Hypertension
  - Renal insufficiency (can be managed with hydration and N-acetylcysteine)
  - Severe cardiac or pulmonary dysfunction
  - Iodinated contrast allergy

1.5 Preoperative Checklist

- *Sign in*: Pause for verification of the identity of the patient, site, and side of intervention.

- *Time out*: Ensure that all of the necessary equipment and staff are available and present within the operating room. Review the patient's allergies and confirm the administration of the proper antibiotics.
- *Time in*: After all staff are in agreement, the surgery can begin.

1.6 Postoperative Checklist

- *Debriefing*: Review of the operation including preoperative and postoperative diagnoses, including any complications or equipment failures encountered during the procedure. The final instrument and sponge counts are then verified.

1.7 Decision-Making Checklist

Catheter recommendations for selective catheterization of branches of the aortic arch:
- Brachiocephalic trunk/right subclavian/right carotid:
  - *H1 catheter*:

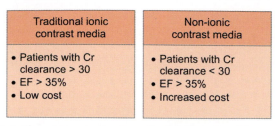

Traditional ionic contrast media	Non-ionic contrast media
• Patients with Cr clearance > 30 • EF > 35% • Low cost	• Patients with Cr clearance < 30 • EF > 35% • Increased cost

Fig. 2.9: Choosing a contrast media. Decision algorithm to help guide choice of contrast media for angiography. (Cr: Creatinine; EF: Ejection fraction).

- Type 1 or possibly Type 2 arch
- Simmons
  - First choice = H1
  - Second choice = Simmons
  - Third choice = Vitek
  - *Simmons catheter*:
    - Type 3 or possibly Type 2 arch
- *Left carotid*:
  - H1 catheter or vertebral catheter
    - Type 1 or possibly Type 2 arch
  - Simmons catheter
    - Bovine arch
- *Left subclavian*:
  - H1 catheter
  - Vertebral catheter
  - Simmons
    - Some Type 3 arches

Contrast choice:
- Complications of contrast include pain on injection, cardiac overload, and renal toxicity.
- Such complications are related to the hyperosmolarity of contrast agents.
- To reduce complications, choose nonionic contrast agents, which have less osmolarity than traditional ionic contrast agents; however, they are more expensive (Fig. 2.9).[9]
- Omnipaque 300 mg/mL is a common nonionic contrast media used in aortic arch angiography.[9]

Access site choice:
- If femoral access is not possible, due to aortoiliac disease, consider a brachial approach (Fig. 2.10).

1.8 Pearls and Pitfalls

Pearls:
- It is preferable to use less than 300 mL of contrast.
- *Useful formula*: Cockroft-Gault to calculate

Advantages of femoral artery access	Advantages of brachial artery access
• Forehand positioning • Ease of guidewire and catheter placement • Equal femoral pulses: right hand operator usually punctures the right common femoral artery • If diminished femoral artery pulses, use least diseased side	• Aortic occlusion • Bilateral critical/diffuse iliac occlusive disease • Bilateral common femoral artery occlusion or severe stenosis • Presence of recent surgery, infection, aneurysm, or pseudoanuerysm in femoral artery

Fig. 2.10: Choosing an access site. Decision algorithm to help guide choice of access site during aortic arch and four-vessel angiography.

$$GFR = \frac{(140-age) \times weight\,(kg)}{Creatinine\,(mg/dL) \times 72}$$

- *Note for females*: Use 0.85 × weight.
- Minimize injections within the arch vessels, to minimize the risk of air embolism.
- Minimize the risk of forming a clot within the catheter by being vigilant about flushing all catheters with heparinized saline and systemically anticoagulating the patient.
- Evaluate bilateral femoral arteries with physical examination and/or duplex ultrasound to assess for best access site prior to the procedure.
- Patients with contrast allergies should undergo pretreatment with Prednisone and Benadryl to decrease the likelihood of further kidney insult during angiography.

Pitfalls:
- Carbon dioxide should not be used in cerebral and aortic arch angiography due to a high risk of stroke.
- Patients with elevated creatinine are at an increased risk of renal failure.
- Patients with significant arch atherosclerotic disease are at an increased risk of embolic stroke.
- Excess manipulation of catheters within the arch increases the risk of embolic stroke.

1.9 Surgical Anatomy

Access Technique:
- Identify the common femoral artery pulse below the inguinal ligament (Fig. 2.11).
- Access of the femoral artery at its proximal portion overlying the femoral head.
- The level of the femoral head can be best identified under fluoroscopy and marked with a clamp (e.g. hemostat) (Fig. 2.12).
- Access artery via a 22-gauge needle or a micropuncture kit as described in Section 2.1.

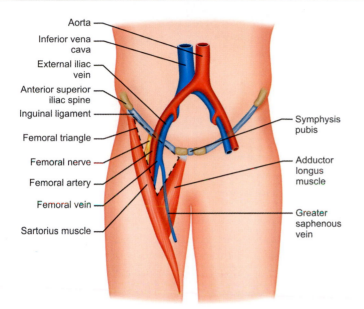

Fig. 2.11: Anatomy of a femoral artery. Access of the femoral artery is desired at the proximal portion where it overlies the femoral head. Begin by identification of the inguinal ligament and palpation of the femoral artery.

1.10 Positioning

- Patient should be comfortably positioned on operating room table in supine position with head cradle, safety straps, and side restraints.

1.11 Anesthesia

- Local anesthesia with 1% lidocaine at access site.
- Sedation should be minimized to allow for breath holding and assessment of neurologic status.
- General anesthesia should be avoided, as procedure can adequately be performed under light sedation.
- Intravenous Fentanyl or Versed are often used for sedation.
- Continuous electrocardiographic tracing and vital sign monitoring should be used.

2 PERIOPERATIVE

2.1 Incision

- Choose access site; the most common is a retrograde femoral puncture (alternative choice is brachial access).
- Identify the proper anatomical landmarks and palpate femoral pulse.

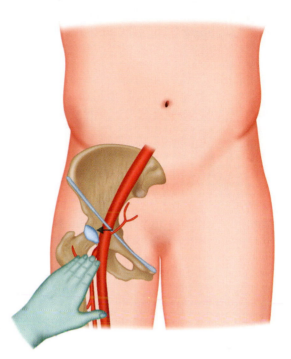

Fig. 2.12: Ideal access point of common femoral artery. The access needle should pierce the common femoral artery where it overlies the femoral head. This location should be identified by landmarks and, possibly, ultrasound. It should also be confirmed with fluoroscopy.

- Mark the patient's groin with a clamp as a reference point over the femoral head.
- Administer 1% lidocaine as a local anesthetic in the skin and subcutaneous tissue over the common femoral artery.
- Create a small stab incision with a No. 11 scalpel blade overlying the common femoral artery.
- Use puncture needle to access common femoral artery at a 45° angle to the skin.
- When pulsatile back bleeding is achieved, thread the guidewire through the puncture needle and advance the wire into the iliac artery under fluoroscopy.
- Remove the puncture needle, pinning the wire in place, and place a 4-Fr or 5-Fr sheath.
- Flush the sheath with heparinized saline.

2.2 Steps

Arch aortogram:
- Advance an exchange length wire through the abdominal aorta toward the aortic arch.
- Park the wire in the ascending aorta and advance a pigtail catheter over the wire until it reaches the proximal ascending aorta.

- Remove the guidewire, flush the catheter with heparinized saline, and connect the power injector to the catheter (confirm air is absent from the catheter and tubing).
- Position the image intensifier to capture the aortic arch and the origin of the arch vessels. This can be best achieved at 30–45° in the left anterior oblique projection.
- Ask the patient to hold respiration to decrease motion artifact.
- Inject contrast at 15 mL/s for 2 seconds under digital subtraction angiography.

Selective catheterization:
- Choose the catheter to perform selective catheterization of the aortic arch vessels to be studied. *See* Section 1.7 Decision-Making Algorithm.
- Systemic heparin is given before selective catheterization of the arch vessels.
- If a complex-curve catheter (e.g. Simmons) is selected, manipulation of the catheter and reforming of the catheter tip should be performed in the descending aorta to decrease embolic risk.
- Perform cannulation of the desired arch vessel.
- Most often, hand injection of contrast is used to perform selective angiography of the vessel of interest.
- Vertebral artery arteriography can often be performed by simple injection into the proximal subclavian artery.

2.3 Closure

- Remove sheath and apply pressure over the site of arterial entry for 15–30 minutes.
- Consider application of a pressure dressing at completion of pressure application.
- The patient should remain on bed rest in supine position for at least 4–5 hours before ambulating with assistance.
- Evaluate access site regularly for evidence of hematoma.
- A closure device may be considered with larger sheath sizes (greater than 5-Fr) to decrease postprocedural time until ambulation.
- Examples of closure devices are Angio-Seal Perclose, Mynx, and Starclose.

3 POSTOPERATIVE

3.1 Complications

Most common complications:
- Neurologic complication (reversible or nonreversible cerebral ischemia)
- Arterial access site hematoma
- Iodinated contrast allergic reaction
- Arterial access site pseudoaneurysm or arteriovenous fistula
- Contrast induced nephropathy/renal failure
- Extremity thrombosis resulting from access arterial dissection, injury, or embolus
- Congestive heart failure
- Myocardial infarction

3.2 Outcomes

- Identification of aortic arch type and arch vessel anatomy
- Identification of disease or lesions of the aortic arch, subclavian arteries, carotid arteries, vertebral arteries, and intracranial arteries

3.3 Follow-Up

- Immediate postprocedural complete neurological examination
- Evaluation of access site for evidence of hematoma after ambulation and prior to discharge
- Perform vascular examination in limb distal to access site
- Evaluation of renal function if patient is at risk for renal insufficiency/failure.
- Office visit within 2 weeks to assess the arterial access site.

3.4 E-mail an Expert

- *E-mail address*: jason.slaikeu@spectrumhealth.org and Lindsey.korepta@grmep.com

3.5 Web Resources/References

- http://my.clevelandclinic.org/services/angiography/hic_angiography_test.aspx
- http://www.vascularweb.org/vascularhealth/pages/angiogram.aspx
- http://www.radiologyinfo.org/en/info.cfm?pg=angiocath

REFERENCES

1. North American Symptomatic Carotid Endarterectomy Trial Collaborators. Beneficial effect of carotid endarterectomy in symptomatic patients with high-grad stenosis. N Engl J Med. 1998;339:1415-25.

2. Asymptomatic Carotid Artherosclerosis Study Group. Carotid endarterectomy for patients with asymptomatic internal carotid artery stenosis. JAMA. 1995;273:1421-8.
3. Hankey GJ, Warlow CP, Sellar RJ. Cerebral angiographic risk in mild cerebrovascular disease. Stroke. 1990;21(2):209-22.
4. Ergun E, Simsek B, Kosar PN, et al. Anatomical variations in branching pattern of arcus aorta: 64-slice CTA appearance. Surg Radiol Anat. 2013;35(6):503-9. Epub 2012 Dec 28.
5. Jakanani GC, Adair W. Frequency of variations in aortic arch anatomy depicted on multidetector CT. Clin Radiol. 2010;65:481-7.
6. Uchino A, Saito N, Okada Y, et al. Variation of the origin of the left common carotid artery diagnosed by CT angiography. Surg Radiol Anat. 2013;35(4):339-42. Epub 2012 Nov 6.
7. Muller M, Schmitz BL, Pauls S, et al. Variations of the aortic arch—a study on the most common branching patterns. Acta Radiol. 2011;52:738-42.
8. Schneider PA, Bohannon WT, Silva MB, (Eds). Carotid Interventions, 1st edition. New York: Marcel Dekker; 2004.
9. Schneider PA. Endovascular skills. Guidewire and Catheter Skills for Endovascular Surgery, 2nd edition. Danvers: Informa Healthcare USA; 2007;80-5,90-8,148-9.

QUIZ

Question 1: CarContra-indications to aortic arch and four vessel angiography include all of the following EXCEPT:
a. Pregnancy
b. Obesity
c. Inability to lie supine
d. Severe PAD that limits access

Question 2: If cost is not prohibitive, in aortic arch and four vessel angiography, it is preferable to use:
a. High doses of iodinated contrast media
b. Either iodinated or non-iodinated contrast media
c. Moderate doses of non-iodinated contrast media
d. Carbon dioxide as contrast media

Question 3: Commonly used methods of anesthesia for aortic arch and four vessel angiography include:
a. General sedation
b. Light conscious sedation with local anesthesia
c. Local anesthesia only
d. No anesthesia needed

Question 4: In a Type 3 aortic arch, which catheters might be useful in accessing the cerebrovascular branches?
a. H1 headhunter catheter
b. Simmons catheter
c. Vertebral catheter
d. Vitek catheter

ANSWERS:

1. a   2. c   3. b   4. b

Carotid Angioplasty and Stent

Jennifer J Watson, Christopher M Chambers

1 PREOPERATIVE

1.1 Indications

Indications

Carotid stenosis identified on color-flow duplex scan or other imaging modality, >50% stenosis by NASCET criteria in a symptomatic patient, or >80% stenosis in an asymptomatic patient. In general, consideration for endarterectomy should be considered; however, if one or more conditions identified below are present, the patient is considered high-risk surgical candidate:

- Prior neck surgery, radiation, tracheostomy or neck immobility
- Prior open-carotid surgery with recurrent stenosis
- Pre-existing vocal cord or cranial nerve injury
- Severe cardiopulmonary comorbidities that increase the risk of general or regional anesthesia
- High lesions that are difficult to access with open surgery (at or above the level of C2)

Contraindications

- *Tortuous arch anatomy*: Tortuosity often increases with patient age and as the arch becomes more tortuous it becomes more difficult to select major vessels (Type 3 arches can be prohibitive in some cases) (Fig. 3.1).
- Extensive aortic calcification and extensive wall irregularities increase the risk of embolization and may be prohibitive in some cases.
- *Carotid artery considerations*: Heavy circumferential calcifications, tortuosity, unstable plaque, fresh thrombus, string sign, and lack of landing zone for placement of a cerebral protection device.

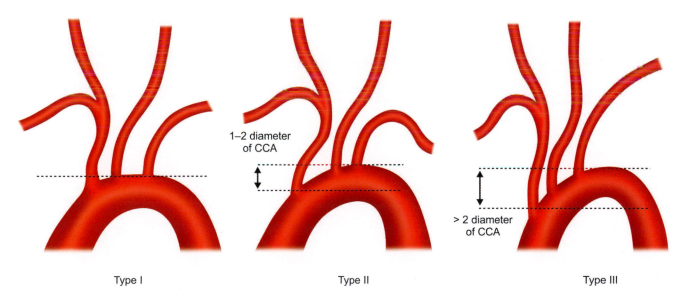

1–2 diameter of CCA

> 2 diameter of CCA

Type I   Type II   Type III

Fig. 3.1: The aortic arch is classified into three types. Type I the apex of the arch is at the same level as the take of the arch vessels. In a Type II arch one of the target vessels is below the level of the arch apex. In a Type III arch two or more of the target vessels are below the level of the arch. Type II and III arches can make cannulation and establishing a stable platform for stenting difficult.

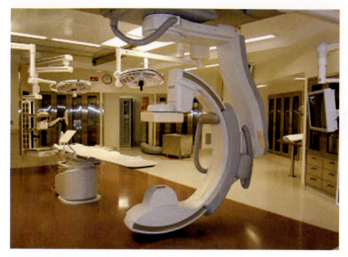

Fig. 3.2: Hybrid operating room.

- Inability to take clopidogrel (due to allergy or prior bleeding events) or dual antiplatelet regimen.

Relative Contraindications

- Congenital vascular anomalies that increase difficulty
- Chronic renal insufficiently (consider contrast-induced nephropathy prophylaxis)
- Contrast allergy (consider premedication with steroids and antihistamines)

1.2 Evidence

- Carotid stenting is feasible and has an acceptable complication rate when performed by experience operators in selected patients. Indications are similar to that of carotid endarterectomy with both asymptomatic (usually >80% internal carotid artery stenosis) and symptomatic (usually >50% internal carotid artery stenosis) disease being treated. In rare circumstances, dissections and ulcerated plaques with lesser degrees of stenosis have also been treated with stenting.[1]
- Carotid stenting has not been demonstrated to be superior to carotid endarterectomy. The SAPPHIRE trial results approached statistical significance ($p = 0.053$) for superiority with a composite endpoint of stroke, death, and myocardial infarction (MI). However, this trial has been criticized because the definition of MI was based solely on the elevation of CPK-MB, with or without symptoms or ST-T changes.[2,3]
- SPACE, EVA-3S and CREST all failed to demonstrate noninferiority for carotid stenting with the endpoint

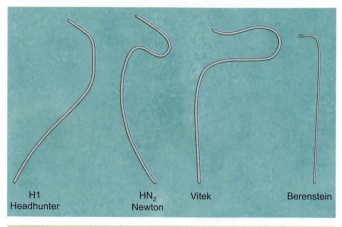

	Type 1 Arch	Type II Arch	Type III Arch
1st choice	Angled glidecath	Headhunter H1	Vitek
2nd choice	Headhunter H1	JB2	Simmons 2
3rd choice	Vertebral	Simmons 2	JB2

Fig. 3.3: This is a sample of currently available catheters for cannulation of target vessels. Selection is based on arch type and surgeon preference.

of stroke at 30 days. The periprocedural stroke rate in EVA-3, SPACE and CREST was higher in the carotid artery stenting group than in the open-surgery group making open surgery the better option for many patients.[4-6]

- In selected patients, carotid stenting has a role and is an important alternative to open surgery for patients with significant comorbid conditions such as high lesions, recurrent stenosis after open surgery, cervical spine immobility, prior neck surgery, and neck irradiation.

1.3 Materials Needed

- Appropriate radiographic equipment (preferably a hybrid operating room, interventional radiology suite or cardiac catheter laboratory) (Fig. 3.2)
- Access supplies (access needle, local anesthetic, knife, 5-Fr short sheath, etc.)
- Sheath 58 Fr (delivery system dependent)
- Contrast material (see chapter on carotid angiography)
- Guidewires (Benson 180-cm floppy tip 0.035 in and glidewire 260 cm, angled tip 0.035 in.)
- Flush catheters (Pigtail 100 cm 5 Fr)
- Cerebral selection catheters—Multiple options depending on arch anatomy (Vertebral, Headhunter, Simmons, Vitek, use 100–125 cm lengths) (Fig. 3.3)

- Selected stent and deployment system (see stent selection section)
- Selected cerebral protection device (see cerebral protection device section)
- Femoral closure device if indicated

1.4 Preoperative Risk Assessment

Low risk:
- All patient undergoing carotid artery stenting will fall into the intermediate- or high-risk categories.

Intermediate risk (if two or more of the following consider the patient high risk):
- Prior MI with stable cardiac function
- Stable angina
- Controlled diabetes mellitus (DM)
- Advanced age >80 years
- Female gender

High risk:
- Ejection factor (EF) <30%, Unstable angina, poorly controlled coronary heart failure
- Poorly controlled DM
- Forced expiratory volume <30% predicted, need for home O_2
- Restenosis of prior CEA
- Renal insufficiency (creatinine >3.0).

1.5 Preoperative Checklist

Sign in:
- Patient identification via two patient identifiers, confirm surgical site.
- Confirm preoperative anticoagulation, antibiotic administration, β-blockers when indicated and contrast dye allergy prophylaxis if indicated.
- Verify necessary equipment is available and ready for use.
- Introduce all members or operating room team.

Time out:
- Final patient confirmation
- Laterality confirmation
- Review available imaging.

Sign out:
- Procedure preformed
- Patient disposition
- Postoperative concerns and postoperative anticoagulation.

1.6 Decision-Making Algorithm

Carotid artery angioplasty and stenting has not been proven to be superior to the open approach. In light of

Flowchart 3.1: Clinical decision-making algorithm.

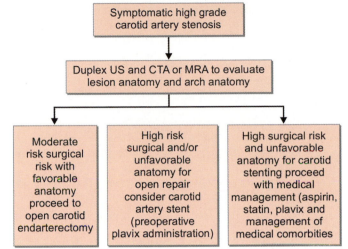

this each patient's symptoms, comorbid conditions and anatomy must be considered on an individual basis. Carotid artery angioplasty and stenting is an important part of the vascular surgeon's armamentarium and in selected cases can provide benefit.

When considering endovascular carotid interventions preoperative imaging with computed tomography angiography or magnetic resonance angiography is essential to evaluate arch anatomy, severity of stenosis, type of plaque, length of target lesion, and the diameter of common and internal carotid artery for device selection. Aortic arch tortuosity increases with age and as the arch becomes more tortuous it becomes more difficult to select the major vessels. The lower the target vessels in relation to the height of the arch the more difficult cannulation will be. Extensive aortic calcification or extensive wall irregularities increase the risk of embolization and thus stroke. The anatomy of the carotid artery itself is also important with heavy circumferential calcifications, tortuosity, and unstable plaque or fresh thrombus, making stenting unfavorable. Access vessels should also be assessed by physical examination and in some cases require further imaging.

See Flowchart 3.1.

1.7 Pearls and Pitfalls

Pearls:

- *Preoperative anticoagulation*:
  - *Aspirin*: 81–325 mg daily for a minimum 4 days before the procedure unless urgent (if urgent a single dose can be given prior to surgery)

- *Clopidogrel*: loading dose of 300–600 mg on the day of the procedure OR 75 mg daily for 4 days before the procedure Continue aspirin and clopidogrel for a minimum of 4 weeks after procedure. Consider lifelong treatment if no contraindications
  - Consider statins in all patients
- *Preoperative considerations*:
  - Hydration and contrast premedication for renal protection.
  - Have atropine available during the procedure for carotid bulb manipulation with stent deployment and balloon angioplasty. Significant bradycardia and hypotension may occur
  - Vasodilators such as nitroglycerin should be available for direct administration into the carotid artery in the case of vasospasm.
- *Early heparinization*:
  - May reduced embolic events
  - Monitor activated clotting time to ensure systemic heparinization throughout the procedure
  - Use continuous heparin flush in the sheaths to avoid thrombus formation on the tip or in the lumen of the catheter
- *Negotiating tortuous anatomy*:
  - In cases with severe tortuosity, the 0.014 wires may not be stiff enough to allow advancement of the embolic protection device (EPD) or the stent. A "buddy wire", usually an angled glide wire is sometimes necessary to help advancing the EPD-stent.
  - It is sometimes necessary to "predilate" the stenosis to be able to deliver the stent.
- *Be prepared for potential complications*:
  - *Distal embolization*: prepare for intracranial lysis
  - EPD becomes plugged with debri and no flow seen distally: prepare for retrieval and place another filter if the stent is not deployed yet.

Pitfalls:

- Avoid unnecessary flushing into the arch or cerebral system, always back bleed sheaths and catheters before flushing.
- Avoid excessive wire manipulation which likely increases the risk of embolic events.
- "Puff" contrast to confirm the location of sheaths and catheters before pressure injection.

1.8 Surgical Anatomy

- *See* Figures 3.4A to C.

1.9 Positioning

An imaging system with the ability to achieve the appropriate fluoroscopic angles for arch and cerebral angiograms is required. We recommend the use of a hydride operating room when possible. The patient should be placed in the spine position with a squeeze toy secured in the contralateral hand. His or her arms should be tucked at the side with all lines, leads, and wires out of the fluoroscopic field. The patient's head should be comfortably extended on a support with a shoulder roll. The patient may be asked to turn his or her head to the contralateral side during portions of the procedure. At least two potential access sites should be sterilely prepped and draped (usually bilateral groin sites).

1.10 Anesthesia

- The patient should be alert enough to follow commands such as breath holding and squeezing the plastic squeeze toy in contralateral hand.
- An arterial line catheter should be inserted for blood pressure monitoring and frequent phlebotomy.
- The patient should receive preoperative β-blockers and antibiotics.
- Atropine should be available during angioplasty and stent deployment.

2 PERIOPERATIVE

2.1 Instructions

- *Access*: retrograde right common femoral percutaneous access with placement of a 5–8 Fr introducer (left common femoral access and brachial access are also options)
- Administer systemic heparin after access is achieved and prior to arch manipulation.
- Perform arch angiogram using a pigtail catheter, C-arm angled 45°–60° left arterial oblique.
- Select the common carotid artery; both sheath-based platforms and guiding catheter-based platforms are available:
  - When using a sheath-based platform a pre-shaped 5-Fr catheters (Simmons 1, Headhunter, Judkins 4, etc.) is used to select the common carotid artery and a stiff 0.035-in. guidwire is placed in the external carotid artery. A 6F 90 cm Shuttle Sheath (Cook, Inc.) is then advanced over the wire and placed in the distal common carotid artery.
  - When using a guiding catheter based platform the common carotid artery is selected with preshaped catheter (vertebral or reverse-angle Vitek catheter) and a 7–8 Fr is positioned in the common carotid artery and left in place. Intermittent heparinization of the catheter throughout the procedure is preformed via a side port.

- Next perform a selective angiogram via the sheath or catheter. Use the optimal C-arm angle to open the angle between the external carotid artery and internal carotid artery.
- Next select the appropriate cerebral protection device. We most commonly use a distal embolic protection device. For placement, cross the internal carotid artery with a 0.014 wire and deploy the protection device just before C3/petrous portion of the internal carotid artery in a straight segment of artery.
- Consider predilatation in selected cases such as those with severe (>90%) stenosis. A 2.5–4.0 mm coronary balloon can be used at low inflation (4–6 atm).
- Take measurements based on the angiogram and preoperative CT and select the appropriate stent. Position a self-expanding 6–10 mm, 2–4 cm length sent across the lesion. This will cross the carotid bifurcation in most cases. The stent should be size to largest portion of the common carotid artery plus 1 mm. Multiple varieties of stents are available (Fig. 3.5).
- Next postdilate with a 2-cm (5–6 mm) balloon, taking care never to exceed the diameter of the internal carotid artery. Take care to keep balloon within the stent during inflations and fully deflate the balloon prior to removal as not to disrupt the stent.
- Perform a completion angiogram and ensure flow beyond protection device.
- Remove protection device (device specific).
- Perform completion cerebral angiogram.
- Access site closures maybe preformed with a closure device or manual pressure. Systemic heparin reversal is rarely necessary.

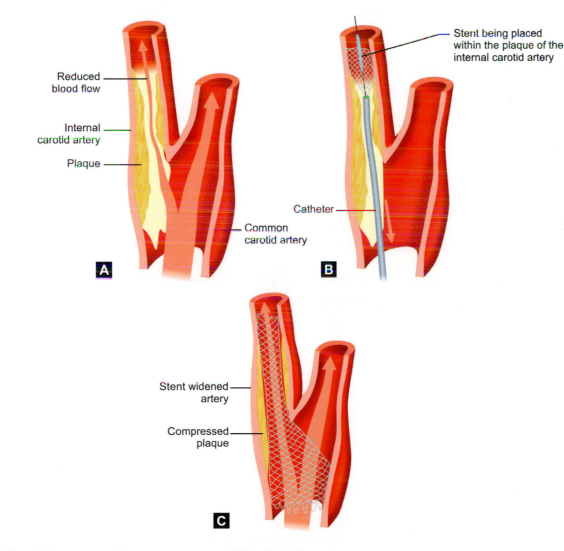

Figs. 3.4A to C: Internal carotid artery anatomy and flow dynamics.

2.2 Cerebral Protection Devices Embolic Protection Devices (EPD)

There are three classifications of cerebral protection devices. The first in use were distal occlusion balloons. These devices are rarely the first choice today. The occlusive balloon is placed distal to lesion, inflated and frequently flushed and suctioned to remove plaque and debris. Major disadvantages include the need to cross the lesion unprotected, vasospasm, dissection or wall damage, and complete interruption of carotid flow (Figs. 3.6A and B).

The second type, distal filters, is commonly used and there are multiple types commercially available. They are umbrella like devices designed for placement in the distal internal carotid artery. These devices are mounted on a

guidewire or their own delivery system. They are then retrieved at the end of the procedure using a dedicated retrieval system. Major advantages include allowing for continued flow and ease of use. While disadvantage include the need to cross the lesion unprotected, the possibility of clogging with debris, and difficultly in placement if the distal internal carotid artery lacks a straight segment.

Lastly, proximal occlusion or flow reversal device are made of two compliant balloons. One is placed in common carotid artery and one is place in the external carotid artery. Reversal of flow from the internal carotid artery occurs by continuous shunting of blood through a side post of the introducer and a separate femoral venous access. Advantages include no unprotected crossing of the lesion and disadvantages include technically difficultly, need for additional venous access and intolerance in some patients. Surgeons should select the protection device that suites their patient and with which they are most familiar.

2.3 Stent Selection

Multiple stents are commercially available with a range of sizes and configurations. They are constructed of stainless steel or nitinol and are available in open- and closed-cell designs. The open-cell design provides additional flexibility, while the closed-cell design may decrease embolic events. Hybrid configurations also exist with closed central portions and open proximal and distal portions. Tapered stents may be selected for cases with large discrepancies in proximal and distal diameters (Fig. 3.5)

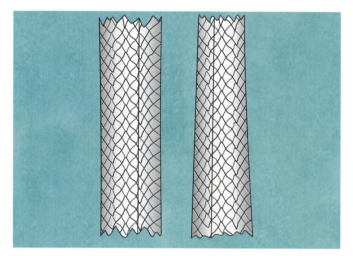

Fig. 3.5: Sample carotid stents, tapered and nontapered.

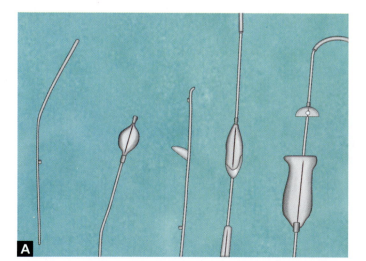

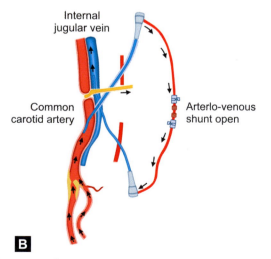

Figs. 3.6A and B: (A) Cerebral protection devices. (B) An example of flow reversal.

3 POSTOPERATIVE

3.1 Complications

Most common complications (1–10%):
- Transient ischemic attack or ischemia stroke (at risk patients include those with difficult arch anatomy, advanced age and long lesions)
- Access site complications including bleeding, hematoma, and pseudoaneurysm (1–3%)
- Bradycardia or hypotension with carotid bulb manipulation (can be prolonged beyond 24 hours in rare cases)
- Cardiac events (ischemia, MI).

Least common complications (<1%):
- Bleeding from arch trauma or local vessel injury
- Dissection, in the arch or carotid
- Jaw claudication (associated with coverage of the external carotid artery).

3.2 Outcomes

- Immediate postoperative hypotension, hypertension, or bradycardia requiring ICU admission is seen in approximately 10% of patients
- Average 30-day stroke rate is 2% to 5%
- 30-day combined stroke, MI, and death rate is 4–7%
- 5–15% restenosis at 2 years.

3.3 Follow-Up

- Patients should initially have 24 hours of in-hospital neurologic and cardiovascular monitoring.
- Outpatient follow-up plans differ but we suggest physical examination and duplex US imaging at 6 weeks, 6 months, 1 year, and annually thereafter
- The contralateral carotid artery may require monitoring depending on the degree of stenosis
- Consider lifelong aspirin and statin administration. Clopidogrel should be continued for 3 months postoperatively and lifelong in some cases.

3.4 E-mail an Expert

- *E-mail address:* christopher.chambers@spectrumhealth.org

REFERENCES

1. Brott TG, Hobson RW, Howard G, et al. Stenting versus endarterectomy for treatment of carotid-artery stenosis (CREST). NEMJ. 2010;363:11-23.
2. Eckstein HH, Ringleb P, Allenberg JR, et al. Results of the stent-protected angioplasty versus carotid endarterectomy (SPACE) study to treat symptomatic stenoses at 2 years: a multinational, prospective, randomised trial. Lancet Neurol. 2008;7:893-902.
3. Yadav J, SAPPHIRE investigators. Stenting and angioplasty with protection in patients at high risk for carotid endarterectomy: the SAPPHIRE trial. Circulation. 2002;106:2986-689.
4. EVA-3S Investigators. Endarterectomy vs. angioplasty in patients with symptomatic severe carotid stenosis. Cerebrovasc Dis. 2004;18(1):62-5.
5. Ederle J, Featherstone RL, Brown MM. Randomized controlled trials comparing endarterectomy and endovascular treatment for carotid artery stenosis: a Cochrane systematic review. Stroke. 2009;40(4):1373-80.
6. Yadav JS, Wholey MH, Kuntz RE, et al. Protected carotid-artery stenting versus endarterectomy in high-risk patients. NEJM. 2004;351(15):1493-501.

QUIZ

Question 1: Which of the following patients is most likely to benefit from carotid artery stenting
a. 55-year male smoker with symptomatic high grade stenosis of his internal carotid artery and a prior coronary artery bypass graft and an EF of 55%
b. 88-year female with asymptomatic 60–79% carotid stenosis and prior neck radiation
c. 60-year male with symptomatic high-grade stenosis and a prior radical neck dissection
d. 75-year female with asymptomatic high-grade stenosis and poorly controlled DM

Question 2: The best time to administer systemic heparin when performing carotid artery stenting is
a. Prior to starting the procedure
b. After gaining initial access via the common femoral artery
c. After placement of a sheath within the common carotid artery
d. Five minutes before stent deployment

Question 3: When planning to perform carotid artery stenting a preoperative CT angiogram of the neck can provide information regarding which of the following:
a. Aortic arch anatomy including grade and degree of calcifications
b. Severity of stenosis
c. Diameter of common and internal carotid artery for device selection
d. All of the above

ANSWERS: 1. c   2. b   3. d

Vertebral Artery Transposition

Mark D Morasch, M Ashraf Mansour

1 PREOPERATIVE

1.1 Indications

- Treatment for occlusive lesions involving the origin of the vertebral artery (V1 segment) is undertaken in patients with demonstrable posterior brain circulation ischemia.
- It is important to evaluate the carotid arteries.

1.2 Evidence

- When selected appropriately, more than 80% of patients will have relief of their symptoms after proximal surgical reconstruction.[1,2]
- Due to the relatively low incidence of VBI, there are no prospective studies.

1.3 Materials Needed

See Figure 1.1 in Chapter 1.
- Self-retaining retractors
- Silk ligatures
- Micro-bulldog clamps, Satinski Clamp, Angled Cooley vascular clamps
- 5-mm cardiac punch
- 7-0 monofilament vascular suture

1.4 Preoperative Risk Assessment

Significant cardiorespiratory disease:
- Older age
- Prolonged history of steroid use
- Vertebral artery entrance into the transverse process foramina below C6
- Inability of patients to hyperextend their necks
- Arteritis from prior radiation therapy
- *See* risk factors in Chapter 1.

1.5 Preoperative Checklist

- Sign in
- Time out
- Sign out

1.6 Decision-Making Algorithm

- *See* Flowchart 4.1.

1.7 Pearls and Pitfalls

Pearls:
- On the left side, the thoracic dust will be encountered. On the right side, there are multiple lymphatic channels. All must be meticulously tied prior to division to prevent chylous leak.
- Freeing up as much vertebral artery as possible, up to its entry into the transverse process of C6, will facilitate transposition.

Flowchart 4.1: Decision-making algorithm.

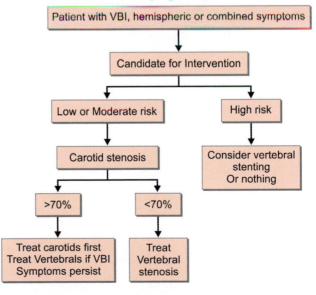

- Preservation of the sympathetic fibers that surround the proximal vertebral will prevent significant Horner's syndrome postoperatively.

Pitfalls:

- A vertebral artery that enters the transverse foramina below C6 as can often be seen when the vertebral artery takes origin from the aortic arch may be impossible to transpose. It is important to verify this anatomy prior to surgery.
- A redundant vertebral artery may need to be shortened to prevent kinking.

1.8 Surgical Anatomy

- The surgical anatomy of the paired vertebral arteries has traditionally been divided into four segments.
  - The V1 segment originates at the posterior surface of the first segment of the subclavian artery and extends to the transverse foramina of either the fifth or sixth cervical vertebrae.[3]
  - The V2 segment courses through the bony canal of the transverse foramina from C2-C6 and is buried deep within intertransversarium muscle.
  - The V3 segment continues as the artery exits the transverse foramina at C2 and ends as the vessel passes through the foramen magnum and penetrates the dura matter.
  - The V4 segment is entirely intracranial beginning at the atlantooccipital membrane and terminating as the two vertebrals converge to form the basilar artery.
- The V1 segment takes origin from the posterior aspect of the middle third of the subclavian artery. This

segment of the vertebral artery lies deep to the thoracic duct on the left and lymphatic channels on the right and also deep to the vertebral vein.

- The artery is intimately surrounded by nerves of the sympathetic plexus.
- *See* Figure 4.1.

1.9 Positioning

- The patient is positioned in a slight chair position to decrease venous pressure and to allow optimal viualization of the anatomy at the base of the neck.
- *See* Chapter 1 Positioning for carotid surgery.
- *See* Figure 4.2.

1.10 Anesthesia

- General anesthesia is preferred.

2 PERIOPERATIVE

The incision and approach described are for treatment of the more common V1 segment.

2.1 Incision

- The incision is placed transversely about a finger's breadth above the clavicle and directly over the two heads of the sternocleidomastoid.
- *See* Figure 4.3.

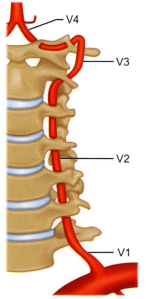

Fig. 4.1: Surgical anatomy.

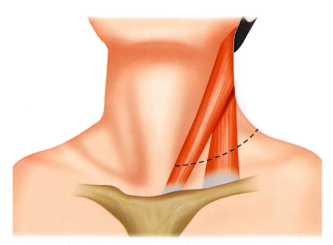

Fig. 4.2: Preferred incision for exposure of V1 segment.

2.2 Steps

- Subplatysmal skin flaps are created and dissection is carried down directly between the two bellies of the sternocleidomastoid.
- The omohyoid muscle is divided with electocautery.
- The jugular vein is mobilized laterally and the vagus nerve is retracted medially with the common carotid artery.
- The carotid should be exposed proximally as far as possible and well behind the ipsilateral clavicle.
- On the left side, the thoracic duct is divided between ligatures.
- Accessory lymph ducts, often seen on the right side of the neck, are also meticulously identified, ligated, and divided (Fig. 4.3).
- The entire dissection is confined medial to the prescalene fat pad that covers the scalenus anticus muscle and phrenic nerve. These structures are left unexposed lateral to the field (Figs. 4.4 and 4.5).
- The vertebral vein emerges from the angle formed by the longus colli and scalenus anticus and overlies the proximal vertebral artery. It is ligated and divided.
- The vertebral and subclavian vessels are now visible.
- It is important to identify and avoid injury to the adjacent sympathetic chain.
- The vertebral artery is dissected superiorly up to the level of the tendon of the longus colli and inferiorly to its origin from the subclavian artery, exposing 2–3 centimeters of length.
- The vertebral artery is freed from the sympathetic trunk resting on its anterior surface without damaging the trunk or the ganglionic rami (Fig. 4.6).
- After dividing the vertebral artery at its origin it can be transposed to a position anterior to the sympathetic trunk without causing them harm.
- Once the artery is fully exposed, an appropriate site for reimplantation in the common carotid artery is selected.
- The patient is given systemic heparin.
- The distal portion of the V1 segment of the vertebral artery is clamped below the edge of the longus colli.
- The proximal vertebral artery is ligated immediately above the stenosis at its origin using a small monofilament suture as a transfixion stitch. The artery is divided at this proximal level.
- The carotid artery is then cross-clamped.
- An elliptical 5 to 7 mm arteriotomy is created in the posterolateral wall of the common carotid artery with an aortic punch (Fig. 4.7).
- The anastomosis is performed in parachute fashion with a continuous 7-0 polypropylene suture, avoiding any tension on the vertebral artery, which may tear easily.
- Before completion of the anastomosis, standard flushing maneuvers are performed, the suture is tied, and flow is re-established.

See Flowchart 4.1 and Figures 4.4 and 4.5.

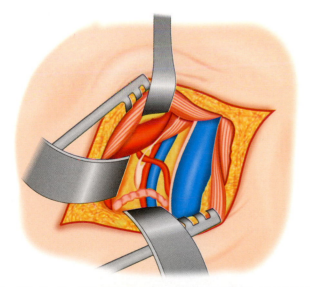

Fig. 4.3: On the left side, the thoracic duct will be encountered between and behind the common carotid and jugular vein.

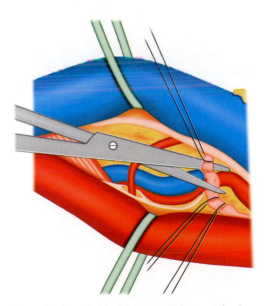

Fig. 4.4: Thoracic duct divided to expose the vertebral artery and vein.

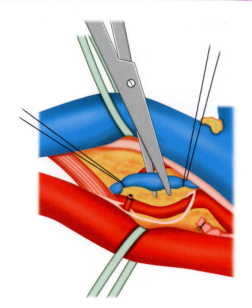

Fig. 4.5: Left vertebral vein being divided prior to reaching the vertebral artery.

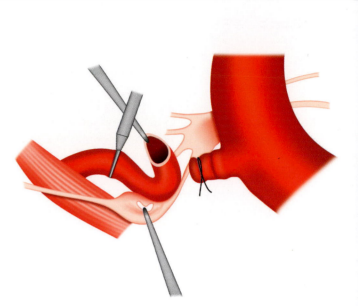

Fig. 4.6: Left vertebral artery divided and being prepared for transposition into the left common carotid artery.

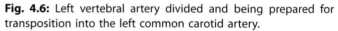

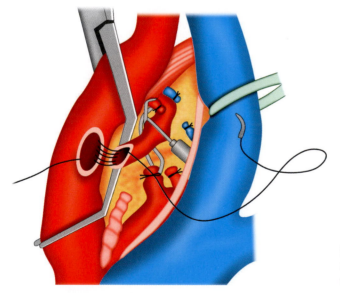

Fig. 4.7: The anastomosis is performed in parachute fashion with continuous 7-0 polypropylene suture, avoiding any tension on the vertebral artery.

2.3 Closure

- The skin incision is closed by reapproximating the platysma with an absorbable suture, followed by a subcuticular monofilament stitch.
- *See* Figures 4.6 to 4.7.

3 POSTOPERATIVE

3.1 Complications

- Thrombosis: <3%
- Stroke rate: <2%

- Death rate: <1%
- Combined stroke and death: <3%
- Chylous leak, bleeding, pneumothorax: <8%
- Cranial nerve injury: <3%

3.2 Outcomes

- Five-year patency rate: 80%
- Five-year survival: 70%
- In survivors, 97% are stroke free

3.3 Follow-Up

- Postoperative chest radiograph in PACU
- Global neurologic function testing
  - Remove drain on POD #1
- Return to adls within 1-week postdischarge

- Surgical follow-up visit in 3 weeks to inspect surgical site

3.4 E-mail an Expert

- *E-mail address*: Mark.morasch@svh-mt.org

REFERENCES

1. Berguer R, Flynn LM, Kline RA, et al. Surgical reconstruction of the extracranial vertebral artery: management and outcome. J Vasc Surg. 2000;31:9-18.
2. Berguer R, Morasch MD, Kline RA. A review of 100 consecutive reconstructions of the distal vertebral artery for embolic and hemodynamic disease. J Vasc Surg. 1998;27:852-9.
3. Lee V, Riles TS, Stableford J, et al. Two case presentations and surgical management of Bow Hunter's syndrome associated with bony abnormalities of the C7 vertebra. J Vasc Surg. 2011;53:1381-5.

Carotid—Carotid Bypass

M Ashraf Mansour

1 PREOPERATIVE

1.1 Indications

- Symptomatic carotid stenosis or occlusion involving a segment or the entire length of the common carotid artery proximal to the bifurcation.
- A more common indication now is to perform a "debranching" procedure to prepare patients who are undergoing TEVAR (thoracic aorta endografts for any indication) with intended coverage of the origin of the left common carotid artery.

1.2 Evidence

- For symptomatic carotid stenosis see the European carotid surgery trial (ECST), North American Symptomatic Carotid Endarterectomy Trial (NASCET), and Veterans administration (VA) trial (*See* Chapter 1).

1.3 Instruments Needed

- Picture of back table (Fig. 5.1)

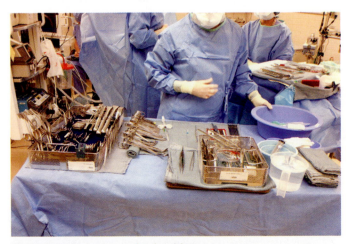

Fig. 5.1: Instruments at back table.

- Vascular instruments and clamps
- Suture material 5.0 or 6.0 monofilament
- Back pressure line, shunt (*see* Chapter 1)
- PTFE or Dacron 6- or 8-mm grafts (depending or native vessel diameter, usually 6 mm for women and 8 mm for men)

1.4 Preoperative Planning and Risk Assessment

Planning:
- *Diagnostic studies*: Carotid duplex from an accredited vascular laboratory, CT angiogram, magnetic resonance angiography (MRA) or digital subtraction angiogram showing the carotid bifurcation and must include the common and internal carotid, proximal and distal to the lesion, respectively.
- Is the patient for general or regional anesthesia?
- Is the patient fit for *surgery*: good cardiopulmonary reserve?
- Previous operations or radiation to the neck make dissection more difficult.
- Osteoarthritis of the cervical spine and morbid obesity make positioning the neck in surgery difficult.
- The donor carotid is usually the right side for debranching, and could be either side for occlusive disease. The donor vessel ought to be relatively free of disease to place a clamp. The recipient (or target vessel) should have a patent carotid bifurcation or at least a patent and accessible internal carotid artery.

Risk assessment:
- *Low risk*: No cardiopulmonary disease, no anatomical risks, e.g. previous radiation or neck surgery, degenerative disease of the spine precluding rotation, and extension.
- *Intermediate risk*: Low cardiac or pulmonary risk, comorbid disease such as obesity, poorly controlled

hypertension and hyperlipidemia, tobacco use, and mild chronic obstructive pulmonary disease (COPD).
- *High risk*: Poor ejection fraction (<20%), angina or recent MI, oxygen dependent COPD, previous radical neck dissection or neck radiation, tracheostomy, frozen neck (consider carotid stenting).

1.5 Preoperative Checklist

- Preoperative β-blockers, statins, and aspirin should be started preoperatively.
- There is no contraindication for maintaining Plavix preoperatively; however, there is an increased risk of bleeding.
- Special considerations for diabetic patients:

Sign in	Time out	Sign out
Patient confirms: Identity Site Procedure Appropriate consent form	Team members introduction	Procedure performed Instrument and needle final count Labeling specimen Equipment problems to address
Site marked	Verbal confirmation from surgeon, anesthesiologist, and nurse	Anesthesia and surgeon report key concerns to Postanaesthesia care unit (PACU)
Anesthesia safety checklist	Anticipated critical events	
Allergy, special considerations	Antibiotic prophylaxis Preoperative imaging	

1.6 Decision-Making Algorithm

- *See* Flowchart 5.1.

1.7 Pearls and Pitfalls

Pearls:
- Planning the incision is very important. For occlusive disease, two separate neck incisions or a "U" shaped incision can be used.
- The length of the incision can be shortened if the carotid bifurcation is located preoperatively by duplex scan. An experienced operator with an ultrasound machine in the operating room can do this in less than a minute.
- An oblique incision in a skin crease is cosmetically more acceptable to patients.

Flowchart 5.1: Decision-making algorithm.

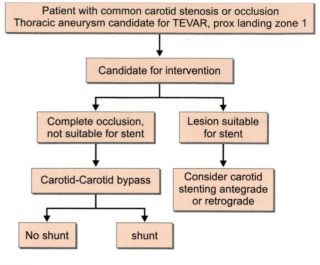

- If a left subclavian transposition or bypass are being performed, as is a frequent situation for debranching prior to TEVAR, a single transverse supraclavicular left neck incision is made to be used for both the subclavian and carotid–carotid bypass.
- The ideal position to access the neck fully is having the patient semisitting (30–45° Fowler) with the arms tucked in at the sides after insertion of arterial lines and proper intravenous access.
- In a large neck, the mini Omni retractor can be very helpful.
- If the occlusion is at the origin of the common carotid and the rest of the vessel is relatively normal, a carotid transposition can be performed.
- The neck tunnel for the graft may be created anteriorly in a subcutaneous position (will be prominent and look like a necklace in a thin neck) or a retropharyngeal plane, directly anterior to the spine.

Pitfalls:
- Identify and treat the vagus nerve with utmost respect. A bilateral recurrent nerve injury will cause bilateral vocal cord paralysis and potential need for a tracheostomy immediately postoperatively.
- On preoperative imaging, the arch and origin of the donor carotid must be clearly visualized to avoid any intraoperative surprises.
- Be careful with dividing the facial vein, the hypoglossal can be adherent to it.
- Vigorous retraction can cause marginal mandibular nerve injury.
- To avoid cerebral ischemia or stroke on the donor side, a side-biting clamp is preferred, and minimize clamp time, keep blood pressure elevated (avoid hypotension).

1.8 Surgical Anatomy

- The best exposure to the carotid bifurcation is from the anterior approach.
- Beware of nerves, vagus, hypoglossal, descendens hypoglossi.
- Ligation of common facial vein to provide exposure.
- Occasionally, ligation of a tethering vessel posterior to the hypoglossal is required for high exposure.
- Injection of lidocaine in the bifurcation is necessary to treat bradycardia that occurs with carotid manipulation.

1.9 Positioning

- I prefer a modified Fowler position, which is semi-sitting, with knees resting on a pillow and a small shoulder role behind the shoulders and have the neck turned to the opposite side.

1.10 Anesthesia

- Most surgeons and anesthesiologists prefer general endotracheal anesthesia. A cervical block may be considered in selected patients.
- Clamp time, anticoagulation and blood pressure should be strictly monitored.

2 PERIOPERATIVE

2.1 Incision

See Figure 5.2.
- The most common type of incision is bilateral oblique or longitudinal incisions along the anterior border of the sternocleidomastoid.
- If a left subclavian transposition or bypass is being performed simultaneously, a transverse left supraclavicular incision can be used.

2.2 Steps

- Exposure of the carotid bifurcation and/or the common carotid artery.
- Avoid manipulation of the vessels because a plaque may be dislodged causing a neurological complications
- Clamp the distal internal or common carotid artery first.
- Decision to shunt or not is based on back pressure (*See* Flowchart 5.1).

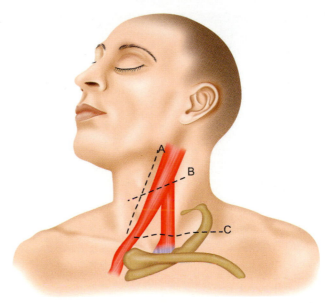

Fig. 5.2: Three types of incisions may be used: longitudinal anterior to sternocleidomastoid (A), oblique (B) or transverse (C) just above the clavicle.

- If a shunt is to be used on the donor carotid, Rummel tourniquet with indwelling straight shunt introduced after creating an opening in the common carotid with aortic punch.
- Arteriotomy on the common carotid should be created on the medial side of both sides, beware of possible twist or rotation.
- Create the tunnel for the graft before administering heparin.
- The donor anastomosis should be created first, and minimize clamp time.
- The carotid–carotid graft configuration can be straight, or slightly curved to allow spatulation of the anastomosis.
- Flush the graft before allowing forward flow.
- The proximal recipient carotid can be ligated or oversewn so the anastomosis can be done end to end.

2.3 Closure

- The anastomosis is sewn with 5.0 or 6.0 Prolene.
- Dacron or ePTFE ringed graft is used, 6 mm for a woman and 8 mm for a man.
- A subcuticular closure is preferred for skin closure. Most patients can be discharged on postoperative day 1 and do not need to be seen for 1 or 2 weeks if they have no surgical complications (no cranial nerve injury or hematoma interfering with swallowing).

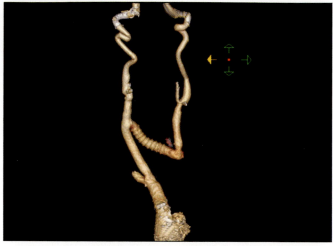

Fig. 5.3: Computed tomography angiogram (CTA) of neck after carotid–carotid bypass performed for debranching prior to TEVAR.

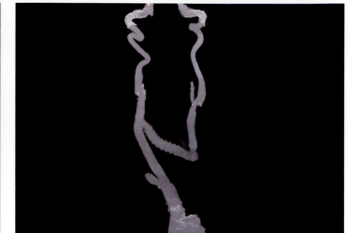

Fig. 5.4: Computed tomography angiogram (CTA) picture.

- Some surgeons use closed suction drains, either routinely or selectively; however, there is no evidence this decreases the incidence of wound hematoma.

3 POSTOPERATIVE

3.1 Complications
- The most serious and feared complication is stroke.
- Stroke rate is higher for symptomatic lesions.
- Cranial nerve injury may be vagus, hypoglossal, marginal mandibular, or rarely glossopharyngeal.
- With bilateral cervical incisions, bilateral recurrent laryngeal nerve injury can lead to complete vocal cord paralysis, hoarseness and stridor. An emergent tracheostomy will be needed.
- Wound hematoma requires re-exploration.
- Wound infection or graft infection is quite rare in carotids.
- Graft occlusion is usually a technical problem with inflow, outflow, or graft tunnel.

3.2 Outcomes
- The ideal stroke rate is 1–2% in centers of excellence.
- The incidence of myocardial infarction should be <5%.
- Some patients mild temporary dysphagia from swelling in the tunnel, whether the graft is tunneled retropharyngeal or anteriorly.

3.3 Postoperative Hospitalization
- After a period of 2–4 hours of close monitoring in a postanesthesia care unit, most patients may go to a vascular ward for neurological checks and vital signs every 4 hours.
- Patients with blood pressure lability require monitoring in an ICU with vasopressors if hypotensive and antihypertensive drips if hypertensive (*See* Chapter 1).
- We prefer to stage the 24–48 hours after bypass.

3.4 Discharge Instruction
- Patients should monitor their blood pressure postoperatively, and continue to take their medications (especially statins, antihypertensives and antiplatelet agents).
- We counsel patients not to drive for a week and avoid strenuous activity and heavy lifting.
- Wound infection is rare, but routine wound care, keeping the wound clean and avoid contamination is good advice.

See Figures 5.3 and 5.4.

3.5 Follow-Up
- A follow-up visit in the office 2–4 weeks postoperative is recommended for wound and neuro check.

3.6 E-mail an Expert
- *E-mail address*: ashraf.mansour@spectrumhealth.org

SUGGESTED READINGS

Antoniou GA, El Sakka K, Hamady M, et al. Hybrid treatment of complex aortic arch disease with supra-arotic debranching and endovascular stent graft repair. Eur J Vasc Endovasc Surg. 2010;39:683-90.

European Carotid Surgery Trial: Interim results for symptomatic patients with severe (70–99%) or with mild (0–29%) carotid stenosis. Lancet. 1991;337:1235-43.

Ferrero E, Ferri M, Viazzo A, et al. Is total debranching a safe procedure for extensive arotic arch disease? A single experience of 27 cases. Euro J CardioThorac Surg. 2012;41:177-82.

Hobson RW, Weiss DG, Fields WS, et al. Efficacy of carotid endarterectomy for asymptomatic carotid stenosis. N Engl J Med. 1993;328:221-7.

North American Symptomatic Carotid Endarterectomy Trial Collaborators. Beneficial effect of carotid endarterectomy in symptomatic patients with high-grade carotid stenosis. N Engl J Med. 1991;325:445-53.

QUIZ

Question 1: Carotid–carotid bypass is indicated when:
a. There is complete occlusion of the common carotid artery and the external carotid is patent.
b. There is complete occlusion of the common carotid artery and the internal carotid is patent to the brain.
c. There is a stenosis in the common carotid that can be stented.
d. There is a stenosis in the ipsilateral internal carotid artery.
e. There is vertebral artery stenosis.

Question 2: The most common indication for carotid–carotid bypass in contemporary practice is:
a. Unilateral common carotid occlusive disease.
b. Failure of common carotid stenting.
c. In a debranching procedure prior to thoracic stent graft deployment.
d. In radiated necks when revascularization is indicated.
e. When the right subclavian is occluded.

Question 3: When performing carotid–carotid bypass:
a. Only autogenous vein may be used.
b. The retropharyngeal tunnel is the only route.
c. The anterior cervical tunnel is preferred.
d. The incidence of stroke is >5%.
e. A prosthetic graft, usually ePTFE, is selected to match the donor common carotid diameter.

ANSWERS: 1. b   2. c   3. e

Endovascular Therapy for Subclavian and Innominate Artery Stenosis

Jordan R Stern, Ross Milner

1 INTRODUCTION

Stenosis of the brachiocephalic (innominate) and subclavian arteries is a relatively rare problem, with the prevalence in the general population estimated at approximately 2%[1] for subclavian lesions, and even lower for the innominate artery. However, complications arising from stenotic proximal vessels can be severe, including vertebrobasilar insufficiency and stroke, cerebral embolism, and debilitating claudication of the upper extremity.[2] Additionally, in patients with a history of coronary artery bypass grafting using the internal mammary artery, subclavian artery stenosis can lead to coronary steal.[3] Stenosis more commonly affects the left subclavian artery than the right, with the majority of lesions on both sides affecting the ostia primarily.[4] Ostial and other proximal stenosis tend to be atherosclerotic in nature,[4] and therefore, perhaps not surprisingly, there is a fivefold increased rate of subclavian and innominate stenosis in patients with peripheral vascular disease.[1] Other identified risk factors include current or past smoking and systolic hypertension, while elevated high-density lipoprotein cholesterol seems to be protective.[1] In contrast, more distal subclavian artery stenoses tend to be caused by mechanical forces such as trauma or external compression, or systemic disease processes such as various forms of arteritis.[4] Historically, management of proximal subclavian and innominate artery stenosis was primarily via surgical bypass from the ipsilateral carotid, at times requiring a large sternotomy or thoracotomy incision.[5] The increased use of endovascular techniques, however, has recently led to a culture shift and this has now become the primary technique utilized in treatment of arterial occlusive disease in the branches of the aortic arch. Here we aim to provide an overview of subclavian and innominate arterial occlusive disease, and describe the current diagnosis and management paradigm in the endovascular era. For reference, the anatomy of the aortic arch and its branches is depicted in Figure 6.1.[6]

2 DIAGNOSIS AND PREOPERATIVE EVALUATION

Most patients with subclavian and innominate arterial stenosis are asymptomatic in their early stages, and therefore screening has been advocated in high-risk groups

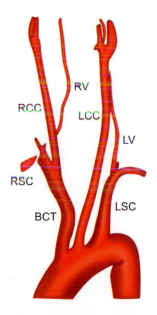

Fig. 6.1: Anatomy of the aortic arch and its branches. This depicts the most common anatomic arrangement of the proximal branches of the aorta. The primary branches are the brachiocephalic trunk (BCT) or innominate artery, the left common carotid artery (LCC), and the left subclavian artery (LSC). The innominate artery bifurcates to become the right common carotid (RCC) and right subclavian (RSC) arteries. The left and right vertebral arteries (LV, RV) come off their respective subclavian arteries.

in order to facilitate early detection and intervention prior to the onset of symptoms. The majority of patients who become symptomatic complain of upper extremity claudication on the affected side, or show signs of arm ischemia or vertebrobasilar insufficiency.[5] Claudication is more commonly seen in patients in whom the dominant hand corresponds to the affected side. These patients tend to be younger, and present with arm pain and fatigue with repetitive use. Rest pain is extraordinarily rare, due to the extensive capacity for collateral circulation in the upper extremity.[4]

Some patients may present with subclavian steal syndrome, which is more worrisome due to the associated cerebrovascular consequences. Hemodynamically significant stenosis of the subclavian or innominate artery proximal to the takeoff of the vertebral artery can lead to retrograde vertebral arterial flow, with insufficient perfusion of the vertebrobasilar territory of the brainstem. Presenting symptoms can range from blurry vision and dizziness to basilar transient ischemic attack and stroke.[7] A variant of the subclavian steal syndrome can occur following harvest of the left internal mammary artery (LIMA) for coronary bypass to the left anterior descending artery (LAD). Here, flow reversal can occur in the LIMA conduit itself, leading to myocardial ischemia and angina pectoris with use of the left arm.[8] This can be not only lifestyle-altering, but indeed life-threatening as the benefit of the coronary bypass may be subverted. These syndromes are outlined in Figure 6.2.

In evaluating a patient for subclavian and innominate artery occlusive disease, a thorough history should be taken with regard to symptoms of vertebrobasilar insufficiency and claudication. The presence of any significant risk factors should be identified, in particular a personal history of peripheral arterial disease and tobacco use. Physical examination should include auscultation for bruits in the supraclavicular and cervical areas, as well as a thorough pulse exam. Bilateral blood pressure measurement in the upper extremities is the simplest and least invasive screening test available, but a positive result is very nonspecific; up to 50% of all patients may have >10 mm Hg difference between arms, the majority of which have no underlying pathology.[9] Moreover, patients with bilateral disease may have equal arm pressures. History, physical examination and noninvasive blood pressure measurement should therefore be taken together to form an overall clinical risk profile in the mind of the examining practitioner.

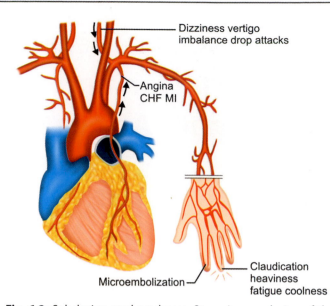

Fig. 6.2: Subclavian steal syndrome. Stenosis or occlusion of the subclavian artery proximal to the vertebral takeoff causes reversal of flow in the vertebral artery. This may lead to neurologic symptoms of vertebrobasilar insufficiency, as well as symptoms in the affected limb. A variant syndrome, which occurs when flow is reversed in the internal mammary artery following coronary artery bypass, leads to myocardial ischemia and is termed the coronary steal syndrome.

For these reasons, the use of duplex ultrasound screening in some populations has been advocated, particularly those undergoing examination of the extracranial vasculature for cerebrovascular symptoms.[10] Arterial velocity measurements above 300 cm/s are indicative of a hemodynamically significant stenosis, and may be accompanied by biphasic or monophasic waveforms.[4] With regard to the vertebral artery, flow reversal is progressively graded. Grade I lesions demonstrate decreased peak systolic velocity with antegrade flow, grade II lesions result in retrograde systolic flow with preserved antegrade flow during diastole, and grade III lesions result in complete reversal.[11] Grade II-III lesions have a statistically higher incidence of associated neurologic symptoms.[11]

The use of computed-tomography and magnetic resonance angiography (CTA/MRA) is generally limited to those patients for whom suspicion of stenosis is high, as well as for operative planning in order to properly delineate the pertinent anatomy and extent of disease. MRA in particular has shown to be an excellent diagnostic tool in these patients, with a reported specificity and sensitivity of 100% and 99.3%, respectively, in the detection of stenosis.[12] This compares favorably to the gold-standard digital subtraction angiography, and where available, these noninvasive tools should be strongly considered as part of the preoperative workup.

3 ANATOMICAL CONSIDERATIONS

The proximal branches of the aortic arch include the brachiocephalic (innominate), left common carotid and left subclavian arteries (*See* Fig. 6.1). The innominate artery gives rise to the right subclavian and right common carotid arteries. The vertebral arteries originate from the proximal subclavian arteries bilaterally. These vessels lie within the thoracic outlet, deep to the sternum and clavicular heads, making direct access difficult. For the most proximal or bilateral lesions this will require a median sternotomy, while more peripheral lesions may be amenable to a supra- or infraclavicular approach.

4 TECHNIQUE

Access is obtained primarily through the common femoral artery, in a retrograde fashion. Alternatively, if femoral access is not feasible or the lesion cannot be crossed from the femoral approach, then the brachial artery may be used as an access site. Some treating physicians perform the brachial access in a percutaneous fashion, while others prefer to perform a cutdown and to directly repair the artery. This decision is more commonly made when the artery is pulseless.

Interventionalists prefer different wires and catheters to successfully accomplish wire access past the stenosis or occlusion. It is important to be facile with both 0.035- and 0.014-in. wires to treat these lesions. In addition, a variety of catheters need to be in your treatment "bag". Straightforward anatomy can be approached using simple catheters such as a vertebral catheter or MPA. More challenging anatomy may require a reversed catheter such as a Headhunter, VTK, or SIM catheter. Protection devices are not commonly utilized for left subclavian artery interventions, but may have a role in the percutaneous treatment of the innominate artery. A combination of hydrophilic wires to traverse the stenosis and stiffer wires for the treatment are employed. A long, stiff sheath (usually 6 or 7 Fr and 90 cm in length) is selected to deliver the balloons and stents. Balloon-expandable stents are more commonly selected to treat these great vessel lesions (Figs. 6.3A to C). And, there seems to be an

increasing role in choosing covered stent technology to decrease the risk of recurrent stenosis.

When using the brachial approach, similar techniques are needed. The main difference between the two approaches is that shorter sheaths can be selected. In addition, this approach minimizes manipulation in the aortic arch and allows for more "pushability" to treat an occlusion that originates directly at the aortic arch.

5 OUTCOMES

The durability of endovascular angioplasty and stenting in the proximal aortic branches has been questioned since the first use of the procedure for subclavian lesions in the early 1980s.[13] However with advancements in endovascular technique, patency rates have steadily improved over time. Early studies indeed confirmed feasibility and good technical and patency outcomes,[14,15] and endovascular therapy has since become the primary treatment modality. The largest series examining 166 patients undergoing subclavian artery stenting demonstrated a technical success rate of 98%, with 83% primary patency and 96% secondary patency at 3 years.[16] Multiple other studies have consistently shown technical success in >90% of patients, and similar patency rates over 5 years.[17-19] Factors predicting restenosis included the use of multiple stents (i.e. long segment stenosis), smaller stent diameter, and persistent upper extremity systolic blood pressure difference postprocedure.[20]

6 ENDOVASCULAR VS OPEN REPAIR

Historically, surgical bypass was the standard of care for stenosis of the innominate and subclavian arteries, with generally good outcomes and acceptable complication rates.[21,22] Patency rates in two of the largest series were 94% and 98% at 5 years and 88% and 96% at 10 years, respectively.[23,24] However, with the advent of endovascular surgery, and given the inherent anatomic constraints of open surgery, there was much interest in applying these minimally invasive techniques to proximal aortic branch disease. Although no randomized, prospective data exists, two retrospective studies have directly compared endovascular therapy to open surgery (primarily carotid-subclavian bypass) within the past 10 years. In one study, endovascular primary patency rates were 78%, 72%, and 62% at 1, 3, and 5 years, respectively, with assisted primary patency of 84%, 76%, and 76% at the same intervals.[25]

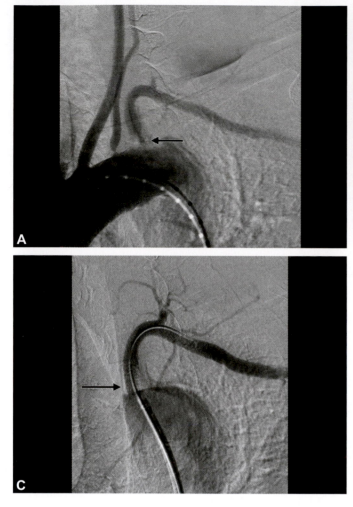

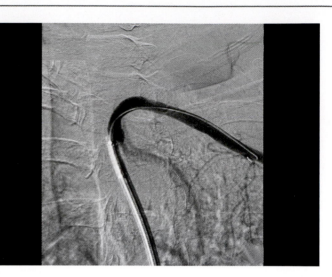

Figs. 6.3A to C: Stenting of a proximal left subclavian stenosis. (A) The initial digital subtraction angiogram demonstrates an endovascular wire traversing a significant subclavian stenosis (black arrow). (B) A stent is placed across the lesion. (C) Completion angiogram demonstrates successful stenting with resolution of the stenosis.

The second demonstrated endovascular primary patency of 93%, 78%, and 70% at 1, 3, and 5 years.[26] In both of these studies, the open surgical groups had significantly higher patency rates of >90% at 5 years, as well as longer freedom from recurrent symptoms. However, the endovascular patency rates in these studies are lower than those demonstrated in the noncomparison studies of endovascular therapy alone noted above where these data compare more favorably. Although open surgery seems to provide a more durable result, there is a still a major role for endovascular therapy. One of the major advantages of primary endovascular intervention is that is does not preclude future endovascular re-intervention, nor salvage surgical bypass for those with significant restenosis. Moreover, the data suggest that in a large proportion of patients, long-term durability can be achieved. For these reasons, endovascular therapy should be the first-line treatment in a significant number of patients with symptomatic subclavian and innominate artery stenoses. The exception to this would be younger patients without significant comorbidities; for these patients an up-front, single, durable repair would likely be preferable.

7 COMPLICATIONS OF ENDOVASCULAR REPAIR

Complications arising from endovascular surgery can generally be divided into three groups: (1) local complications related to access sites, (2) lesion-associated complications such as intimal dissection or perforation, and (3) systemic complications including neurologic sequelae and emboli. Access site issues often arise in the setting of atherosclerotic or calcified vessels. With femoral artery access, a calcified anterior wall may preclude percutaneous access, and in severe disease may preclude use of the artery altogether. For patients with known peripheral arterial disease who are likely to have calcified common femoral arteries, a cut-down technique is preferred to obtain proper vascular control and properly gain luminal access. Or, an alternative access site can be utilized. Other local complications include hematoma, acute thrombosis with or without distal emboli, pseudoaneurysm, dissection, and arterial-venous fistula. Complication rates associated with femoral arterial access are reported between 2% and 9%,[4] with brachial access site complications up to five times more likely to occur.[19] Perforation during stenting or wire dissection are iatrogenic in nature and, fortunately, quite rare. Both ischemic and embolic stroke are also uncommon, with rates reported at 0–2%.[5,20,27] Embolic events involving the vertebrobasilar system may be protected against by the reversed vertebral arterial flow.

8 CONCLUSION

Open-surgical bypass has long been the gold-standard for treatment of proximal aortic branch stenosis. However, as with much of vascular surgery in general, the tide is shifting in favor of less invasive endovascular techniques. It appears as though angioplasty and stenting of the subclavian and innominate arteries is safe, technically feasible, and provides long-term patency and freedom from symptoms in a large number of patients. Although retrospective data suggest that long-term patency rates are lower with endovascular repair than with open surgery, this is not always the primary objective of the intervention. Patients with subclavian and innominate stenoses tend to have multiple vascular and nonvascular comorbidities which place them at high risk for a major operation such as a sternotomy. The primary goal is often to relieve symptoms, especially cardiac ischemia in the setting of subclavian steal syndrome. The high technical success rate and initial patency, along with the significantly lower perioperative morbidity favors the use of endovascular interventions in the majority of patients as first-line therapy. Indeed, the primary advantage may lie in the fact that endovascular repair does not preclude future open repair, and will still result in long-term patency in the majority of patients, obviating the need for open surgery. Those patients who undergo angioplasty and/or stenting do require more procedures in the long term.[25,26,28] For this reason, open-surgical bypass should still be considered as primary therapy for young, otherwise healthy patients who would benefit from definitive repair up-front, as well as for those patients in whom endovascular repair has failed.

REFERENCES

1. Shadman R, Criqui MH, Bundens WP, et al. Subclavian artery stenosis: prevalence, risk factors, and association with cardiovascular diseases. J Am Coll Cardiol. 2004;44(3):618-23.
2. Yamamoto M, Hara H, Shinji H, et al. Endovascular treatment of innominate artery stenosis via the bilateral brachial approach. Cardiovasc Revasc Med. 2010;11(2):105-9.
3. Takach T, Reul GJ, Cooley DA, et al. Myocardial thievery: the coronary-subclavian steal syndrome. Ann Thorac Surg. 2006;81(1):386-92.
4. Stone P, Srivastiva M, Campbell JE, et al. Diagnosis and treatment of subclavian artery occlusive disease. Exp Rev Cardiovasc Ther. 2010;8(9):1275-82.
5. Woo E, Fairman RM, Velasquez OC, et al. Endovascular therapy of symptomatic innominate-subclavian arterial occlusive disease. Vasc Endovasc Surg. 2006;40(1):27-33.
6. Müller M, Schmitz BL, Pauls S, et al. Variations of the aortic arch—a study on the most common branching patterns. Acta Radiol. 2011;52(7):738-42.
7. Alcocer F, David M, Goodman R, et al. A forgotten vascular disease with important clinical implications. Subclavian steal syndrome. Am J Case Rep. 2013;14:58-62.
8. Rogers J, Calhoun RF 2nd. Diagnosis and management of subclavian artery stenosis prior to coronary artery bypass grafting in the current era. Angiology. 2007;22(1):20-25.
9. Singer AJ, Hollander JE. Blood pressure. assessment of interarm differences. Arch Intern Med. 1996;156(17):2005-8.
10. Ruegg W, VanDis FJ, Feldman HJ, et al. Aortic arch vessel disease and rationale for echocardiographic screening. J Am Soc Echoardiogr. 2013;26(2):114-25.
11. Thomassen L, Aarli JA. Subclavian steal phenomenon. Clinical and hemodynamic aspects. Acta Neurol Scand. 1994;90(4):241-4.
12. Willinek W, von Falkenhausen M, Born M, et al. Noninvasive detection of steno-occlusive disease of the supra-aortic arteries with three-dimensional contrast-enhanced magnetic resonance angiography: a prospective, intra-individual comparative analysis with digital subtraction angiography. Stroke. 2005;36(1):38-43.
13. Bachman D, Kim RM. Transluminal dilatation for subclavian steal syndrome. Am J Roentgenol. 1980;135(5):995-6.
14. Millaire A, Trinca M, Marache P, et al. Subclavian angioplasty: immediate and late results in 50 patients. Cathet Cardiovasc Diagn. 1993;29:8-17.
15. Mathias K, Luth I, Haarmann P. Percutaneous transluminal angioplasty of proximal subclavian artery occlusions. Cardiovasc Interv Radiol. 1993;16:214-8.
16. Patel S, White CJ, Collins TJ, et al. Catheter-based treatment of the subclavian and innominate arteries. Catheter Cardiovasc Interv. 2008;71(7):963-8.
17. De Vries J, Jager LC, Van den Berg JC, et al. Durability of percutaneous transluminal angioplasty for obstructive lesions of proximal subclavian artery: long-term results. J Vasc Surg. 2005;41(1):19-23.

18. Bates M, Broce M, Lavigne PS, et al. Subclavian artery stenting: factors influencing long-term outcome. Catheter Cardiovasc Interv. 2004;61(1):5-11.

19. Sullivan T, Gray BH, Bacharach JM, et al. Angioplasty and primary stenting of the subclavian, innominate, and common carotid arteries in 83 patients. J Vasc Surg. 1998;28(6): 1059-65.

20. Przewlocki T, Kablak-Ziembicka A, Pieniazek P, et al. Determinants of immediate and long-term results of subclavian and innominate artery angioplasty. Catheter Cardiovasc Interv. 2006;67(4):519-26.

21. Wylie E, Effeney DJ. Surgery of the aortic branches and vertebral arteries. Surg Clin North Am. 1979;59:669-80.

22. Edwards W, Mulherin JL Jr. The surgical reconstruction of the proximal subclavian and vertebral artery. J Vasc Surg. 1985;2:634-42.

23. Kieffer E, Sabatier J, Koskas F, et al. Atherosclerotic innominate artery occlusive disease: early and long-term results of surgical reconstruction. J Vasc Surg. 1995;21(2):326-36.

24. Berguer R, Morasch MD, Kline RA, et al. Cervical reconstruction of the supra-aortic trunks: a 16-year experience. J Vasc Surg. 1999;29(2):239-46.

25. Palchik E, Bakken AM, Wolford HY, et al. Subclavian artery revascularization: an outcome analysis based on mode of therapy and presenting symptoms. Ann Vasc Surg. 2008; 22(1):70-78.

26. AbuRahma A, Bates MC, Stone PA, et al. Angioplasty and stenting versus carotid-subclavian bypass for the treatment of isolated subclavian artery disease. J Endovasc Ther. 2007;14(5):698-704.

27. Hüttl K, Nemes B, Simonffy A, et al. Angioplasty of the innominate artery in 89 patients: experience over 19 years. Cardiovasc Interv Radiol. 2002;25(2):109-14.

28. Farina C, Mingoli A, Schultz RD, et al. Percutaneous transluminal angioplasty versus surgery for subclavian artery occlusive disease. Am J Surg. 1989;158(6):511-4.

Endovascular Treatment of Iatrogenic and Penetrating Subclavian Artery Injury

Michelle C Kosovec, Robert F Cuff

1 PREOPERATIVE

1.1 Indications

- Iatrogenic placement of central line or sheath into subclavian artery
- Penetrating trauma to subclavian artery
  - Pseudoaneurysm
  - Laceration
  - Arteriovenous fistula

1.2 Evidence

- Once there is cannulation of the subclavian artery with a sheath from a central line, blind removal of the sheath with manual pressure has high rate of mortality.[1]
- Blind sheath removal or unrecognized traumatic injury can lead to complications of hematoma, airway obstruction, stroke, and false aneurysm.[1,2]
- Balloon tamponade can be useful to control bleeding in traumatic hemorrhage in conjunction with covered stent placement.[2]
- Arterial closure devices have been used with success in select cases.[3,4]
- Endovascular repair of iatrogenic subclavian artery or penetrating injury with stenting has shown excellent technical success rates with low perioperative morbidity from the procedure.[5-9]
- Covered stent placement has also been used successfully in the setting of failed closure device attempt.[10]

1.3 Equipment

- *Exposure*:
  - *Percutaneous*: 19-gauge standard needle, Bentson or J-wire, short 5-Fr sheath, Glidewire, longer 8- to 12-Fr sheath to accommodate stents

  - *Open*: Standard common femoral artery approach with scalpel, electrocautery, metzenbaum scissors, vascular clamps, and vessel loops
    - May be preferable if using larger sheath.
  - Heparinize patient when larger sheath inserted or before clamping common femoral artery with open approach.
- *Endovascular*:
  - *Exchange length wires*: Bentson or J-wire, Glidewire
  - *Short 5-Fr sheath, longer sheaths*: 8–12 Fr
  - Covered stents (Viabahn, iCast)

1.4 Preoperative Planning and Risk Assessment

- *Comorbidities of patient*:
  - Iatrogenic injury occurs more often in patients with severe injuries that can be life-threatening necessitating emergent central line.
  - Risk factors include obesity, emergency puncture, and lack of ultrasound guidance.[11]
  - Traumatic injury to subclavian may also be part of multiple injuries in trauma patient.
- *If iatrogenic injury occurs with arterial catheter in position, do not immediately remove catheter*:
  - Catheter can be left in place until patient is stable enough for planned repair if patient critically ill from other injuries.[8]
- Traumatic injury with active exsanguination requires emergent repair.
- *Timeout*:
  - Correctly identify patient, side of injury, surgical approach.
  - Ensure appropriate wires, sheaths, and stents are available.
  - Confirm plan for removal of sheath at time of deployment of stent if iatrogenic central line injury with sheath left in position.

1.5 Contraindications

- Injury is at bifurcation of the innominate artery.
- Stenting would result in coverage of vertebral artery or other major arterial branch.
- Inability to place wire across site of injury.
- Shaggy aorta or significant intraluminal thrombus with common femoral artery approach, which could risk stroke, consider brachial approach.
- Severe renal insufficiency, risk of contrast-induced nephropathy.
- If contraindication present to endovascular repair, open repair may be necessary.
  - Open cutdown onto subclavian artery
  - Thoracotomy or median sternotomy for more proximal innominate injury
  - Video-assisted thoracic surgery technique has been described in one case.[12]

1.6 Surgical Anatomy

- *See* Figure 7.1.

1.7 Positioning

- The patient should lie supine on the operating table in an endovascular suite, with both groins exposed for planned access or arm exposure if brachial approach is anticipated (be prepared).

1.8 Anesthesia

- Local anesthetic is injected into site overlying needle access location.
- Monitored anesthesia care with sedation is also given unless patient already intubated with general anesthesia.

2 PERIOPERATIVE

2.1 Vascular Access

- 19-gauge needle access into common femoral artery overlying common femoral head in groin or into brachial artery under ultrasound guidance.
- A standard common femoral artery exposure or brachial exposure may be required for arterial access if using a larger sheath, ± a counter incision to ensure smooth entry of wires and catheters.

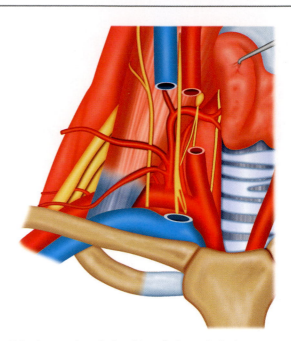

Fig. 7.1: Anatomic relationship of the subclavian artery and vein. The subclavian artery lies posterior to the anterior scalene muscle, while the subclavian vein lies anterior to the anterior scalene muscle. Both lie behind the clavicle.

2.2 Steps

- *See* Figures 7.2 to 7.8.

3 POSTOPERATIVE

3.1 Possible Complications of Stent Placement

- Technical failure
- Coverage of a vertebral artery—posterior circulation stroke
- Stroke from manipulation of wires/catheters in proximal arch.
- Contrast-induced nephropathy
- Groin infection rate higher if performing open cutdown technique for arterial exposure.
- Restenosis or occlusion of stent
- Migration of stent or stent fracture
- Limb-threatening ischemic events
- Stent infection

3.2 Outcomes

- Patients treated with endovascular repair of iatrogenic subclavian artery injury have excellent technical success rates without significant morbidity or mortality related to procedure.[8,10]

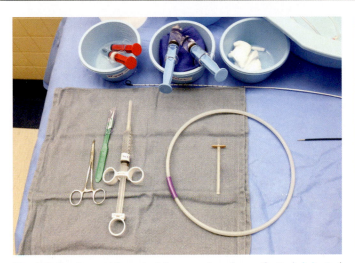

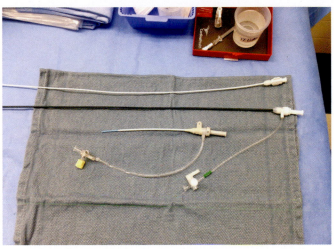

Fig. 7.2: Equipment for arterial access. Local anesthetic is injected into planned area of needle insertion. Standard 19-gauge standard needle access is used to common femoral artery overlying femoral head. A Bentson or J-wire is then guided through the wire under fluoroscopic guidance through the iliacs. A small 11 blade skin nick is sometimes needed for insertion of a short 5-Fr sheath (not pictured).

Fig. 7.3: Different sheaths needed during common femoral artery access. A 5-Fr sheath (foreground) is exchanged for a 19-gauge needle over Bentson or J-wire. A Glidewire (not pictured) is then guided through the 5-Fr sheath up into the proximal descending thoracic aorta. The short 5-Fr sheath is then exchanged for a longer, larger 8- to 12-Fr sheath (black, pictured in background) in order to guide in the covered stent and obtain further angiography for planned placement.

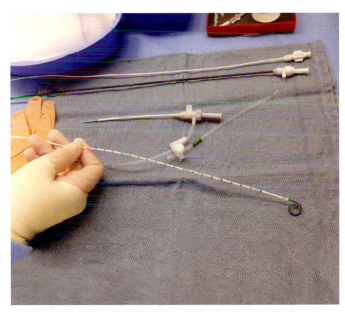

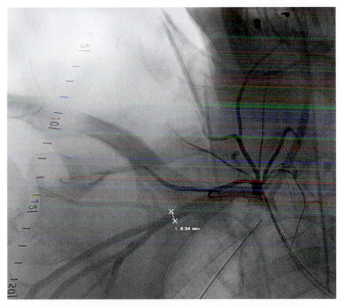

Fig. 7.4: Pigtail catheter for use during angiography. A catheter is then guided through the sheath over the wire in order to perform an angiogram and locate the site of injury to the subclavian artery (pigtail catheter, illustrated above). This is also used to determine the length of stent needed to treat the injury.

- Endovascular covered stent treatment for traumatic penetrating injury has also been shown to be safe and effective in small series for control of hemorrhage and

Fig. 7.5: Right subclavian artery injury as illustrated by angiography. Area noted for planned stent placement is in white.

exclusion of pseudoaneurysm, laceration, or arteriovenous fistula.[6]
- Meta-analysis conducted from 1990 to 2012 by DuBose et al. found no mortalities related to endovascular intervention and only 1 out of 160 patient had a new neurologic deficit (intraprocedural stroke).[7]

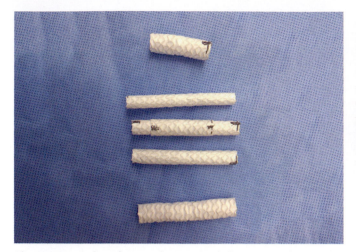

Fig. 7.6: Examples of covered stents (Viabahn, iCAST) that can be used for adequate coverage of the site of injury. Prompt removal of the existing sheath is required in timely fashion.

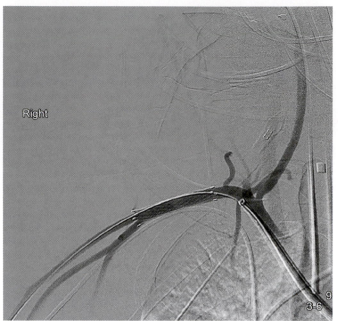

Fig. 7.7: Deployment and confirmation of stent placement. Once the stent has been successfully deployed in position, completion angiogram is performed to rule out any extravasation of contrast and seal of leak.

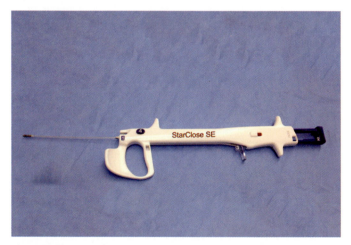

Fig. 7.8: Closure of access site. If there is significant atherosclerotic disease in the common femoral artery, manual pressure should be held after sheath removal over the access site for 10–15 minutes. If the arterial access site does not have significant atherosclerotic disease, a formal closure device may be used, such as Starclose (pictured), Perclose, or Mynx in standard fashion.

3.4 E-mail an Expert

- *E-mail address*: michelle.kosovec@gmail.com or robert.cuff@spectrumhealth.org

3.5 Web Resources/References

- Journal of Vascular Surgery: www.jvascsurg.org
- Society of Vascular Surgery: www.vascularweb.org

3.3 Follow-up

- Short-term follow-up is promising—meta-analysis with average follow-up of 70 months revealed patency rate of 84.4% of covered stents.[7]
- Other case-series demonstrate similar encouraging patency results without significant morbidity complications.[1,2,5,6,8,9]
- Literature thus far mostly consists of retrospective case reports and small case-series. Long-term follow-up results of endovascular stent placement are not known.

REFERENCES

1. Guilbert MC, Elkouri S, Bracco D, et al. Arterial trauma during central venous catheter insertion: case series, review and proposed algorithm. J Vasc Surg. 2008;48(4):918-25.
2. Yamagami T, Yoshimatsu R, Tanaka O, et al. A case of iatrogenic subclavian artery injury successfully treated with endovascular procedures. Ann Vasc Dis. 2011;4(1):53-5.
3. Kirkwood ML, Wahlgren CM, Desai TR. The use of arterial closure devices for incidental arterial injury. Vasc Endovasc Surg. 2008;42(5):471-6.
4. Tran V, Shiferson A, Hingorani AP, et al. Use of the StarClose device for closure of inadvertent subclavian artery punctures. Ann Vasc Surg. 2009;23(5):688
5. Cayne NS, Berland TL, Rockman CB, et al. Experience and technique for the endovascular management of iatrogenic subclavian artery injury. Ann Vasc Surg. 2010;24(1):44-7.
6. Cohen JE, Rajz G, Gomori JM, et al. Urgent endovascular stent-graft placement for traumatic penetrating subclavian artery injuries. J Neurol Sci. 2008;272(1-2):151-7.

7. DuBose JJ, Rajani R, Gilani R, et al. Endovascular management of axillo-subclavian arterial injury: a review of published experience. Injury. 2012;43:1785-92.

8. Kosovec MC, Mansour MA, Chambers CM, et al. Treatment of iatrogenic arterial injury during placement of a central venous line. [Abstract]. Society for Clinical Vascular Surgery 42nd Annual Symposium, Carlsbad, CA, Mar 18–22, 2014.

9. Rocha L, Dalio M, Joviliano E, et al. Endovascular approach for peripheral arterial injuries. Ann Vasc Surg. 2013;27 (5):587-93.

10. Abi-Jaoudeh N, Turba U, Arslan B, et al. Management of subclavian arterial injuries following inadvertent arterial puncture during central venous catheter placement. J Vasc Int Radiol. 2009;20:396-402.

11. Pikwer A, Acosta S, Kölbel T, et al. Management of inadvertent arterial catheterization associated with central venous access procedures. Eur J Vasc Endovasc Surg. 2009; 38(6):707-14.

12. Tam J, Atasha A, Tan A. Video-assisted thoracic surgery repair of subclavian artery injury following central venous catheterization: a new approach. Interact Cardiovasc Thorac Surg. 2013;17:13-15.

QUIZ

Question 1: All of the following are possible complications of stent placement EXCEPT:

a. Migration of stent or stent fracture
b. Posterior circulation stroke
c. Middle cerebral artery distribution stroke
d. Pulmonary embolism
e. Limb-threatening ischemic events

Question 2: The subclavian artery lies:

a. Anterior to the anterior scalene muscle and posterior to the subclavian vein
b. Anterior to the anterior scalene muscle and anterior to the subclavian vein
c. Posterior to the anterior scalene muscle and anterior to the subclavian vein
d. Posterior to the anterior scalene muscle and posterior to the subclavian vein

Question 3: A central line is placed on a patient in the Intensive Care Unit, and the monitor demonstrates arterial waveforms. The following are all contraindications to endovascular repair of the subclavian artery injury, EXCEPT:

a. Days of time from initial injury recognition to treatment
b. Shaggy aorta with femoral access
c. Close proximity of vertebral artery to injury site
d. Renal insufficiency
e. Inability to cross lesion with wire

ANSWERS:

1. d   2. d   3. a

Carotid Body Tumor Excision

Shonda Banegas, Jason D Slaikeu

1 PREOPERATIVE

1.1 Indications and Contraindications

Indications
- Any carotid body tumor identified should be resected.
- Any recurrent carotid body tumor should be resected if able.

Contraindications
- Poor surgical candidate for resection

1.2 Evidence

- Incidence of cranial nerve injury can be up to 50% with 70% to 80% resolution of clinically significant deficits in the first postoperative year.
- Incidence of stroke increases with Shamblin classification and need for arterial reconstruction.
- Recent studies show no significant benefit in the use of preoperative embolization to reduce the incidence of cranial nerve injury, operative time, stroke, death, or postoperative length of stay.
- Only 8–12% of tumors are malignant.

1.3 Materials Needed

- *Bipolar cautery forceps*: Ideal for dissecting along nerves (Fig. 8.1)
- *Harmonic Scalpel-Focus handle/Ligasure device*: Facilitates dissection in the subadventitial plane (Fig. 8.2).
- Have grafts available for bypass, patches available for any arterial injury requiring repair with patch (Fig. 8.3).

1.4 Preoperative Planning and Risk Assessment

- Perform full cranial nerve examination preoperatively.
- Laboratory evaluation to determine functionality including serum catecholamines and urine metanephrines and VMA.
- Consider subluxation of mandible with nasotracheal intubation.
- Shamblin Classification serves as a predictor for operative blood loss and need for arterial reconstruction (Fig. 8.4).

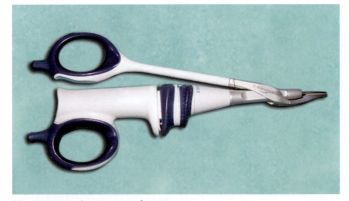

Fig. 8.1: Bipolar cautery forceps.

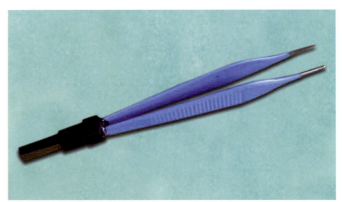

Fig. 8.2: Harmonic scalpel.

Low risk:
- *Shamblin type I*: Lower blood loss, excision with relative ease

Moderate risk:
- *Shamblin type II:* Larger, more arterial attachment, can be removed with care

High risk:
- *Shamblin type III*: Direct involvement with the artery and/or nerves. Higher likelihood of vascular reconstruction

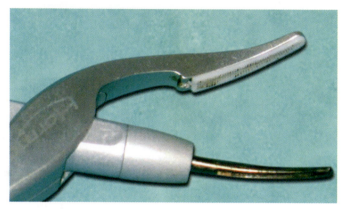

Fig. 8.3: Have grafts available for bypass.

1.5 Preoperative Checklist

Sign in:
- Blood availability
- Positioning
- α-Blockade available if patient becomes hypertensive
- Equipment available
- Imaging available

Time out:
- Consent for carotid body tumor excision with possible reconstruction.
- Preoperative antibiotics necessary with possibility of reconstruction.

Sign out:
- Specimen sent to laboratory, including any lymph nodes.
- Neurologic examination upon patient wakening.

1.6 Decision-Making Checklist

Pertinent history:
- *Symptoms of functional tumors*: Hypertension, tachycardia, palpitations
- *Symptoms of anatomical compression*: Hoarseness, neck pain, stridor, dysphonia, dysphagia, odynophagia, jaw stiffness, sore throat

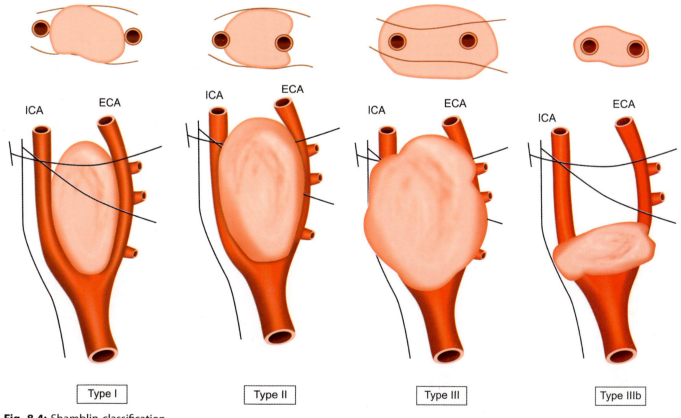

Fig. 8.4: Shamblin classification.

- *Family history*: Familial associated tumors and those associated with succinate dehydrogenase mutations are more likely to be functional and multifocal

Imaging:
- Angiography is the gold standard, but CT/MR angiography more acceptable now.
- Benefit of angiography is concurrent embolization and balloon occlusion evaluation if concerned for need to ligate internal carotid artery during the resection.

1.7 Pearls and Pitfalls

Pearls:
- Maintain meticulous hemostasis by careful dissection and use of bipolar cautery and Harmonic Scalpel or Ligasure.
- Identify and control inflow vessel(s) prior to aggressively resecting from the carotid.
- Identify cranial nerves prior to dissecting tumor.
- Sample cervical lymph nodes seen to evaluate for metastatic disease.

Pitfalls:
- Anatomy will be distorted and the tumor will be more adherent to adjacent structures as the tumor size increases. Proceed cautiously to minimize risk for nerve injury.
- If preoperative embolization is performed, do not wait >2–3 days before proceeding with the resection.
- During dissection, take care to stay in the subadventitial plane and not violate the media.

1.8 Surgical Anatomy

- *Important structures to identify*: Common, internal, and external carotid arteries; hypoglossal, vagus, superior laryngeal, and glossopharyngeal nerves.

See Figure 8.5.

1.9 Positioning

- Supine
- Shoulder roll in place
- Neck flexed as much as tolerated
- Head rotated to the contralateral side

1.10 Anesthesia

- Potential need for nasotracheal intubation if higher lesion with planned mandibular subluxation.
- Preparation for blockade if patient becomes hypertensive and/or tachycardic.

2 PERIOPERATIVE

2.1 Incision

- Oblique incision along anterior border of the sternocleidomastoid.
- Curve posteriorly once 1 cm below the angle of the mandible and inferior to the parotid gland.

2.2 Steps

- After the incision is made, carry the dissection through the subcutaneous tissues and platysma.
- Once the sternocleidomastoid is encountered, reflect the sternocleidomastoid muscle and internal jugular vein laterally. With silk suture, ligate any medial branches of the internal jugular vein that are overlying the tumor, but not those draining the tumor.
- With silk ties or the Harmonic Scalpel/Ligasure, ligate and sample any overlying lymphatic tissue.
- Identify the external carotid artery and any branches that are supplying the tumor. These can be ligated with the Harmonic Scalpel or silk ties.
- Identify the hypoglossal nerve and carefully dissect this free from the tumor. Can use bipolar cautery to facilitate removal without excessive bleeding.
- Identify the vagus nerve laterally and reflect the tumor anteriorly off the nerve through its course. Take the dissection to the most superior extent of the tumor along the internal carotid artery.

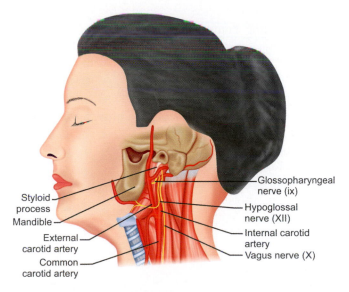

Fig. 8.5: Anatomy of carotid artery.

- Dissect in a lateral to medial/posterior to anterior direction. This will allow for identification of the superior laryngeal nerve. This will be left posterior to the artery.
- Once all nerves have been identified and dissected from the tumor, then dissect the tumor directly off of the carotid artery staying in the subadventitial plane. The Harmonic Scalpel/Ligasure works nice in this area to maintain hemostasis.
- Direct the dissection toward the carotid bulb.
- If the tumor is fixed along the artery, consider resection of the artery with either patch or bypass reconstruction. Can also ligate the internal or external carotid artery if the anatomy does not allow for repair.

2.3 Closure

- Irrigate the wound and check for hemostasis.
- Bring out a 7-Fr flat Jackson-Pratt drain through a separate stab incision and secure with suture.
- Close the platysma with 3–0 absorbable suture.
- Close the skin with a running subcuticular suture.

3 POSTOPERATIVE

3.1 Complications

Most common complications:
- Nerve injury
- Stroke or transient ischemic attack
- Bleeding (higher likelihood with arterial reconstruction)

Least common complications:
- Infection
- Cardiac (patient population is usually younger and healthier)
- Baroreceptor failure syndrome (only after bilateral resection, very rare)

3.2 Outcomes

- Tumors resected at Shamblin I and II classifications have lowest morbidity.
- Most cranial nerve injuries are due to stretch injury and resolve over time.
- Long-term control of the tumor is gained in up to 94% of patients that receive surgical intervention.

3.3 Follow-Up

- Yearly clinical examination for evidence of recurrence.
- PET scan if malignant on final pathology.
- Patients with bilateral, familial, and incompletely resected tumors need to be followed for life.

3.4 E-mail an Expert

- *E-mail address*: jason.slaikeu@spectrumhealth.org.

3.5 Web Resources/References

- Journal of Vascular Surgery: www.jvascsurg.org

SUGGESTED READING

Kruger A, Walker P, Foster W, et al. Important observations made managing carotid body tumors during a 25-year period. J Vasc Surg. 2010;52(6):1518-24.

Power A, Bower T, Kasperbauer J, et al. Impact of preoperative embolization on outcomes of carotid body tumor resections. J Vasc Surg. 2012;56(4):979-89.

Vogel T, Mousa A, Dombrovskiy V, et al. Carotid body tumor surgery: management and outcomes in the nation. Vasc Endovascular Surg. 2009;43(5):457-61.

Zhang W, Cheng J, Li Q, et al. Clinical and pathological analysis of malignant carotid body tumor: a report of nine cases. Acta Otolaryngol. 2008;43(8):591-5.

QUIZ

Question 1: The Shamblin classification serves as an indicator for:
a. Intraoperative blood loss
b. Risk of cranial nerve injury
c. Need for arterial reconstruction
d. All of the Above

Question 2: The blood supply of a carotid body tumor comes from the:
a. Common carotid artery
b. Internal carotid artery
c. External carotid artery
d. Vertebral artery

Question 3: The most common complication following carotid body tumor excision is:
a. Cranial nerve injury
b. Stroke
c. Bleeding
d. Infection

1. a   2. c   3. a

ANSWERS:

Thoracic Aorta

Thoracic Aneurysm Repair

Basel Ramlawi, Michael J Reardon

1 PREOPERATIVE

1.1 Indications

- Symptomatic TAA must be resected regardless of size. Symptoms may be due to pain, compression of adjacent organs, or significant aortic insufficiency (Figs. 9.1A and B).
- Asymptomatic patients with degenerative thoracic aneurysm, chronic aortic dissection, intramural hematoma, penetrating atherosclerotic ulcer, mycotic aneurysm, or pseudoaneurysm who are otherwise suitable candidates and for whom the ascending aorta or aortic sinus diameter is 5.5 cm or greater should be evaluated for surgical repair.
- Patients with bicuspid aortic valve (BAV), genetically mediated disorders, or familial history of thoracic aortic disease should undergo elective operation at smaller diameters (4.0–5.0 cm depending on the condition) to avoid acute dissection or rupture.
- Patients with an aneurysm growth rate of >0.5 cm/year in an aorta that is <5.5 cm in diameter should be considered for operation.

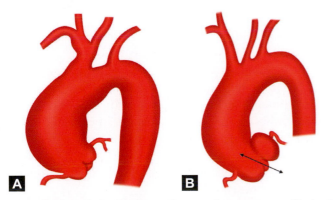

Figs. 9.1A and B: (A) Ascending aortic aneurysm. (B) Aortic insufficiency with ascending aneurysm.

- Patients undergoing cardiac surgery and who have an ascending aorta or aortic root of >4.5 cm should be considered for concomitant repair of the aortic root or replacement of the ascending aorta (Fig. 9.2).
- Aortic imaging is recommended for first-degree relatives of patients with thoracic aortic aneurysm (TAA) and/or dissection. If one or more first-degree relatives of a patient with known TAA and/or dissection are found to have TAA, then imaging of second-degree relatives is advised (Fig. 9.3).

1.2 Evidence

- Studies of the natural history of ascending aortic aneurysms indicate that aneurysms exceeding 6 cm in maximum diameter are associated with a particularly high risk of complications.
- The yearly risk of rupture increased 11-fold for aneurysms 5.0–5.9 cm in diameter compared with those <4.0 cm in maximum size, and it increased 27-fold for those over 6.0 cm.
- The annual risk of the composite endpoint of dissection or death was 15.6% for aneurysms >6.0 cm. By the time a patient's ascending aortic size reaches 6 cm, that patient has incurred a cumulative 34% risk of rupture or dissection.
- These recommendations for surgical intervention were comprehensively addressed in the 2010 Guidelines for the Diagnosis and Management of Patients with Thoracic Aortic Disease.

1.3 Materials Needed

- Standard cardiac surgical operating setup and instruments.
- Cardiopulmonary bypass.
- Hybrid operating room required where intraoperative fluoroscopy is needed for combined open surgical and

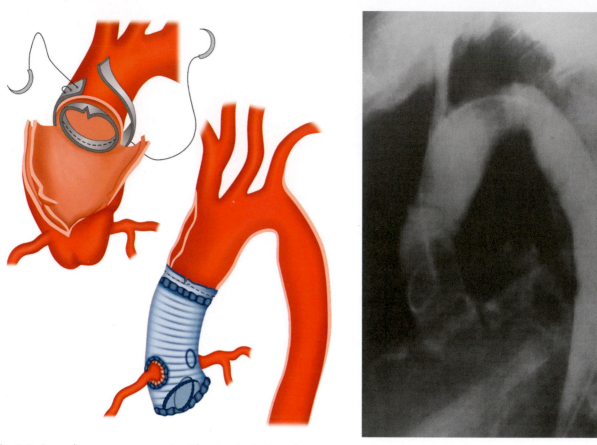

Fig. 9.2: Ascending aneurysm repair with reimplantation of coronary arteries.

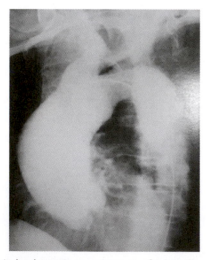

Fig. 9.3: Digital subtraction angiogram of ascending aneurysm.

thoracic aortic endograft placement (aortic endografting). Standard endovascular tools including soft and stiff wires, catheters, and balloons.

- Various size coated Dacron grafts for aortic replacement (26–34 mm diameter) as well as 8 mm Dacron graft for use during axillary artery cannulation (used for repair of thoracic aortic arch or distal ascending thoracic aorta).
- Neuromonitoring equipment (electroencephalogram (EEG), transcranial Doppler, cerebral oximetry, etc.) needed for thoracic aortic arch repair.

1.4 Preoperative Planning and Risk Assessment

Planning:
- Computed tomography (CT) of entire aorta and ileofemoral access with/without contrast or dynamic aortic magnetic resonance imaging with cardiac imaging (CMR increasingly more useful).
- Transthoracic echocardiogram with assessment of aortic valve morphology (tricuspid vs bicuspid).
- Cardiac catheterization or coronary CT scan (for low-risk patients).
- Cardiology consult and preoperative cardiac clearance.
- Pulmonary function tests.
- Complete physical examination with emphasis on neurologic assessment and peripheral vascular supply.

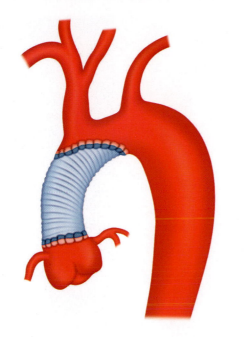

Fig. 9.4: Ascending aneurysm repair above the coronary sinus.

- Basic blood tests including renal and hepatic panel.

Risk assessment:

- Low-risk patients generally <5% risk of mortality for ascending aortic or aortic root repair procedures (Fig. 9.4).
- Risk of death, stroke and renal insufficiency increases significantly (10–20%) with involvement of aortic arch requiring debranching or thoracoabdominal aneurysm repair (Figs. 9.5A to D).
- Factors that increase perioperative risk:
  – Advanced age
  – Calcified aorta
  – History of stroke
  – Comorbidities (renal, liver, lung disease)
  – Need to replace long segments of aorta
  – Concomitant cardiac disease
  – Coagulopathy
  – Frailty

1.5 Preoperative Checklist

- Adequate blood pressure control
- Cessation of blood thinners and antiplatelet medications
- Cardiac clearance
- Confirmation of imaging studies including all aortic anatomy involved and branch vessels (carotids, vertebrals, subclavians, and visceral vessels).

- Review operative plan with team members including anesthesiologist, perfusionist, and nursing staff

1.6 Decision-Making Checklist

- Thoracic aortic aneurysm repaired if:
  – Symptomatic (chest pain)
  – Meets size criteria (>5.5 cm in tricuspid aortic valve or >5.0 cm in BAV or family history of aortic complications)
  – Undergoing other cardiac surgery with size >4.5 cm.
- Thoracic endovascular repair (TEVAR) has become the preferred approach for descending aortic pathology with adequate proximal and distal landing zones (>2.0 cm) (Figs. 9.6A and B).
- Aortic arch repair procedures can now be performed with excellent outcomes using hybrid arch vessel debranching from ascending aorta followed by TEVAR of the aortic arch (Fig. 9.7).

1.7 Pearls and Pitfalls

Pearls:

- Axillary artery cannulation for cardiopulmonary bypass preferred in context of aortic arch and distal ascending aortic pathology, as it allows for most flexibility and easy antegrade cerebral perfusion during periods of circulatory arrest.
- Proximal and distal control of the aorta and any relevant branches is mandatory.
- Always fill the right ventricle and aorta prior to determining location or right coronary ostium anastomosis, as this will avoid kinking of right carotid artery.
- If performing an aortic arch debranching as part of a hybrid aortic arch repair, always place the proximal component as low as possible on ascending aorta (close to sinotubular junction) in order to allow for adequate proximal endograft landing zone.
- Complete deairing is critical for neuroprotection.
- Most needle-hole bleeding stops with protamine reversal. Extrasutures in weak aortic tissue can lead to more bleeding. Topical surgical sealants are often used as valuable adjuncts.

Pitfalls:

- Beware of coronary ostial bleeding during coronary reimplantation (modified Bentall procedure), as visualization of these will be challenging once distal aortic anastomosis is completed.
- Beware of large collateral vessel bleeding in context descending thoracic aortic repair for coarctation.

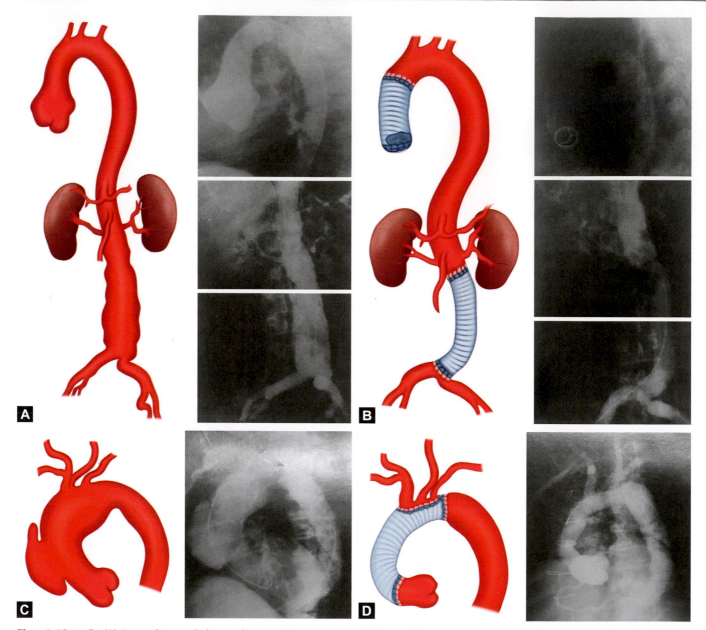

Figs. 9.5A to D: (A) Ascending and descending aortic aneurysms. (B) Ascending aneurysm repair with Dacron graft and infrarenal aortic aneurysm repair with tube Dacron graft. (C) Ascending and transverse thoracic aortic aneurysm (D) Debranching procedure with separate grafts to the innominate, left common carotid and left subclavian arteries.

1.8 Positioning

- Ascending aorta and aortic arch procedures performed in the supine position through a standard sternotomy approach (Fig. 9.8).
- Repair of the descending thoracic aorta or thoracoabdominal procedures performed in the right lateral decubitus position (left side up), left arm above the head and left groin exposed. This allows for exposure of the left hemithorax from the vertebrae to the sternum as well as the abdomen. Groin is exposed in case femoral vessel cannulation is required for cardiopulmonary bypass.

1.9 Anesthesia

- All procedures generally performed under general anesthesia.

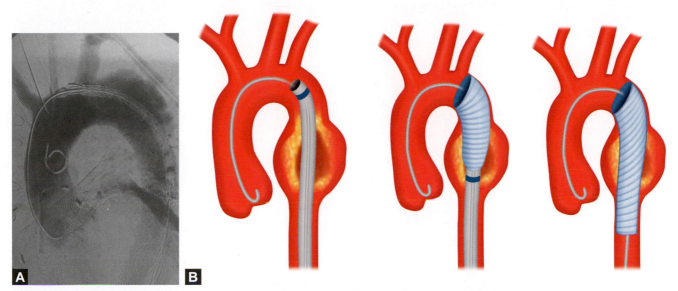

Figs. 9.6A and B: Digital subtraction angiography of descending thoracic aneurysm, endograft predeployment.

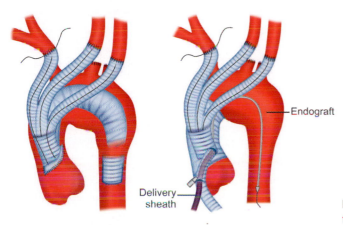

Fig. 9.7: Debranching of the ascending and transverse aneurysms followed by thoracic endovascular repair.

- Double lumen endotracheal tube used for thoracotomy or thoracoabdominal incision.
- Cerebrospinal fluid drain is inserted for descending thoracic aortic repair procedures where a long segment of aorta is involved.
- High thoracic epidural may be inserted for postoperative analgesia.

2 PERIOPERATIVE

2.1 Incision

- Midline sternotomy incision for all ascending thoracic aorta and aortic arch procedures (Fig. 9.8).
- 5 cm axillary incision in right deltopectoral groove for subclavian artery cannulation (via 8 mm Dacron graft)

used in aortic arch or high ascending aortic aneurysm cases.
- Full posterolateral thoracotomy position used for descending thoracic aortic aneurysms at the 6th to 8th intercostal space depending on location of aortic pathology. Incision extended to umbilicus through rectus abdominis muscle for thoracoabdominal incision (retroperitoneal exposure).

2.2 Steps

- Midline sternotomy, suspension of pericardium, and insertion of sternal retractor.
- Axillary cannulation is performed through a 5 cm incision in the deltopectoral groove followed by splitting the pectoralis major muscle along the fibers and

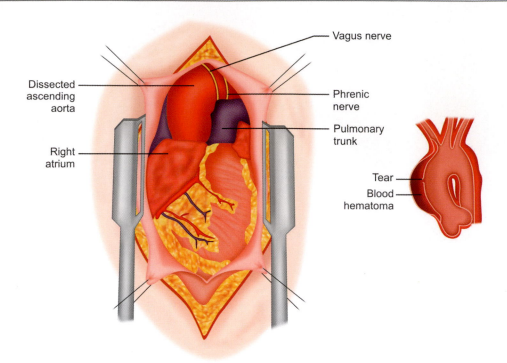

Fig. 9.8: Median sternotomy with suspension of the pericardium.

transecting the pectoralis minor muscle at its insertion. The artery is readily visualized and care should be taken when mobilizing the subclavian artery to not retract or injure the brachial plexus. Heparin (5,000 units) is administered, artery is opened longitudinally, and 8 mm Dacron graft is anastomosed to the subclavian artery using 5-0 or 6-0 Prolene suture. Graft is then attached to arterial limb of cardiopulmonary bypass machine.

- Administration of systemic heparinization (activated clotting time >480 s) and cannulation for cardiopulmonary bypass. Typically, this is done by cannulation of right atrium through two-stage venous cannula for venous drainage. If axillary cannulation is not performed, then usual arterial cannulation at level of aortic arch can be done for ascending and root procedures.
- Antegrade and retrograde cardioplegia catheters are inserted. LV vent is inserted via right superior pulmonary vein. Cardiopulmonary bypass is initiated.
- If procedure is to be performed under circulatory arrest, then cooling is initiated to 18°C for approximately 30 minutes. This can also be monitored with EEG and bispectral index neuromonitoring to ensure brain protection.
- Circulatory arrest is begun and distal aortic anastomosis is performed at level of aortic arch (using 4-0 or 3-0 Prolene).

- Antegrade cerebral perfusion through the axillary cannula by clamping innominate artery and initiating flow at 10 mL/kg/min.
- Cardioplegia is administered via coronary ostial cannulae or via retrograde through the coronary sinus every 15 minutes.
- Graft and aorta are desired. Graft is clamped and full systemic perfusion is restored. Rewarming of the patient is begun to normothermia.
- Aortic graft is tailored to the appropriate length (excessive length leads to kinking). Proximal aortic anastomosis is performed at the level of the sinotubular junction. If aortic root procedures are to be performed (e.g. modified Bentall or aortic valve repair), this is done during the rewarming process (Fig. 9.9).
- Aortic cross clamp is removed, ending cardiac ischemia.
- Suture lines are inspected and any bleeding repaired.
- Patient is weaned from cardiopulmonary bypass and protamine is administered. Cannulas and catheters are removed.
- Transesophageal echocardiography is performed to ensure adequate aortic valve and ventricular function.
- Mediastinal drainage tubes are inserted and chest is closed in routine fashion.

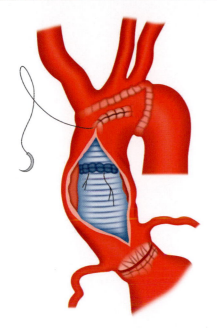

Fig. 9.9: Ascending and transverse repair.

3 POSTOPERATIVE

3.1 Complications

- The most serious complications following thoracic aortic repair are bleeding (intra-operative), stroke and myocardial infarction (perioperative).
- The circulatory arrest process often leads to coagulopathy that can be reversed with transfusion of blood products.
- Stroke can be minimized through deairing, decreasing circulatory arrest time, increasing perfusion pressure, removal of potential calcified debris and use of cerebral perfusion and monitoring techniques.

- The risk of paraplegia increases significantly in descending thoracic aortic aneurysm repair procedures, where pathology involves long segments of the aorta. Reimplantation of spinal arteries and use of cerebrospinal fluid drain improve outcomes.

3.2 Outcomes

- Thoracic aortic aneurysm repairs can be performed with excellent outcomes and minimal complications using modern, commonly used techniques.
- Isolated ascending and root aortic aneurysm repairs carry <5% risk of mortality, stroke or myocardial infarction. Risk increased with aortic arch involvement requiring circulatory arrest (5–15% mortality or major morbidity).

3.3 Follow-Up

- Patients with open thoracic aortic aneurysm repair require routine postoperative clinic follow-up at 30 days. Further imaging follow-up is required on an annual or biannual basis to assess remaining aortic segments.
- Hybrid and endovascular aortic repair procedures need close imaging follow-up (3–6 months) to ensure aneurysm sac decreases in size and ensure lack of endoleak.

3.4 Web Resources/References

- Hiratzka et al. 2010 ACCF/AHA/AATS/ACR/ASA/SCA/SCAI/SIR/STS/SVM Guidelines for the Diagnosis and Management of Patients with Thoracic Aortic Disease. Circulation. 2010;121:e266-e369
- CTSNet.org

QUIZ

Question 1: A 64-year-old male patient, otherwise healthy, presents with incidental finding of a 5.6 cm asymptomatic ascending aortic aneurysm extending from the level of the aortic sinuses to the proximal arch (4.5 cm). Aneurysm tapers off in midarch to 3.6 cm. Echocardiography reveals the presence of a BAV. What management option would you offer this patient?

a. Blood pressure control (medical management)
b. Replacement of ascending aorta
c. Replacement of ascending aorta and root
d. Replacement of aortic root, ascending and hemiarch with circulatory arrest
e. Replacement of aortic root, ascending and total arch with circulatory arrest

ANSWER:

1. c

Thoracic Endovascular Aortic Repair for Traumatic Aortic Injury

Ali Azizzadeh, Sapan S Desai, Kristofer M Charlton-Ouw, Anthony L Estrera, Hazim J Safi

1 PREOPERATIVE

1.1 Indications

- Medical therapy
  - *Grade 1 injury*: Intimal tear without external contour abnormality
- Thoracic endovascular aortic repair (TEVAR; urgent vs delayed)
  - *Grade 2 injury*: Intramural hematoma with an external contour abnormality
  - *Grade 3 injury*: Pseudoaneurysm
- TEVAR (emergent)
  - *Grade 4 injury*: Free rupture
- Contraindications
  - Anatomically unsuitable candidates due to location of injury (ascending aorta or transverse arch) or inadequate access
  - Patients with allergy to nickel or titanium alloys

See Figure 10.1.[1]

1.2 Evidence

- For the 2011 clinical practice guidelines of the society for vascular surgery (SVS) on endovascular repair of traumatic thoracic aortic injury, an expert panel was assembled and a meta-analysis of the literature was performed.[2] Based on an overall very low quality of evidence, the committee found that TEVAR was associated with "better survival and decreased risk of spinal cord ischemia, renal injury, graft, and systemic infections compared with open repair or nonoperative management."[2]
- In the 2011 systematic review of the literature involving 7,768 patients from 139 studies, the SVS reported a significantly higher early mortality rate for nonoperative

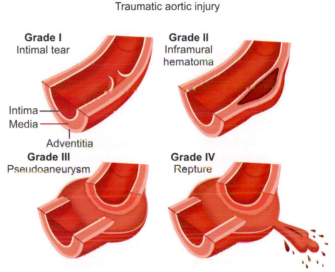

Classification of Traumatic aortic injury

Grade I Intimal tear

Grade II Inframural hematoma

Intima
Media
Adventitia

Grade III Pseudoaneurysm

Grade IV Repture

Fig. 10.1: Classification of traumatic aortic injury. *Adapted from* Azizzadeh et al.

management and open repair compared to TEVAR (nonoperative 46%; open repair 19%, and TEVAR 9%; $p < 0.01$).[3]

- In a prospective multicenter study conducted by the American Association for the surgery of trauma (AAST) that included 193 patients from 18 centers, the mortality was 23.5% in the open repair group compared to 7.2% in the TEVAR group ($p = 0.001$).[4]

See Figures 10.2A and B.

1.3 Materials Needed

- Operating room equipped with mobile or fixed fluoroscopy imaging equipment
- Adequate supply of needles, wires, catheters, sheaths, and balloons
- Radiopaque intravenous contrast

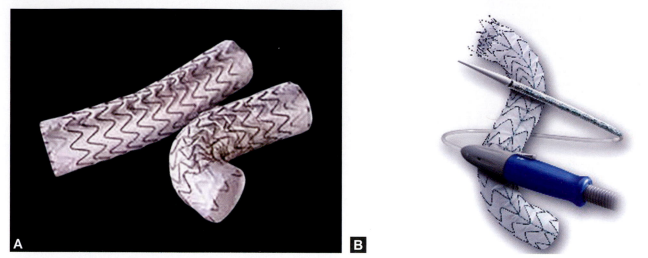

Figs. 10.2A and B: Current devices approved for treatment of traumatic aortic injury include (A) C-TAG (WL Gore, Flagstaff, AZ) and (B) Valiant (Medtronic, Santa Rosa, CA).

- Endovascular thoracic stent-graft selected based on computed tomographic angiography (CTA) measurements of the aorta
- Device oversizing is based on the manufacturer's instructions for use (IFU)
- Covered stent grafts to treat access complications as needed
- Intravascular ultrasound (IVUS) as needed

1.4 Preoperative Risk Assessment

Low risk:
- Low-injury severity score
- Adequate proximal and distal landing zone
- Satisfactory access vessels
- No major cardiovascular disease
- No renal disease

High risk:
- High injury severity score
- Required left subclavian artery (LSCA) coverage and/or revascularization
- Inadequate access requiring adjunct procedures
- Major cardiovascular disease
- Renal disease

1.5 Checklist

Sign in:
- Patient supine on a fluoroscopy table
- Availability of C-arm, contrast media, radiology technician, and supplies
- Patient prepped xiphoid process to knees

Time out:
- Plan for aortogram, possible intravascular ultrasound, possible TEVAR
- Possible LSCA revascularization
- Possible adjunctive access procedure (endovascular or retroperitoneal conduit)

Sign out:
- No type I or III endoleaks on completion angiogram
- Satisfactory lower extremity pulses
- Hemodynamically stable patient

1.6 Decision-Making Checklist

Diagnosis:
- Diagnosis is based on CTA (Fig. 10.3).
- The grade of injury (1–4) has both prognostic and therapeutic significance.
- IVUS is useful in delineating injury grade in patients with equivocal CTA.[5]
- Traditional angiography is primarily performed at the time of repair.

Timing of repair:
- The timing and sequence of repair in patients with multiorgan trauma is individualized based on the hemodynamic status of the patient, the grade of traumatic aortic injury (TAI), and the presence and severity of the associated injuries.
- Patients with TAI who undergo delayed repair should be started on anti-impulse (β-blockade) medical therapy if possible.

- Patient with concomitant traumatic brain injury who benefit from increased mean arterial pressures should undergo early repair if possible.

LSCA coverage:[6,7]

- Selective revascularization of the LSCA is safe in patients with TAI.
- Indications for LSCA revascularization include:
  - *Preoperative*:
    - Left internal mammary artery coronary bypass graft
    - Left vertebral artery terminating in the posterior inferior cerebellar artery
    - Stenotic or occluded right vertebral artery
    - Dominant left vertebral artery
    - Left upper extremity hemodialysis access
    - Spinal protection (relative indication in patients who are at high risk for paraplegia).
  - *Postoperative*:
    - Left upper extremity ischemia evidenced by claudication or rest pain
    - Vertebrobasilar insufficiency.

See Figure 10.3.

1.7 Pearls and Pitfalls

Pearls:

- Some forward tension on the stiff wire prior to deployment can ensure appropriate apposition of the stent-graft along the outer curvature of the aorta, especially in patients with a tight aortic arch (Fig. 10.4).
- In some patients with tight aortic arches, intentional coverage of the subclavian artery will place the proximal end of the device in a more straight and desirable segment of aorta. This will avoid the curved "no man's land" in zone 3 and help achieve good inner curvature apposition.
- Three-dimensional reconstructions may aid in device sizing and identifying whether left subclavian coverage and/or revascularization may be necessary
- Use of local intra-arterial vasodilators and Surgilube can be helpful in placement of small and/or borderline iliacs. Young patients are especially prone to vasospasm.

Pitfalls:

- An aortogram is recommended after device delivery and prior to deployment to confirm proper placement. Micro-adjustments can be done if necessary. The assistant can hold forward tension on the wire with the device in a "locked-in" position, while the surgeon does the deployment (or vice versa).
- Postdeployment angioplasty can be avoided in most patients who have an adequate seal after device placement.
- Significant oversizing of the device can lead to endoleaks and device failure.

1.8 Surgical Anatomy

- The ascending aorta begins within the pericardial sac, gives off the right and left coronary arteries at the root

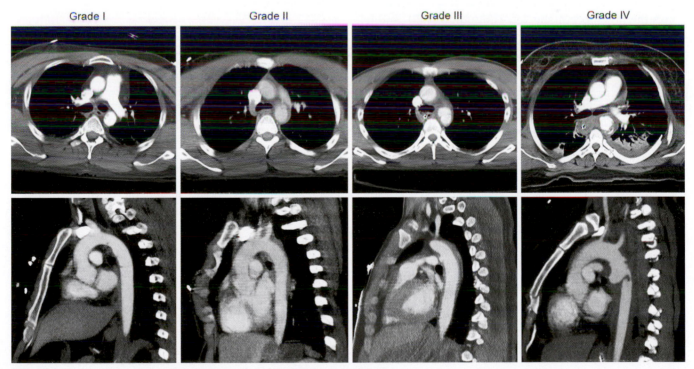

Fig. 10.3: Computed tomographic angiography of traumatic aortic injury.

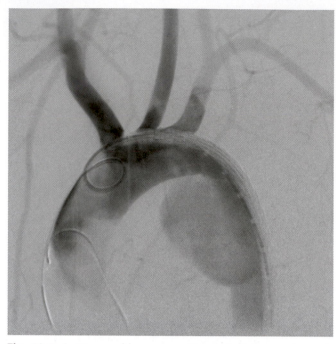

Fig. 10.4: A 17-year-old woman with grade 3 traumatic aortic injury. Forward tension on the stiff wire prior to deployment ensures appropriate apposition of the stent-graft along the outer curvature of the aorta.

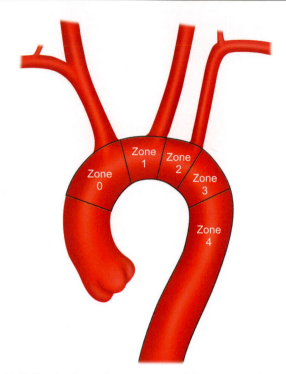

Fig. 10.5: Proximal attachment zones of the aortic arch.

of the aorta, and travels approximately 5 cm before giving off the branches of the aortic arch.
- The arch consists of the segments of the aorta that give off the brachiocephalic, left common carotid, and left subclavian arteries.
- The descending aorta begins distal to the LSCA and travels to the aortic hiatus at the level of the diaphragm near the T12 vertebra, where it becomes the abdominal aorta.
- The proximal attachment of the thoracic device is classified into Zones 0–4.[8,9]
- A variety of congenital alterations to the transverse arch and proximal descending thoracic aorta exist. These include the bovine variation, aortic spindle, ductus diverticulum, and bronchointercostal artery (*see* Figure 10.5).

1.9 Positioning

- The patient should be positioned supine.
- The patient should be prepped from the sternal notch to the knees.
- Access to the chest may be required for a tube thoracostomy in patients with Grade 4 injuries.

- Access to the retroperitoneum be required if an adjunctive access procedure (retroperitoneal conduit) becomes necessary.

1.10 Anesthesia

- General endotracheal anesthesia is preferred for TEVAR in patients with TAI.

2 PERIOPERATIVE

2.1 Incision

- Either percutaneous or open femoral artery access is acceptable. The choice should be based on patient's anatomy and the experience of the surgeon.

2.2 Steps

- Diagnostic arch aortogram is completed in a left anterior oblique projection using a marker diagnostic catheter.
  - Cerebrovascular and arch anatomy should be evaluated to determine if LSCA coverage is necessary, and whether revascularization will be required.

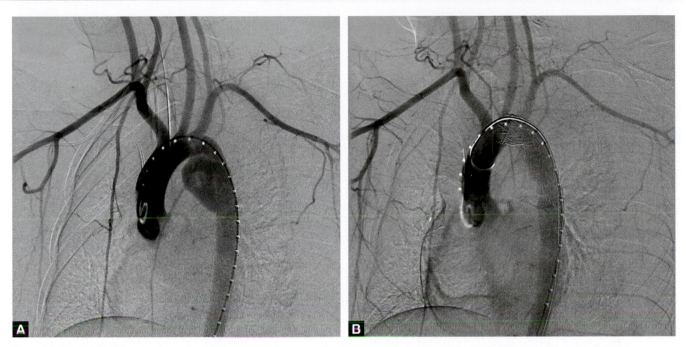

Figs. 10.6A and B: Diagnostic and completion angiogram of a 17-year-old woman with grade 3 traumatic aortic injury.

- The patient should be anticoagulated with reduced-dose heparin at 0.5 mg/kg in multiorgan trauma cases.
- A thoracic stent-graft is delivered via the femoral access.
- A follow-up angiogram is obtained to identify the location of the injury as well as the arch vessels in relation to the device.
- Microadjustments are made and a repeat angiogram is performed if necessary.
- The device is deployed using standard technique according to the manufacturer's IFU.
- A completion aortogram should be performed to ensure satisfactory placement and to rule out endoleaks.
- Selective balloon angioplasty can be performed if there is concern about graft apposition.
- The heparin should be reversed with protamine.

See Figures 10.6A and B.

2.3 Closure

- Standard percutaneous or open closure of the groin should be performed.
- We prefer to use two Proglide (Abbott) devices for percutaneous closure.
- A piece of rubber tubing can be used with the sutures similar to a Rummel tourniquet for hemostasis.

See Figure 10.7.[12]

3 POSTOPERATIVE

3.1 Complications

- *Most common complications*:
  - Trauma to access vessels
  - Device malapposition (especially to inner aortic curve)
  - Endoleak
- *Uncommon complications*:
  - Stroke
  - Device compression/collapse
  - Renal failure
  - Respiratory failure
  - Neurologic deficit (paraplegia/paraparesis)
  - Migration of the stent-graft
  - Device maldeployment
  - Retrograde aortic dissection
  - Death

3.2 Outcomes

- In our 15-year institutional experience on 338 patients with TAI, the early mortality was 41%.[10]
- The mortality for patients undergoing TEVAR was 4% compared to 17% for open repair.

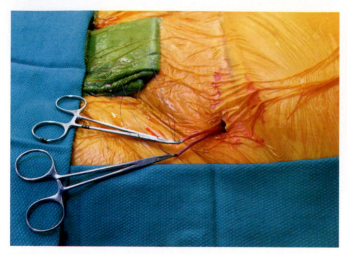

Fig. 10.7: Rubber tubing used with percutaneous closure similar to a Rummel tourniquet.

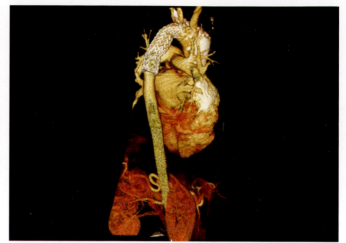

Fig. 10.8: One-year follow-up computed tomographic angiography of the patient shown in Figure 10.6 demonstrates healing of the traumatic aortic injury.

- One- and five-year survival after TEVAR is 92% and 87% compared to 76% and 75% after open repair.
- Variable costs for TEVAR are higher compared to open repair, but total cost of care is similar.[11]

3.3 Follow-Up

- The patient should be monitored in the trauma ICU.
- The patient may be discharged after treatment of associated injuries.
- The patient should follow-up in clinic in 1 month with CTA imaging.
- The patient will require annual clinic visit and CTA to monitor for delayed complications.

See Figure 10.8.

3.4 E-mail an Expert

- *E-mail address*: Ali.Azizzadeh@uth.tmc.edu

REFERENCES

1. Azizzadeh A, Keyhani K, Miller CC, et al. Blunt traumatic aortic injury: initial experience with endovascular repair. J Vasc Surg. 2009;49(6):1403-8.
2. Lee WA, Matsumura JS, Mitchell RS, et al. Endovascular repair of traumatic thoracic aortic injury: clinical practice guidelines of the Society for Vascular Surgery. J Vasc Surg. 2011;53(1):187-92.
3. Murad MH, Rizvi AZ, Malgor R, et al. Comparative effectiveness of the treatments for aortic transaction: a systematic review and meta-analysis. J Vasc Surg. 2011; 53(1):193-9.e1-21.
4. Demetriades D, Velmahos GC, Scalea TM, et al. Operative repair or endovascular stent graft in blunt traumatic thoracic aortic injuries: results of an American association for the surgery of trauma multicenter study. J Trauma. 2008;64:561-70; discussion 570-571.
5. Azizzadeh A, Valdes J, Miller CC, et al. The utility of intravascular ultrasound compared to angiography in the diagnosis of blunt traumatic aortic injury. J Vasc Surg. 2011;53(3):608-14.
6. Matsumura JS, Lee WA, Mitchell RS, et al. The Society for Vascular Surgery Practice Guidelines: management of the left subclavian artery with thoracic endovascular aortic repair. J Vasc Surg. 2009;50(5):1155-8.
7. Antonello M, Menegolo M, Maturi C, et al. Intentional coverage of the left subclavian artery during endovascular repair of traumatic descending thoracic aortic transection. J Vasc Surg. 2013;57(3):684-90.
8. Balm R, Reekers JA, Jacobs MJHM. Classification of endovascular procedures for treating thoracic aortic aneurysms. In: Jacobs MJHM, Branchereau A (Eds). Surgical and Endovascular Treatment of Aortic Aneurysms. New York: Futura Publishing Company; 2000. pp. 19-26.
9. Mitchell RS, Ishimaru S, Ehrlich MP, et al. First international summit on thoracic aortic endografting: roundtable on thoracic aortic dissection as an indication for endografting. J Endovasc Ther. 2002;9(Suppl 2):II98-105.
10. Estrera AL, Miller CC, Salinas-Guajardo G, et al. Update on Blunt thoracic aortic injury: 15-year single-institution experience. J Thorac Cardiovasc Surg. 2013;145:S154-8.
11. Azizzadeh A, Charlton-Ouw KM, Chen Z, et al. An outcome analysis of endovascular vs. open repair of blunt traumatic aortic injuries. J Vasc Surg. 2013;57(1):108-14.
12. Furlough CL, Desai SS, Azizzadeh A. Adjunctive technique for the use of ProGlide vascular closure device to improve hemostasis. J Vasc Surg. 2014 Oct 1. pii: S0741-5214(14)01670-X.

QUIZ

Question 1: Which of the following is the best management option for a 25-year-old hemodynamically stable patient who has a blunt thoracic aortic injury (pseudoaneurysm, grade 3) that is located 1 cm distal to the takeoff of the LSCA?
a. Left carotid-subclavian artery bypass followed by elective TEVAR
b. Urgent TEVAR with LSCA coverage
c. Urgent TEVAR without LSCA coverage
d. Open repair through a left lateral thoracotomy

Question 2: Which of the following is the most common site of trauma in blunt thoracic aortic injury?
a. Aortic isthmus   b.   Ascending aorta
c. Transverse aortic arch
d. Descending thoracic aorta

Question 3: Which of the following conditions should warrant repair using TEVAR?
a. Pseudoaneurysm   b.   Ductus diverticulum
c. Aortic spindle   d.   Intimal tear

ANSWERS:

1. b   2. a   3. a

Thoracic Endovascular Aneurysm Repair

Allan W Tulloch, David Rigberg

1 PREOPERATIVE

1.1 Indications

- Thoracic aortic aneurysm (TAA) >5.5 cm or enlarging by 0.5 cm or greater in 6 months
- Symptoms of chest pain and/or discomfort attributed to TAA
- Rupture of TAA
- Penetrating aortic ulcer when symptomatic or expanding with intramural hematoma
- Traumatic aortic transection
- Acute type B aortic dissection with end-organ ischemia (evolving indication)
- Chronic type B aortic dissection with aneurysmal degeneration
- There are few contraindications to thoracic endovascular aneurysm repair (TEVAR) except for unfavorable anatomy described below. The one exception is patients with connective tissue disorders (Marfan's, Ehlers–Danlos, etc.), where TEVAR is a relative contraindication and open repair should be considered.

1.2 Evidence

- TEVAR was originally developed for patients who were not candidates for open operations. Its advantages include small or no incisions, no aortic cross clamping, less blood loss, and decreased end-organ ischemia, with a quicker postoperative recovery.
- In clinical trials comparing TEVAR to open repair of TAAs, TEVAR was found to be a safer and more effective alternative with fewer cardiac, pulmonary, and vascular adverse events, but with equivalent neurologic complications compared to open repair.
- Increasing evidence has led to the rapid adoption of TEVAR in the treatment of traumatic aortic transection and it has seen increasing utilization in the management of type B aortic dissections.[1–3]

1.3 Materials Needed

- Ultrasound probe (for percutaneous approach)
- Arteriotomy closure devices (×4)
- 4-Fr micropuncture needle and sheath
- Angled glidewire and catheter
- Pigtail catheter
- Stiff guidewire
- Volcano intravascular ultrasound (IVUS) catheter (recommended)
- Thoracic endograft with associated delivery device

1.4 Preoperative Planning

CTA or MRA imaging of paramount importance:
- Two centimeter proximal and distal landing zone necessary for safe deployment and fixation.
- Shorter landing zones or more angulated necks may require that the endograft cover aortic arch vessels. In these instances, transposition or bypass of aortic arch segments, most notably the left subclavian artery should be performed prior to TEVAR (except in instances of urgent TEVAR for life-threatening aortic syndromes).
- Access vessels of at least 8 mm are necessary to accommodate the large delivery systems for TEVAR (20F smallest currently available delivery system); larger delivery systems will require larger vessels.
- Alternate access sites if the femoral vessels are small or too heavily calcified include the iliac vessels, infrarenal or even ascending aorta. These sites would require placement of an 8–10 mm ePTFE conduit at the beginning of the case.
- Tortuous vessels can lead to decreased pushability of the device necessitating a second buddy wire for stability or brachial cutdown with pullthrough of the device from above. One should plan accordingly.

Risk stratification:
- Should be performed in all patients undergoing TEVAR and depending on cardiac risk and comorbidities locoregional anesthesia may be preferable to general anesthetic.

Cerebrospinal fluid drainage:
- Should be considered when the thoracic aorta is being extensively covered.
- In patients with prior endovascular aortic repair (EVAR).
- In patients with iliac conduits or who will have their left subclavian covered.

Renal Insufficiency:
- Patients with renal insufficiency should be informed of the nephrotoxic nature of contrast agents and the potential risk of contrast nephropathy.

1.5 Preoperative Checklist

Sign in:
- Team introduced.
- Debriefing on procedure with all staff and physicians
- Labs and preoperative assessment reviewed.

Time out:
- Patient identified.
- Procedure defined and critical steps discussed.
- Concerns addressed.
- Blood status identified.
- Prophylactic antibiotics given.

Sign out:
- Discussion of procedure performed.
- Postop plan of care discussed.

1.6 Pearls and Pitfalls

Pearls:
- Proximal and distal neck of at least 2 cm.
- 10% to 15% oversizing of the endograft to prevent type I endoleak and migration.
- Coverage of the left subclavian artery necessitates carotid subclavian bypass except in emergency situations. This is especially in patients with prior CABG using the left internal mammary artery.[4]

Pitfalls:
- Poor graft to vessel apposition can lead to device migration.
- Heavily calcified femoral vessels may necessitate a conduit.
- Highly tortuous vessels may require access from the brachial artery to pull the device up.

1.7 Surgical Anatomy

Figure 11.1 depicts the most common aortic anatomy with the aortic arch vessels coming off in order of innominate,

L carotid, and L subclavian. Not pictured are the numerous spinal arteries lining the aorta and in particular, the Artery of Adamkiewicz, which has a variable origin from T8-L1. Coverage of this vessel increases the risk of paraplegia.

1.8 Positioning

The patient is placed supine with both groins and the entire abdomen prepped and draped. The arms can be prepped and draped as needed in the event that brachial access is required. The left arm can be abducted and medially rotated as well for better exposure of the arch.

1.9 Anesthesia

- The procedure may be performed under general, regional, or local anesthetic depending on preoperative risk assessment.
- Continuous arterial pressure monitoring is needed for the case as perforation or tearing of major vessels can occur. Furthermore, tight blood pressure control especially as the endograft is being deployed will allow it to seat properly. Conversely, hypotension should be avoided as this may exacerbate any spinal cord ischemia associated with endograft coverage.

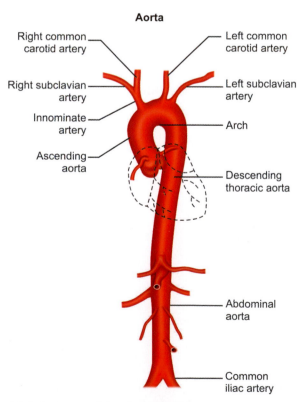

Fig. 11.1: Anatomy of the thoracic aorta.

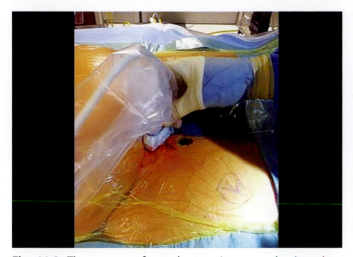

Fig. 11.2: The common femoral artery is accessed using ultrasound guidance of a 4F micropuncture needle.

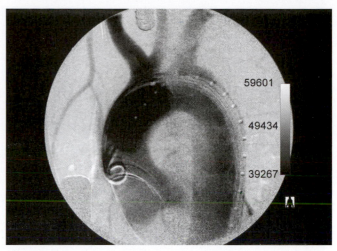

Fig. 11.3: An arch aortogram is performed in the left anterior oblique (LAO) position. In this case a bovine arch is present and the subclavian vessel, which has already undergone carotid subclavian bypass is to be covered by the graft.

- Venous access with two large bore peripheral IVs is sufficient in the majority of cases.

2 PERIOPERATIVE

2.1 Incision

Percutaneous access is achieved by duplex ultrasound guidance of a micropuncture needle (Fig. 11.2). Care is taken to access the common femoral artery below the inguinal ligament in an area with minimal plaque. A 4-Fr sheath is then introduced and fluoroscopy is used to confirm proper placement.

Once percutaneous access is attained, the sheath is upsized to 6 Fr and two arteriotomy closure devices are introduced in the 2 o'clock and 10 o'clock positions for later closure.

Alternatively, an open cutdown on the femoral artery can be performed and the femoral artery directly accessed in this manner.

Under circumstances where the femoral vessels are too small to accommodate a large delivery system, a conduit is required. An 8-mm polytetrafluoroethylene (PTFE) graft can be sewn to the iliac artery or even the infrarenal aorta. In selected cases, antegrade placement of the graft via a conduit to the ascending aorta may be required. The left common carotid approach has also been described.

2.2 Steps

- *See* Figure 11.3.

Following access of the vasculature, a stiff angled glidewire and catheter are introduced. The patient is then therapeutically anticoagulated with heparin and a stiff wire is placed in the aorta and a pigtail catheter used to perform an arch aortogram. This should be performed in the left anterior oblique projection of the image intensifier especially when the proximal landing zone is close to the aortic arch.

A recommended, but often omitted step is to use intravascular ultrasound to confirm the distance of the landing zone proximally between the subclavian and aneurysm/dissection as well as the distal landing zone.

After confirming the size of the landing zone and its proximity to vital structures, the appropriate endograft is opened and the sheath upsized appropriately.

Blood pressure is brought down to a systolic of 100 mm Hg, the device is advanced to the desired location, and if highly precise placement is needed, adenosine can be administered during device deployment.

After deployment, the graft is ballooned to allow for optimal conformation and then a completion angiogram is shot. For imaging of the distal landing zone, a full lateral projection produces the best-quality image.

2.3 Closure

See Figures 11.4A and B.

Closure is dependent on how the patient was accessed at the beginning of the case.

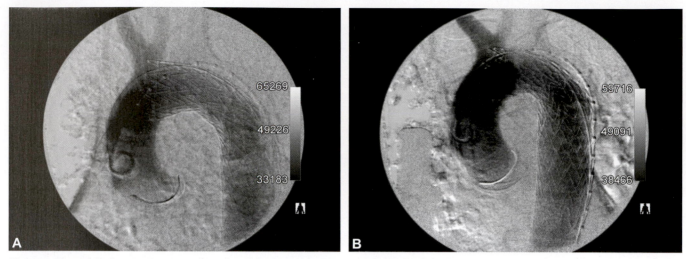

Figs. 11.4A and B: For open access, the artery can be repaired under direct visualization.

For percutaneous access, the arteriotomy closure devices were inserted at the beginning of the case and after removal of all wires and sheaths the sutures can be tied down. In the event of failure of the device knots to produce hemostasis, a femoral cutdown must be performed to repair the blood vessel.

For open access, the artery can be repaired under direct visualization.

3 POSTOPERATIVE

3.1 Complications

Most common complications:

- Peripheral vascular injury (14%)
- Acute kidney injury (14%)
- Endoleak (9%)
- Stroke (4%)
- Paraplegia (3%)

Least common complications:

- Myocardial infarction
- Mesenteric ischemia
- Aortoesophageal and aortobronchial fistula

3.2 Outcomes

Expected outcomes:

- 5-year freedom from aneurysm related mortality 96%
- 5-year freedom from rupture 97%
- 5-year freedom from conversion to open operation 97%
- 5-year rate of further endovascular intervention 14%

3.3 Follow-Up

- Return to ADLs within 1 week postoperatively.
- Repeat CTA is often performed within the first week postoperatively to evaluate for endoleak.
- Postsurgical follow-up at 2 weeks is done to assess the incisions and symptoms.
- Repeat CTA at 6–12 months is recommended followed by annual examinations and imaging.

3.4 E-mail an Expert

- *E-mail address*: drigberg@mednet.ucla.edu

3.5 Web Resources/References

- http://www.vascularweb.org—practice guidelines
- http://www.escardio.org—practice guidelines

REFERENCES

1. Greenburg RK, Lu Q, Roselli E, et al. Contemporary analysis of descending thoracic and thoracoabdominal aneurysm repair: a comparison of endovascular and open techniques. Circulation. 2008;118:808.
2. Matsumura JS, Cambria RP, Dake MD, et al. International controlled clinical trial of thoracic endovascular aneurysm repair with the Zenith TX2 endovascular graft: 1-year results. J Vasc Surg. 2008;4:247-57.
3. Lee AW, Matsumura JS, Mitchell RS, et al. Endovascular repair of traumatic thoracic aortic injury: clinical practice guidelines of the Society for Vascular Surgery. J Vasc Surg. 2011;53:187-92.
4. Matsumura JS, Lee WA, Mitchell RS, et al. The society for vascular surgery practice guidelines: management of the left subclavian artery with thoracic endovascular aortic repair. J Vasc Surg. 2009;50:1155-8.

QUIZ

Question 1: All of the following are true regarding access to the femoral vessels EXCEPT:
a. Access should always be performed using ultrasound.
b. Access should always be above the femoral bifurcation.
c. Placement of two arterial closure devices is recommended at the 2 o'clock and 10 o'clock positions.
d. Access should always be above the inguinal ligament.

Question 2: Which of the following statements about CSF drainage during TEVAR are true?
a. In situations where the subclavian artery will be covered, CSF drainage is recommended.
b. CSF drainage should be performed postoperatively in patients experiencing new onset limb weakness, paresthesia, or paralysis.
c. Prior aortic interventions, either open, or endovascular, predispose patients to spinal ischemia during TEVAR and CSF drainage should be performed.
d. All of the above.

Question 3: Which of the following statements about preoperative planning for TEVAR are true?
a. Femoral vessels that are at least 6 mm in size are sufficient to accommodate the TEVAR catheters.
b. Landing zones of 1.5 cm are adequate for proper deployment and seal during TEVAR.
c. Tortuous and calcified access vessels may necessitate brachial access to pull the device up from above.

d. Planned coverage of the subclavian artery does not necessitate prior carotid subclavian bypass.

Question 4: Which of the following patients meet indications for TEVAR?
a. A 20-year-old man is in a motorcycle accident and is brought to the ED hypotensive, but responds to fluids. A panscan is performed demonstrating an aortic transaction just distal to the left subclavian artery.
b. A 70-year-old woman is referred to you after undergoing a CT scan of the chest for a benign pulmonary nodule and was incidentally found to have a 5-cm TAA.
c. A 58-year-old man comes to your office for evaluation of his chronic and stable type B dissection. He remains normotensive and asymptomatic.
d. An 84-year-old man returns to your clinic with an asymptomatic 5-cm TAA that you have been following. His last CTA 6 months ago showed the aneurysm was 4.4 cm.
e. Both A and D.

Question 5: The most common complication after TEVAR is:
a. Paraplegia
b. Myocardial infarction
c. Stroke
d. Peripheral vascular injury

ANSWERS:
1. d   2. d   3. a   4. e   5. d

Fenestration of Type B Dissection for Visceral Ischemia

S Sadie Ahanchi, Jonathan A Higgins, Jean M Panneton

1 PREOPERATIVE

1.1 Indications

- Aortic dissection with branch vessel compromise, commonly termed malperfusion syndrome.

1.2 Evidence

- Aortic branch occlusion occurs in up to a third of patients with aortic dissection and is associated with increased risk of early death and severe complications.
- The goal of fenestration is to create an opening in the dissection flap that allows egress from the false lumen into the true lumen. This results in false lumen decompression, which then allows perfusion of previously obstructed branch vessels.
- Aortic fenestration can be accomplished using open or minimally invasive endovascular techniques.[1-5]

1.3 Materials Needed

Open repair:
- Omni tract retractor or comparable self-retaining abdominal retractor for exposure
- Cell saver autotransfusion system
- *Open aortic surgical instruments*: curved scissors, long needle drivers, long forceps, etc.
- Nontraumatic aortic clamps, such as fogarty hydragrip covered clamps
- Felt strips/pledgets
- Intraoperative ultrasound

Endovascular repair:
- Hybrid operating room with built in fluoroscopy (preferred)
- Intravascular ultrasound system (IVUS)
- Endovascular snare
- Re-entry catheter or Uchida needle

- Preformed angled sheath
- Endovascular supplies like sheaths, catheters, balloons, etc.
- *Thoracic endografts*: large diameter, self-expanding aortic stents
- Pressure transducer and sterile tubing
- Power injector

1.4 Preoperative Planning and Risk Assessment

Planning:
- Preoperative CT scan of chest, abdomen, and pelvis
- Visceral duplex
- Aortoiliac duplex

Risk assessment:
- Risk stratification is ever-changing and continues to evolve. We view operative risk in these patients as a spectrum:
  - Dynamic true lumen branch vessel compression with mild signs of end-organ ischemia
  - Static true lumen branch vessel compression with moderate signs of end-organ ischemia
  - Static true lumen branch vessel occlusion with thrombosis and severe end-organ ischemic complications
  - Visceral or renal artery compromise
  - Occluded distal aorta
  - Rupture
- End-organ ischemia can present as spinal cord, renal, mesenteric, or lower limb ischemia.
- Risk factors for any surgical aortic patient also apply to aortic fenestration for dissection including unstable cardiac disease, respiratory compromise, renal failure, previous aortic surgery, and extent of aorta removed/repaired.

1.5 Preoperative Checklist

Sign in:
- Patient reidentification
- Informed consent
- Cross-matched blood products available

Time out:
- Briefing on patient position, instruments and equipment needed.
- Confirm patient and procedure
- Antibiotic prophylaxis confirmation

Sign out:
- Name of procedure and wound class
- Completed and correct instrument count
- List of implanted devices
- Debriefing

1.6 Decision-Making Algorithm

- *See* Flowchart 12.1.

1.7 Pearls and Pitfalls

Pearls:
- High index of suspicion and early treatment of suspected ischemic complications of aortic dissection is key to minimizing morbidity and mortality.
- When prepping and draping include all four extremities as well as the neck, chest, and abdomen.
- When performing endovascular fenestration utilize open femoral and brachial exposure liberally to ensure safe introduction of the large sheaths necessary for endovascular repair.
- Measuring the pressure gradient with a central line set up between the true and false lumen can help quantify the severity of the malperfusion and the success of the fenestration.
- Distal aortic perfusion and other adjuncts (e.g. systemic hypothermia, epidural cooling, cerebrospinal fluid drainage, somatosensory, and motor evoked potential monitoring) should be considered if prolonged ischemia time combined with aortic graft replacement is anticipated.

Pitfalls:
- Avoid performing the endovascular repair in an isolated endovascular suite, in case of technical failure and the need for open operative rescue.
- Avoid prolonged aortic cross-clamping with the open repair.
- One of the challenges with operating in an acutely dissected aorta is dealing with the extremely fragile aortic wall, which poses the risk of clamp-induced injury, suture line tears, and bleeding. Utilizing a structurally stabilizing adjunct both inside and outside the aortic wall of the proximal

Flowchart 12.1: Decision-making algorithm.

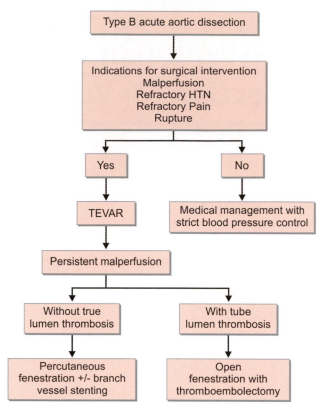

suture line (e.g. felt strips, Teflon pledgets, aortic banding with a Dacron tube graft, adventitial inversion, or hemostatic glues) can help stabilize anastomotic suture line.

1.8 Surgical Anatomy

- *See* Figures 12.1 and 12.2.

1.9 Positioning

- Sterile preparation from chin to knees with brachial and femoral arteries accessible.
- For the transperitoneal open repair and the endovascular repair the patient is placed in the supine position.
- For the retroperitoneal open repair the patient is placed in the jack-knife modified lateral position at up to 45°.

See Figures 12.3A to C.

1.10 Anesthesia

- General anesthesia with endotracheal intubation is routine, use of a double lumen endotracheal tube or

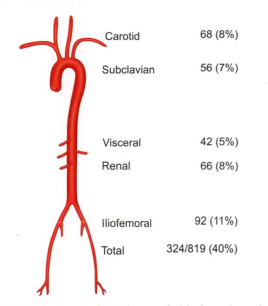

Carotid	68 (8%)
Subclavian	56 (7%)
Visceral	42 (5%)
Renal	66 (8%)
Iliofemoral	92 (11%)
Total	324/819 (40%)

Fig. 12.1: Distribution and incidence of side branch occlusion associated with spontaneous acute aortic dissection.
Source: From Cambria RP et al.[6]

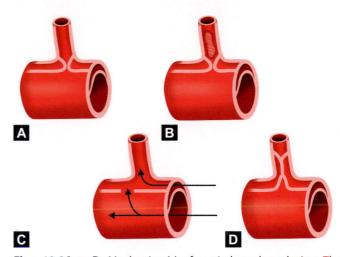

Figs. 12.2A to D: Mechanism(s) of aortic branch occlusion. The most common mechanism is (A) branch vessel compromise caused by bulging of the false lumen resulting in true lumen compression referred to as dynamic obstruction. Alternatively, (B) secondary thrombosis may complicate side branch occlusion, referred to as static obstruction which carries an ominous prognosis. Other mechanisms include (C) an intimal flap blocking flow into the artery or (D) dissection proceeding into the branch and causing narrowing beyond the branch orifice.
Source: Redrawn from the Mayo Clinic.

bronchoscopically placed left main bronchial blocker enhances exposure if thoracic exposure of the aorta is planned.

- The arterial line permits instantaneous evaluation of blood pressure changes, and blood gas sampling can be done when required.
- Several large-bore (16-gauge) catheters should be placed intravenously for adequate control of fluid and blood replacement.
- Spinal drain is advised if plans are to cover or replace a large length of aorta.
- Foley catheter for urine output
- Central venous access
- Warming blankets
- Blood warmer
- Autotransfusion device

2 PERIOPERATIVE

2.1 Incision

Open repair:
- Transperitoneal abdominal aortic exposure through a midline incision from xyphoid to pubic symphysis.
- Transperitoneal or retroperitoneal thoracoabdominal incision starting laterally from fourth, fifth, or ninth interspace (depending on extent of aortic exposure desired) extending inferiomedially toward the pubic symphysis:

  - If the intent is solely to perform a paravisceral fenestration, consider eighth or ninth interspace
  - If proximal thoracic aorta needs replacement, consider fourth interspace

Endovascular repair:
- Open femoral and possibly brachial artery exposure through transverse incisions over the vessel.

2.2 Steps

Open transperitoneal fenestration:
- If aortic diameter is >3.5–4.0 cm proceed to standard aortic replacement with reimplantation of branch vessels as necessary.
- The abdominal aorta and its branches are exposed through a transperitoneal approach because of the advantage of allowing direct visualize of the bowel for ischemia and reperfusion.
- When infrarenal aortic grafting is indicated, a transverse arteriotomy with cephalad extension is preferred over a longitudinal arteriotomy.
- However, a longitudinal aortotomy at the paravisceral level offers better visualization of the celiac, superior mesenteric, and renal artery ostia, in addition to

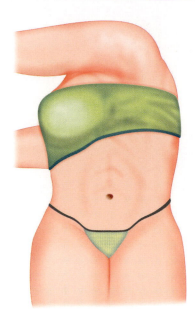

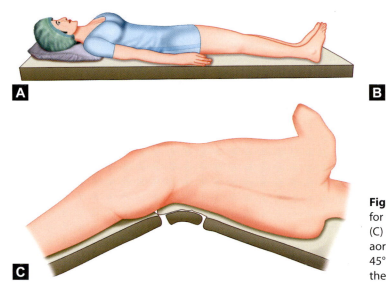

Figs. 12.3A to C: Positioning for (A) standard supine position for transperitoneal exposure and endovascular repair and (B), (C) positioning for retroperitoneal exposure of the visceral aorta with the pelvis horizontal and the left shoulder rotated 45° (B) with the table jack-knifed to widen the space between the costal margin and pelvic brim.

allowing easier access for thrombectomy if the false lumen or aortic branches are filled with thrombus or for resection and tacking of the septum extending into the branch vessel.

- A generous resection of the dissection septum to a level above the celiac trunk is performed in patients with paravisceral thrombosis.
- If there is no evidence of thrombosis or direct branch vessel involvement, fenestration at the infrarenal level might be sufficient to reperfuse the lower limbs distally and the renal and visceral vessels proximally.

Open retroperitoneal fenestration:

- If aortic diameter is >3.5–4.0 cm proceed to standard aortic replacement with reimplantation of branch vessels as necessary.
- A modification of this technique is the "tailored aortoplasty", designed to avoid graft replacement of the thoracoabdominal aorta while removing most of the dissected intima.

- A retroperitoneal approach with aortic clamping at the level of the diaphragm, followed by an extensive longitudinal aortotomy posterior to the origin of the left renal artery.
- The dissected septum is widely excised to connect the true and false lumens.
- The aortotomy is closed in a running fashion with Teflon strip buttresses to create a single aortic lumen 2.5–3 cm in diameter.
- If the dissection extends to the iliofemoral segment, a bifurcated graft may be inserted distally to ensure unimpeded blood flow to the lower extremities.

Endovascular fenestration:

- After vessel access and sheath placement, using a flush catheter, an aortogram is performed.
- Intravascular ultrasound system is used to image the entire aorta and identify true and false lumens by verifying the arch vessel ostia emerging from the true lumen.

- Pressure gradients are measured between the true and false lumens in order to gauge severity of malperfusion and success of treatment.
- Under IVUS guidance, through the same sheath, one wire is placed into the false lumen and one wire is placed into the true lumen (with both wires positioned proximal to the obstructed vessel).
- A Rosch–Uchida introducer set is inserted into the true lumen and the wire is removed and the trocar is quickly advanced to puncture the dissection flap.
- Alternatively, an IVUS directed re-entry catheter can be used to perforate the septum under ultrasound guidance.
- A stiff wire is placed into the false lumen under IVUS and fluoroscopic guidance.
- The fenestration is serially dilated using noncompliant balloons ranging in size from 8 mm to 14 mm.

- Postfenestration equilibration of the true and false lumens should be documented by IVUS imaging and/or resolution of pressure gradients.
- Other techniques to create or enlarge the fenestration have been described, including the use of a snare to have a stiff wire from the arm to the groin across the fenestration or using a double wire/one sheath "push" technique.
- Frequently after fenestration, true lumen stenting of the descending thoracic aorta is completed in a standard fashion.
- If there is evidence of continued compromise of a branch vessel, a self-expanding stent can be deployed across the true lumen of the vessel.

See Figures 12.4 to 12.7.

2.3 Closure

Standard: either open closure, or endovascular vessel closure.

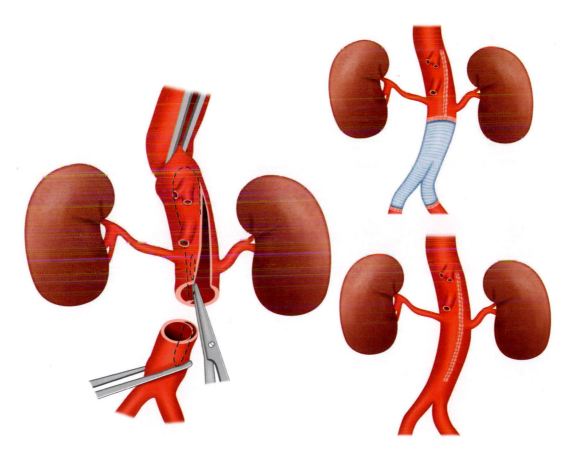

Fig. 12.4: Schematic drawing of open aortic fenestration showing infra renal aortic transection with longitudinal extension and resection of the septum between the false and true lumens (left). After pararenal fenestration, infrarenal aortic replacement with aortobiiliac graft (top right) or primary closure without graft replacement (bottom right).
Source: Redrawn from the Mayo Clinic.

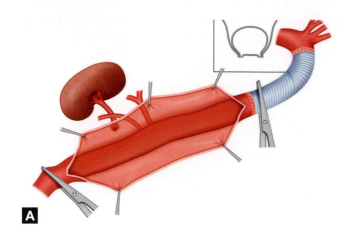

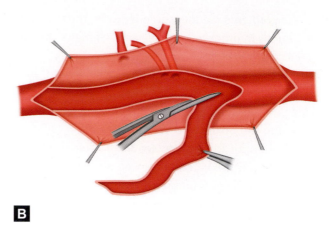

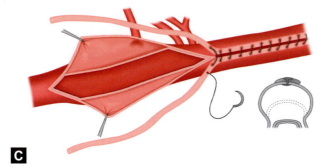

Figs. 12.5A to C: Schematic drawing of the tailored aortoplasty technique. Using a retroperitoneal approach, a long left postero-lateral aortotomy is performed (A). The dissected intima is widely excised and the adherent intima is left in place (B). The aorta is closed primarily using Teflon buttresses to reinforce the thinned adventitia (C).
Source: Redrawn from the Mayo Clinic.

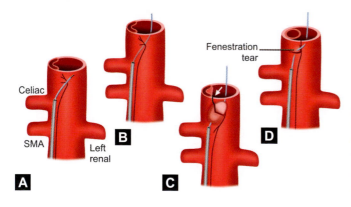

Figs. 12.6A to D: The technique of endovascular aortic fenestration. (A) A puncture is made in the membrane separating the true and false lumens. (B) A wire is advanced through the puncture into the false lumen. (C) The fenestration is dilated with a 14-mm balloon. (D) The resulting fenestration tear.
Source: From Patel H et al.[7]

3 POSTOPERATIVE

3.1 Complications

Most common complications:
- Paraplegia
- Stroke
- Reintervention
- Renal failure

Least common complications:
- Myocardial infarction
- Respiratory failure

- Mesenteric ischemia
- Lower extremity ischemia
- Retrograde dissection

3.2 Outcomes

- Operative mortality rate in the range of 10% to 70%.

3.3 Follow-Up

Immediate postoperative period:
- Admission to vascular intensive care unit

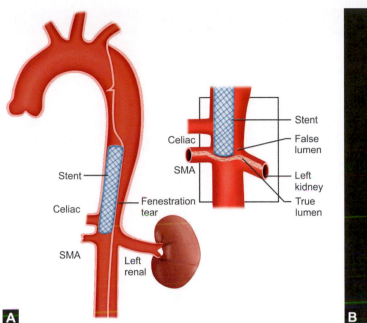

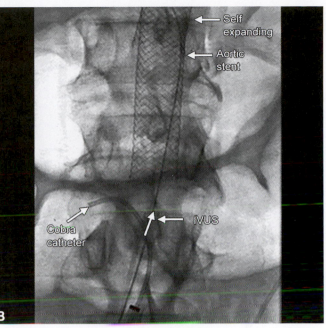

Figs. 12.7A and B: (A) Diagram illustrating the proper placement of a bare metal stent in the true lumen of the aorta. (B) Fluoroscopic image of a self-expanding bare metal stent in the descending thoracic aorta. The IVUS probe and a Cobra catheter can also be seen. (IVUS: Intravascular ultrasound system).
Source: From Patel H et al.[7]

- Continuous arterial line pressure monitoring
- Urine output monitoring with Foley catheter
- *Serial laboratory values*: Complete blood count, basic metabolic panel, lactate level, arterial blood gases, liver function tests, and myoglobin levels
- Serial neurovascular checks
- Visceral, renal, or lower extremity duplex
- Computed tomographic angiography of the chest abdomen and pelvis with reconstruction prior to discharge

Long term:
- Computed tomographic angiography of the chest abdomen and pelvis with reconstruction every 6 months for 2 years then yearly thereafter to evaluate for aneurysm formation and to follow aortic remodeling

3.4 E-mail an Expert

- *E-mail addresses*: pannetjm@emvs.edu or ssahanch@ sentara.com

3.5 Web Resources/References

- http://www.vascualrweb.org/" \t "_blank" www.vascualrweb.org

- http://www.aortarepair.com/type-b-aortic-dissection. html

REFERENCES

1. Oderich GS, Panneton JM. Acute aortic dissection with side branch vessel occlusion: open surgical options. Semin Vasc Surg. 2002;15(2):89-96.
2. Panneton JM, Teh SH, Cherry KJ Jr, et al. Aortic fenestration for acute or chronic aortic dissection: an uncommon but effective procedure. J Vasc Surg. 2000;32(4):711-21.
3. DiMusto PD, Williams DM, Patel HJ, et al. Endovascular management of type B aortic dissections. J Vasc Surg. 2010; 52 (4 Suppl):26S-36S.
4. Williams DM, Lee DY, Hamilton BH, et al. The dissected aorta; percutaneous treatment of ischemic complications-principles and results. J Vasc Interv Radiol. 1997;8:605-25.
5. Rasmussen TE, Panneton JM. Ischemic complications of distal aortic dissections: open surgical or endovascular management. In Gloviczki P, Ascher E (Eds). Perspectives in Vascular Surgery and Endovascular Therapy, Vol. 14, No. 2. New York: Thieme; 2001.
6. Cambria RP, Brewster DC, Gertler J, et al. Vascular complications associated with spontaneous aortic dissection. J Vasc Surg 7:199-209, 1988
7. Patel H, Williams D. Endovascular therapy of malperfusion in acute type B aortic dissection. Op Tech Thor Cardiovasc Surg 2009; 14: 2-11.

QUIZ

Question 1. What is the most common indication for aortic fenestration after dissection:
a. Type B aortic dissection
b. Malperfusion syndrome
c. Type A aortic dissection
d. Uncontrollable hypertension

Question 2. All of the below are viable options for aortic fenestration in a nonaneurysmal aorta except:
a. Open transperitoneal longitudinal aortic fenestration
b. Retroperitoneal tailored aortoplasty
c. Endovascular fenestration
d. False lumen stent graft

Question 3. Aortic dissection with visceral malperfusion and branch vessel thrombosis should be treated with:
a. Aortic replacement
b. Visceral stenting
c. Open fenestration
d. Endovascular fenestration

SECTION

3

Abdominal Aorta

AAA Repair: Transabdominal

Charles Bailey

1 PREOPERATIVE

1.1 Indications

- Symptomatic abdominal aortic aneurysm (AAA) as defined by evidence of rupture or impending rupture, embolic or thrombotic complications, mass effect, and "herald bleeds" via aortoenteric or aortocaval fistulas.
- Asymptomatic AAA with maximal diameter >5.5 cm, or growth rates of >0.5 cm within 6-months or 1.0 cm annually.
- Contraindications to repair include severe cardiac or pulmonary comorbidities prohibiting use of general endotracheal anesthesia.[1-3]

1.2 Evidence

- Two prospective randomized trials, the Aneurysm Detection and Management Veterans Affairs trial and the UK Small Aneurysm trial compared early aneurysm repair versus surveillance for AAA between 4.0 and 5.5 cm. The trials showed no survival benefit between patients receiving early repair and those patients in which AAA repair was reserved for either symptomatic, expanding, or aneurysms >5.5 cm.
- Data from the UK Small Aneurysm trial showed female gender to be an independent risk factor for AAA rupture, suggesting repair in women with AAA >5.0 cm.[4-6]

1.3 Materials Needed

- Major abdominal laparotomy instruments
- Assortment of vascular clamps
- Prosthetic vascular grafts
- Bookwalter (Fig. 13.1A), Omni (Fig. 13.1B), or Thompson (Fig. 13.1C) retractor
- Bovie electrocautery
- Cell Saver

1.4 Preoperative Planning and Risk Assessment

Planning:
- Preoperative CT scanning of chest, abdomen, and pelvis
- Bilateral lower extremity arterial duplex to assess for femoral–popliteal aneurysms
- Cardiopulmonary risk assessment[4]

Risk assessment:
- *Low risk*:
  - Age <80
  - No, or minor, American College of Cardiology (ACC) clinical predictors of increased perioperative cardiovascular risk-abnormal EKG, arrhythmia, history of cerebrovascular accident, low functional capacity, uncontrolled hypertension
  - Noninflammatory infrarenal AAA
- *Intermediate risk*:
  - Age over 80
  - Intermediate ACC clinical predictors—mild angina, previous myocardial infarction or pathological Q waves on EKG, compensated or history of heart failure, diabetes mellitus, renal insufficiency
  - Chronic obstructive pulmonary disease (COPD) with FEV1 >1 L/s
  - Juxtarenal, suprarenal, or inflammatory AAA
- *High risk*:
  - Age over 80
  - Major ACC clinical predictors—unstable coronary syndromes (acute or recent myocardial infarction, unstable or severe angina), decompensated heart failure, significant arrhythmias (high-grade atrioventricular block, symptomatic ventricular arrhythmias, supraventricular arrhythmia with uncontrolled rate), valvular disease[1]

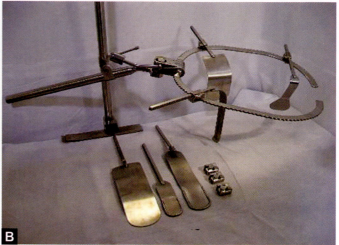

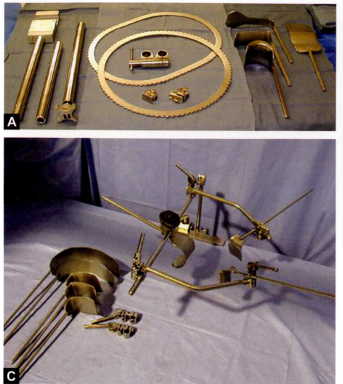

Figs. 13.1A to C: (A) Bookwalter retractor. (B) Omni retractor. (C) Thompson retractor.

– Oxygen-dependent COPD with FEV1 <1 L/s
– Pugh-Child's class B or C hepatic failure

1.5 Preoperative Checklist

• Preoperative administration of β-blockers for risk reduction of cardiovascular events.

Sign in:
• Verify patient identity, operative site, planned procedure and consent.
• Cardiopulmonary risk assessment reviewed by anesthesiology.
• Review patient allergies and use of β-blockers.
• Ensure adequate intravenous access, hemodynamic monitors, availability of blood products.

Time out:
• Team members introduce themselves and role.
• Surgeon, anesthesiologist, and nurse reconfirm correct patient, site, and procedure.
• Surgeon reviews critical steps, operative duration, and estimated blood-loss.
• Anesthesiology reviews any patient-specific concerns.
• Equipment sterility and/or issues are confirmed.
• Verify appropriate antibiotic administration within 60 minutes of incision.

Sign out:
• Nursing confirms procedure performed, correct instrument/sponge/needle counts, labeling of any surgical specimen.
• Surgeon, anesthesiologist, and nurse review tenets of postoperative management.

1.6 Decision-Making Algorithm

• *See* Flowchart 13.1.

1.7 Pearls and Pitfalls

Pearls:
• Aberrant vascular anatomy may be better suited to a retroperitoneal approach.
• If collateral veins remain intact, left renal vein may be divided at the level of the vena cava for added proximal aortic exposure.
• Ligate the inferior mesenteric artery (IMA) from within aneurysm sac away from sigmoid and left colic collaterals.
• Close posterior peritoneum over proximal graft anastomosis.
• Compression of femoral arteries upon release of distal occlusive clamps will help direct debris into the pelvic circulation.

Pitfalls:

- Avoid proximal aortic clamp repositioning if placed above renal arteries.
- Avoid suturing aortic graft into aneurysmal tissue at either proximal or distal anastomoses.
- Avoid circumferential dissection of the aortic bifurcation and proximal common iliac arteries to prevent venous, ureteral, or parasympathetic nerve plexus injury.
- Avoid dissection of AAA off of duodenum in setting of inflammatory aneurysm.
- Reimplant IMA in setting of visceral arterial occlusive disease or poor pelvic collaterals.

1.8. Surgical Anatomy

- *See* Figure. 13.2.

1.9. Positioning

- *See* Figure. 13.3.

1.10. Anesthesia

- In cases of ruptured AAA, position patient on operating room table, secure intravenous access and hemodynamic monitors, and perform sterile preparation and draping of patient prior to induction of anesthesia.

- In elective aneurysm repair, consider epidural analgesia to reduce the surgical stress response and cardiovascular demands.
- Use of a pulmonary artery catheter may assist in the monitoring of patients with coronary atherosclerotic or valvular disease.
- Systemic heparinization (50–100 units/kg) is provided prior to aortic cross-clamping , with coagulation status monitored with frequent measures of activated clotting time (ACT).
- Avoid hypothermia, acidosis, and hypovolemia to offset potential hemodynamic compromise upon restoration of visceral or lower extremity arterial circulation.

2 PERIOPERATIVE

2.1 Incision

- *See* Figure 13.4.

2.2 Steps

- *See* Figures 13.5A to Q.

2.3 Closure

- *See* Figure 13.6.

Flowchart 13.1: Decision-making algorithm.

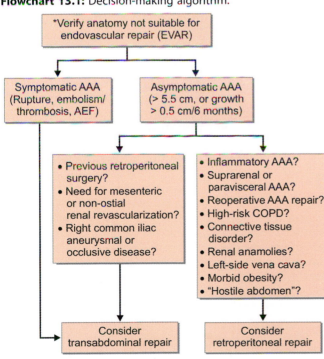

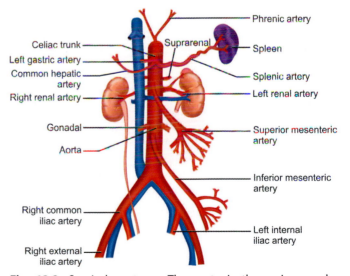

Fig. 13.2: Surgical anatomy. The aorta is the main vascular conduit of the thoracic and abdominal cavities. After entering the abdominal cavity via the diaphragmatic hiatus the aorta lies anterior to the thoracolumbar spine in the retroperitoneum. Aneurysms may develop along any segment of the abdominal aorta and are further classified as infrarenal, juxtarenal, pararenal, or paravisceral based on the aneurysm proximity to named visceral vessels.

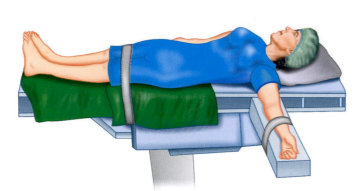

Fig. 13.3: Patient positioning. For a transabdominal approach the patient is placed supine, with either one or both arms adducted. In cases of ruptured aneurysm leaving both arms abducted allows placement of peripheral intravenous and arterial lines.

Fig. 13.4: Surgical incision. Transabdominal repair of an aortic aneurysm can be accomplished via either a standard midline laparotomy incision (T1), or a supraumbilical transverse incision (T2) approximated cephalad to the aortic bifurcation

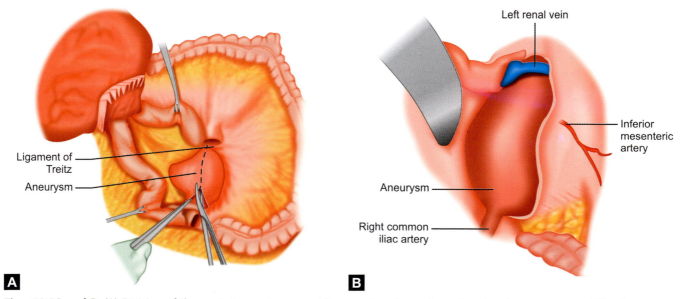

A

B

Figs. 13.5A and B: (A) Division of the posterior peritoneum. After entering the peritoneal cavity via a generous midline laparotomy incision the abdomen is explored to exclude other pathology and assess the abdominal aneurysm. The greater omentum and transverse colon are reflected cephalad, and the ligament of Treitz is divided to facilitate evisceration of the small bowel. Mobilized viscera are wrapped in a moistened surgical towel and left either extracorporeally, or packed into the right upper quadrant. The posterior peritoneum is incised over the aneurysm beginning at the aortic bifurcation and continuing to the inferior border of the pancreas. Care is taken to ligate dilated veins and enlarged lymphatics overlying the aneurysm. (B) Exposure of infrarenal aorta. Aneurysm sac is exposed proximally to the left renal vein and distally to the common iliac arteries. Proximally the dissection continues medial to the inferior mesenteric vein, though lateral enough to the duodenum to allow later closure of the peritoneum over the prosthetic graft. Distally, avoid circumferential dissection at proximal common iliac arteries to prevent iatrogenic injury to ureters, iliac veins, or parasympathetic nerves. Damage to superior hypogastric plexus anterior to the left common iliac artery can result in retrograde ejaculation postoperatively.

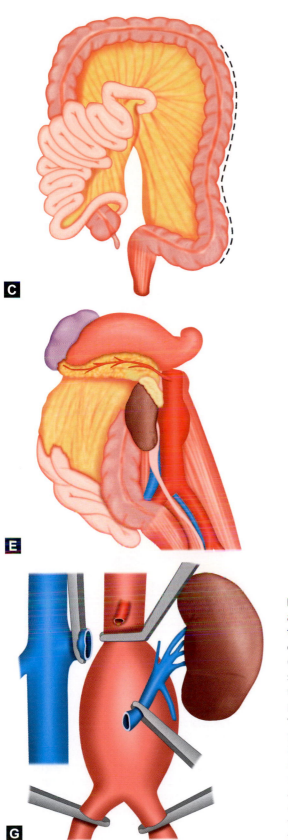

C

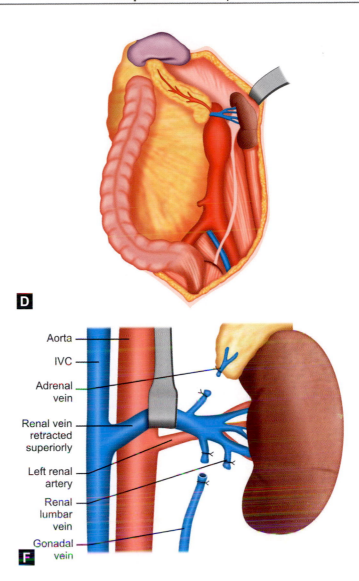

D

E

Aorta

IVC

Adrenal
vein

Renal vein
retracted
superiorly

Left renal
artery

Renal
lumbar
vein

Gonadal
vein

F

G

Figs. 13.5C to G: (C) Left medial visceral rotation. If the aorta is aneurysmal at or above the renal artery orifice greater exposure can be achieved transabdominally via a left medial visceral rotation. Maneuver begins with division of the lateral peritoneal attachments along the white line of Toldt. (D and E) Left medial visceral rotation. After mobilizing the left colon and splenic flexure a retroperitoneal plane may be developed along the left psoas muscle. Medial reflection of the greater curve of the stomach, spleen, and pancreatic body/tail allows exposure of the abdominal aorta at the level of the visceral vessels. The left kidney may be reflected medially, or remain positioned posteriorly in the retroperitoneum. (F) Mobilization of the left renal vein. The infrarenal aorta can be further exposed with isolation of the left renal vein and ligation of the adrenal, renal lumbar, and gonadal venous branches. Rarely, the renal vein may be positioned posterior or even encircle the aorta. Renal venous anomalies must be recognized preoperatively to prevent iatrogenic injury during aortic cross-clamping. (G) Division of the left renal vein. If collateral venous drainage remains intact via adrenal, renal lumbar and gonadal veins, the main left renal vein may be divided at its confluence with the vena cava.

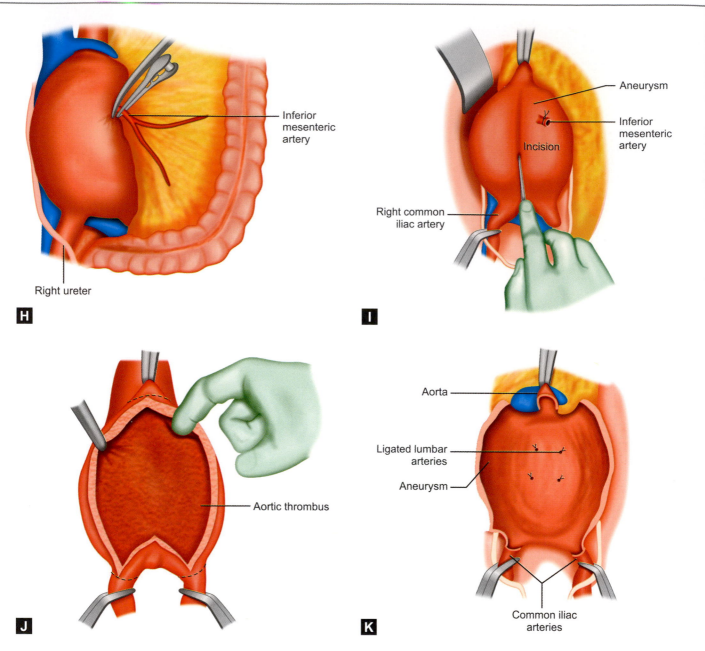

Figs. 13.5H to K: (H) Ligation of inferior mesenteric artery (IMA). If clearly identified, the IMA may be ligated and divided on the surface of the aneurysm sac. Ligation of the IMA from within the opened aneurysm sac is preferred to prevent potential disruption of left colic and sigmoid collaterals. If visceral occlusive disease is present on imaging, or a large meandering mesenteric artery is evident grossly, the IMA should be reimplanted following aortic graft repair. The IMA may be sutured to the aortic graft utilizing a Carrel patch of native aortic wall. (I) Entering the aneurysm. Systemic heparinization (50–100 units/kg) is administered prior to clamping aorta or iliac arteries. Proximal aorta and iliac arteries free of atherosclerotic disease should be isolated for clamp placement to reduce the chance of vessel clamp injury or atheroembolization. Clamps are placed first distally to protect against embolization that may result from proximal aorta cross-clamping. The aneurysm sac is incised at the aortic bifurcation and continued to a point at least 1.0 cm below the proximal aortic cross-clamp. The incision is then carried transversely forming a "T" with division of the lateral aortic wall. Avoid placement of proximal or distal occlusive clamps or creation of anastomoses on aneurysmal tissues as they are at increased risk of continued aneurysmal degeneration. (J) Removal of aortic thrombus. Upon entering the aneurysm sac bluntly dislodge and remove any mural thrombus present. (K) Ligation of lumbar arteries. Back-bleeding from within the aneurysm sac occurs from patent perforating lumbar arteries. Lumbar vessels should be ligated with figure-of-eight interrupted 2-0 silk sutures. Similarly, a patent back-bleeding middle sacral artery at the level of the aortic bifurcation should be suture ligated.

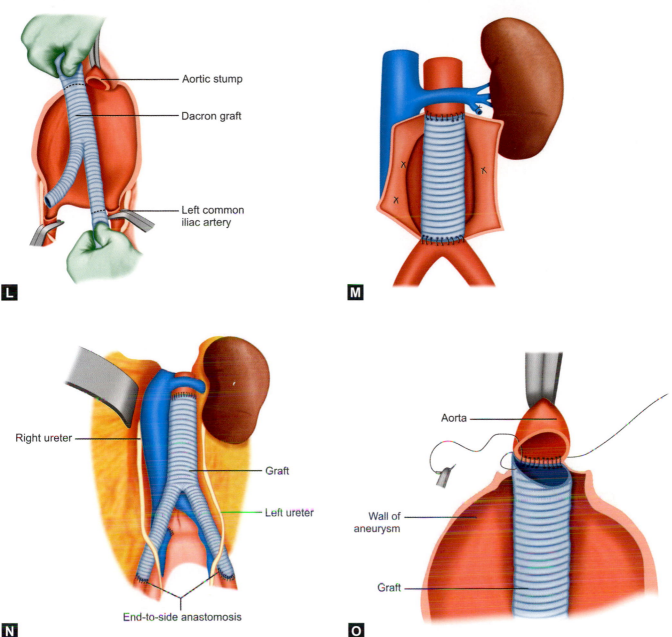

Aortic stump

Dacron graft

Left common
iliac artery

L

M

Right ureter

Graft

Left ureter

End-to-side anastomosis

N

Aorta

Wall of
aneurysm

Graft

O

Figs. 13.5L to O: (L) Sizing of prosthetic graft. Aortic sizers are available for best measure of the appropriate diameter for prosthetic graft sizing. It is important to stretch the graft to length prior to trimming redundant prosthetic material. If a bifurcated prosthetic graft is utilized the redundant length of graft should be removed principally from the graft main body. (M) Aortic tube graft. If the common iliac arteries are free of aneurysmal degeneration or atherosclerotic occlusive disease reconstruction with an aortic tube graft may be performed. The distal anastomosis is sutured to the aortic bifurcation encompassing the lumens of both common iliac arteries. (N) Aortic bifurcated graft. For a bifurcated prosthetic graft the distal iliac anastomoses are created in an end-to-side fashion distal to the aortic bifurcation. It is important to tunnel the iliac limbs posterior to the ureters as they cross over the iliac arteries, as extrinsic compression of the ureters can incite an inflammatory process leading to profound ureteral obstruction and hydronephrosis. (O) Proximal aortic anastomosis. The proximal aortic anastomosis is created at the level of the renal arteries to prevent subsequent aneurysmal degeneration of residual infrarenal aortic tissue. Using 3-0 polypropylene suture, perform running anastomosis with double thickness of posterior aortic wall for increased strength. Teflon or Dacron pledgets may be used if aortic tissue is friable. After completing proximal anastomosis, clamp the prosthetic graft then briefly release aortic cross-clamp to test the integrity of suture line and reinforce as needed.

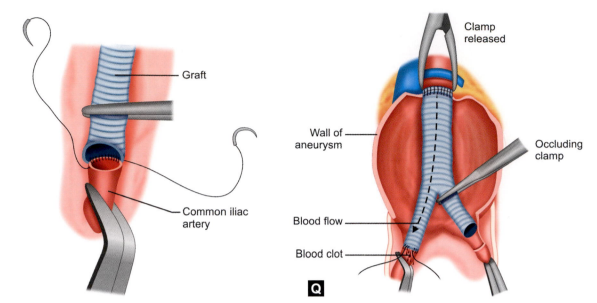

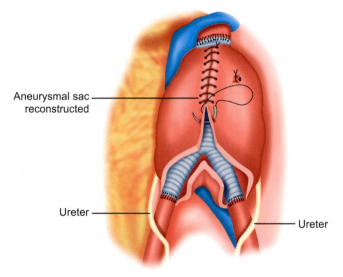

Figs. 13.5P and Q: (P) Distal anastomosis. If prosthetic graft is sutured to distal aorta create distal anastomosis in fashion similar to proximal aorta, encompassing both iliac artery orifices within suture line. Iliac anastomoses are preferred over femoral due to lower rate of infection and pseudoaneurysm formation. Femoral artery anastomoses are indicated for severe iliac atherosclerotic occlusion or extensive aneurysmal degeneration. (Q) Flushing iliac limb. Prior to completion of first iliac limb, release inflow clamp to flush any formed thrombus or debris from within the graft prior to restoring extremity perfusion. When anastomosis if completed, gradually remove outflow clamp to prevent hypotension from release of vasoactive substances. Manual compression of the common femoral artery during limb reperfusion will help direct any residual debris/atheroma into the pelvic circulation. Perform similar steps to flush contralateral limb prior to completion of anastomosis.

Fig. 13.6: Closure. Inspect the descending and sigmoid colon to ensure adequate visceral perfusion prior to wound closure. If bowel appears malperfused, consider reimplantation of the IMA if previously ligated. The prosthetic graft should be concealed with a layered closure of first the aortic aneurysm sac, followed by reapproximation of the incised posterior peritoneum. Midline laparotomy incision is closed in a standard fashion with reapproximation of abdominal wall musculature fascia along the divided linea alba, followed by approximation of skin and subcutaneous tissues. Encompass healthy, well-vascularized tissues within fascial closure as patients are prone to develop incisional hernias following open aortic aneurysm repair. (IMA: Inferior mesenteric artery).

3 POSTOPERATIVE

3.1 Complications

Most common complications:
- Cardiac events (myocardial ischemia, arrhythmias)
- Pulmonary complications (pulmonary edema, pleural effusions, ventilator dependence)
- Renal insufficiency (acute tubular necrosis)
- Ischemic colitis
- Incisional hernia

Least common complications:
- Graft infection or thrombosis
- Spinal ischemia
- Aortoenteric fistula formation

3.2 Outcomes

- Estimated 5- and 10-year survival of 75% and 45%, respectively, with elective repair
- Perioperative mortality of 50% with repair of ruptured AAA
- No significant difference in core outcomes in comparing transabdominal versus retroperitoneal approach for elective repair of AAA

3.3 Follow-Up

- Postsurgery evaluation within 1-month following discharge
- Surveillance cross-sectional imaging at 1-year postoperatively
- Lifelong best medical management of comorbidities

3.4 E-mail an Expert

- *E-mail address*: mshames@health.usf.edu

3.5 Web Resources/References

- www.vascularweb.org
- www.ncbi.nlm.nih.gov
- www.usfvascularsurgery.com

REFERENCES

1. Eagle KA, Berger PB, Calkins H, et al. American College of Cardiology/American Heart Association Guideline Update for Perioperative Cardiovascular Evaluation for Noncardiac Surgery-Executive Summary. Circulation. 2002;105:1257.
2. Cronenwett JL, Johnston KW. Rutherford's Vascular Surgery, 7th edition. Philadelphia; Saunders; 2010.
3. Lederle FA, Wilson SE, Johnson GR, et al. For the Aneurysm Detection and Management (ADAM) Veterans Affairs Cooperative Study Group. Immediate repair compared with surveillance of small abdominal aortic aneurysms. N Engl J Med. 2002;346:1437.
4. Moore WS. Vascular and Endovascular Surgery: A Comprehensive Review, 7th edition. Philadelphia; Saunders; 2006.
5. The UK Small Aneurysm Trial Participants: Mortality results for randomized controlled trial of early elective surgery or ultrasonographic surveillance for small abdominal aortic aneurysms. Lancet. 1998;352:1649.
6. The United Kingdom Small Aneurysm Trial Participants: Long term outcomes of immediate repair compared with surveillance of small abdominal aortic aneurysms. N Engl J Med. 2002;346:1445.

QUIZ

Question 1. Indications for operative treatment of an abdominal aortic aneurysm include all of the following except?
a. Maximal diameter >5.5 cm
b. Aneurysm growth of >0.5 cm in a 6-month time period
c. Aneurysm growth of >1.0 cm in a 6-month time period
d. Aneurysm sac rupture

Question 2. Transabdominal repair of an abdominal aortic aneurysm is the preferred approach for which clinical scenario?
a. Acute AAA rupture with hemodynamic instability
b. 6.5 cm infrarenal aneurysm requiring nonstial renal revascularization
c. 6.0 cm infrarenal aneurysm with atherosclerotic occlusion of the bilateral external iliac arteries
d. All of the above

Question 3. Maneuvers to improve exposure of the proximal extent of an infrarenal AAA include all of the following except?

a. Division of the posterior peritoneum to the Ligament of Treitz
b. Left medial visceral rotation
c. Division of the transverse mesocolon
d. Division of the left renal vein at the confluence of the vena cava

Question 4. Failure to readily identify the left renal vein during exposure of the proximal extent of an infrarenal AAA suggests of which of the following?
a. Congenitally absent left renal vein
b. Aberrant renal venous anatomy
c. Further exposure of the aneurysm neck is required
d. The inferior vena cava should be identified and isolated

Question 5. Reimplantation of the IMA should be considered for which clinical scenario?
a. A patient with high-grade celiac and superior mesenteric artery stenoses
b. Dusky appearing colon at case completion
c. A grossly enlarged, tortuous IMA
d. All of the above

1. c   2. d   3. c   4. b   5. d

ANSWERS:

AAA Repair: Retroperitoneal

Charles Bailey, Murray Shames

1 PREOPERATIVE

1.1 Indications

- Symptomatic abdominal aortic aneurysm (AAA) as defined by evidence of rupture or impending rupture, embolic or thrombotic complications, mass effect, and "herald bleeds" via aortoenteric or aortocaval fistulas.
- Asymptomatic AAA with maximal diameter >5.5 cm, or growth rates of >0.5 cm within 6 months or 1.0 cm annually.
- Contraindications to repair include severe cardiac or pulmonary comorbidities prohibiting use of general endotracheal anesthesia.[1]

1.2 Evidence

- Two prospective randomized trials, the Aneurysm Detection and Management Veterans Affairs trial and the UK Small Aneurysm trial compared early aneurysm repair versus surveillance for AAA between 4.0 and 5.5 cm. The trials showed no survival benefit between patients receiving early repair and those patients in which AAA repair was reserved for either symptomatic, expanding, or aneurysms >5.5 cm.
- Data from the UK Small Aneurysm trial showed female gender to be an independent risk factor for AAA rupture, suggesting repair in women with AAA >5.0 cm.
- In comparison to the transabdominal repair, prospective randomized trials have demonstrated a shorter length of hospital stay, a lower incidence of paralytic ileus, and no significant difference in perioperative cardiac morbidity for the retroperitoneal approach.[2–9]

1.3 Materials Needed

- Major abdominal laparotomy instruments

- Bookwalter (Fig. 14.1A), Omni (Fig. 14.1B), or Thompson (Fig. 14.1C) retractor
- Selection of vascular clamps
- Prosthetic vascular grafts
- Bovie electrocautery
- Cell saver

1.4 Preoperative Planning and Risk Assessment

Planning:
- Preoperative CT scanning of chest, abdomen, and pelvis
- Bilateral lower extremity arterial duplex to assess for femoral-popliteal aneurysms
- Cardiopulmonary risk assessment

Risk assessment:
- *Low risk*:
  - Age <80
  - No, or minor, American College of Cardiology (ACC) clinical predictors of increased perioperative cardiovascular risk- abnormal EKG, arrhythmia, history of cerebrovascular accident, low functional capacity, uncontrolled hypertension[1]
  - Non-inflammatory infrarenal AAA
- *Intermediate risk*:
  - Age over 80
  - Intermediate ACC clinical predictors—mild angina, previous myocardial infarction or pathological Q waves on EKG, compensated or history of heart failure, diabetes mellitus, renal insufficiency
  - Chronic obstructive pulmonary disease (COPD) with FEV1 >1 L/s
  - Juxtarenal, suprarenal, or inflammatory AAA
- *High risk*:
  - Age over 80

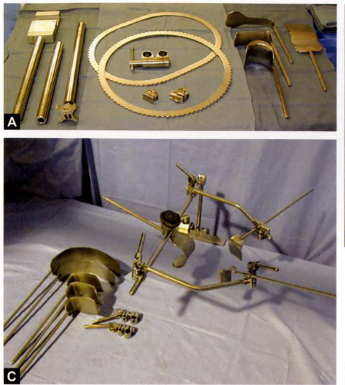

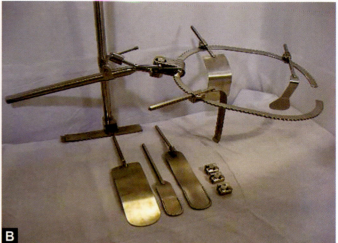

Figs. 14.1A to C: (A) Bookwalter retractor. (B) Omni retractor. (C) Thompson retractor.

– Major ACC clinical predictors—unstable coronary syndromes (acute or recent myocardial infarction, unstable or severe angina), decompensated heart failure, significant arrhythmias (high-grade atrioventricular block, symptomatic ventricular arrhythmias, supraventricular arrhythmia with uncontrolled rate), valvular disease
– Oxygen-dependent COPD with FEV1 <1 L/s
– Pugh-Child's class B or C hepatic failure

1.5 Preoperative Checklist

• Preoperative administration of beta-blockers for risk reduction of cardiovascular events.

Sign in:

• Verified patient identity, operative site, planned procedure and consent.
• Cardiopulmonary risk assessment reviewed by Anesthesiology.
• Review patient allergies and use of beta-blockers.
• Ensure adequate intravenous access, hemodynamic monitors, availability of blood products.

Time out:

• Team members introduce themselves and role.
• Surgeon, anesthesiologist and nurse reconfirm correct patient, site, and procedure.

• Surgeon reviews critical steps, operative duration, and estimated blood-loss.
• Anesthesiology reviews any patient-specific concerns
• Equipment sterility and/or issues are confirmed.
• Verify appropriate antibiotic administration within 60 minutes of incision.

Sign out:

• Nursing confirms procedure performed, correct instrument/sponge/needle counts, labeling of any surgical specimen.
• Surgeon, anesthesiologist and nurse review tenets of postoperative management.

1.6 Decision-Making Algorithm

• *See* Flowchart 14.1.

1.7 Pearls and Pitfalls

Pearls:

• Proper patient positioning is essential for adequate retroperitoneal aortic exposure.
• Aberrant renal vascular anatomy may be better suited to a retroperitoneal approach.
• Left diaphragmatic crus may be divided for exposure of the paravisceral aorta.

- Aortic bifurcated prosthetic grafts must be tunneled posterior to the ureters.
- Left renal artery may be reimplanted either as a Carrel patch or via interposition grafting.

Pitfalls:
- Avoid proximal aortic clamp repositioning if placed above renal arteries.
- Avoid suturing aortic graft into aneurysmal tissue at either proximal or distal anastomoses.
- Avoid circumferential dissection of the aortic bifurcation and proximal common iliac arteries to prevent venous, ureteral, or parasympathetic nerve plexus injury.
- Avoid dissection of aneurysm sac off of duodenum in setting of inflammatory aneurysm.
- Avoid injury to the intercostal nerve in the line of incision to prevent incisional "bulge".

1.8 Surgical Anatomy

- *See* Figure 14.2.

1.9 Positioning

- *See* Figure 14.3.

1.10 Anesthesia

- Following intubation, secure intravenous access and hemodynamic monitors as vessel access will be limited once placed in the right lateral decubitus position.
- Double-lumen endotracheal tubes are often unnecessary, even in retroperitoneal repair of visceral segment Type IV thoracoabdominal aortic aneurysms.
- Use of a pulmonary artery catheter may assist in the monitoring of patients with coronary atherosclerotic or valvular disease.
- Systemic heparinization (50–100 units/kg) is provided prior to aortic cross-clamping, with coagulation status monitored with frequent measures of activated clotting time.
- Avoid hypothermia, acidosis, and hypovolemia to offset potential hemodynamic compromise upon restoration of visceral or lower extremity arterial circulation.

2 PERIOPERATIVE

2.1 Incision

- *See* Figure 14.4.

2.2 Steps

- *See* Figures 14.5A to L.

Flowchart 14.1: Decision-making algorithm.

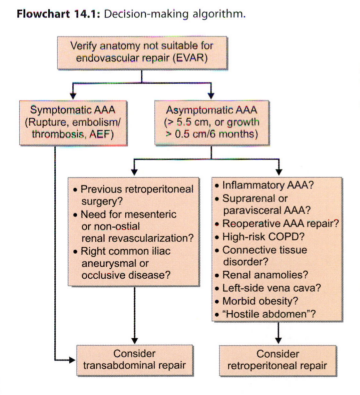

Fig. 14.2: Surgical anatomy. The aorta is the main vascular conduit of the thoracic and abdominal cavities. After entering the abdominal cavity via the diaphragmatic hiatus the aorta lies anterior to the thoracolumbar spine in the retroperitoneum. Aneurysms may develop along any segment of the abdominal aorta and are further classified as infrarenal, juxtarenal, pararenal, or paravisceral based on the aneurysm proximity to named visceral vessels.

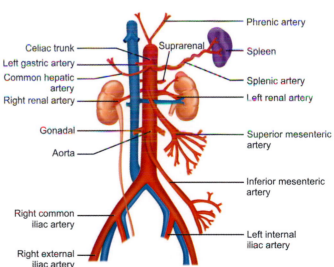

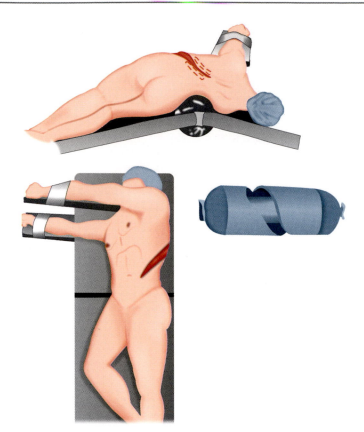

Fig. 14.3: Patient positioning. A vacuum-assisted, self-molding foam bean bag and flexible operating room table are critical to maintaining patient stability. Following endotracheal intubation and establishment of central venous catheters and hemodynamic monitors, the patient is placed in the right lateral decubitus position. The shoulders are placed at a 45° angle, the left arm is extended and supported, the trunk is rotated such that the hips are near-parallel to the table, and the kidney rest is elevated and table flexed to provide maximal separation of the left costal margin and iliac crest.

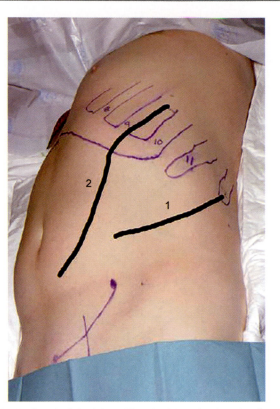

Fig. 14.4: Surgical incision. The incision begins in the 10th interspace and extends medially to the lateral edge of the rectus abdominus at the level of the umbilicus. The external oblique, internal oblique, then transversus abdominus muscles are divided with bovie electrocautery. Lateral border of the rectus muscle may be divided for added pelvic exposure. After dividing the transversalis fascia the retroperitoneal space is entered bluntly mobilizing the peritoneum and its visceral contents medially and superiorly. This incisional approach exposes the infrarenal aorta as well as the distal left external iliac and middle right common iliac arteries.

2.3 Closure

- Retroperitoneal approach does not allow for inspection of the descending and sigmoid colon to ensure adequate visceral perfusion. If needed, the peritoneum may be incised to assess viability of bowel. Tube thoracostomy should be performed if the thoracic cavity is entered during dissection of the diaphragm. The prosthetic graft should be concealed with closure of the aortic aneurysm sac. Lowering the kidney rest and unflexing the operating table facilitates wound closure by narrowing the space between the costal margin and iliac crest. The lateral abdominal wall is closed in two layers using a monofilament suture. The inner layer encompasses the fascia of the transversus abdominis and internal oblique muscles. The external oblique is closed as a single outer layer. Include healthy, well-vascularized tissues within fascial closure as patients are prone to develop incisional hernias following open aortic aneurysm repair.

3 POSTOPERATIVE

3.1 Complications

Most common complications:
- Cardiac events (myocardial ischemia, arrhythmias)
- Pulmonary complications (pulmonary edema, pleural effusions, ventilator dependence)

- Renal insufficiency (acute tubular necrosis)
- Ischemic colitis
- Incisional hernia

Least common complications:
- Graft infection or thrombosis
- Spinal ischemia
- Aortoenteric fistula formation

3.2 Outcomes

- Estimated 5- and 10-year survival of 75% and 45%, respectively, with elective repair.
- Shorter hospital length-of-stay and reduced postoperative paralytic ileus with retroperitoneal approach to aneurysm repair.

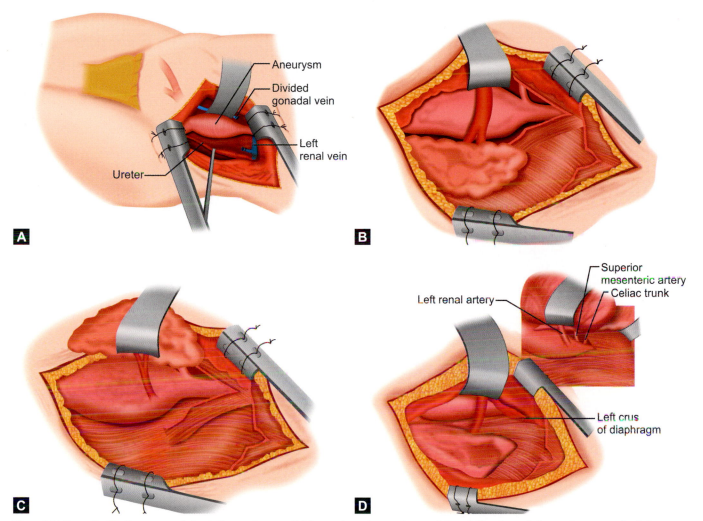

Figs. 14.5A to D: (A) Exposure of the infrarenal aorta. With continued superiormedial mobilization of the peritoneum the left psoas muscle is identified. Dissection continues superiorly in an avascular plane between the peritoneum and Gerota's fascia. Great care is taken to identify and isolate the left ureter along its length from the left iliac artery bifurcation to the renal pelvis. Periureteral fat is mobilized with the ureter to avoid iatrogenic ischemic injury. (B) Posterior position of left kidney. Dissection in the avascular plane between peritoneum and Gerota's fascia allows for posterior positioning of the left kidney in the retroperitoneal bed, full exposure of the left renal vein, as well as the pararenal segment of aorta. (C) Anteromedial position of left kidney. In the setting of pararenal aneurysmal degeneration requiring left renal artery reimplantation, or as a prelude to supraceliac aorta exposure, the left kidney may be positioned anteromedially. Division of the gonadal, adrenal, renal and lumbar veins prevents iatrogenic venous injury with mobilization. (D) Supraceliac aorta exposure. The supraceliac aorta can exposed to the level of the descending thoracic aorta via a retroperitoneal approach. Begin by bluntly sweeping the posterior chest wall extension of the diaphragm away from the retroperitoneal space. As the dissection continues medially toward the aorta, fibers of the left crus of the diaphragm should be divided with electrocautery widening the diaphragmatic hiatus and in doing exposing the supraceliac aorta.

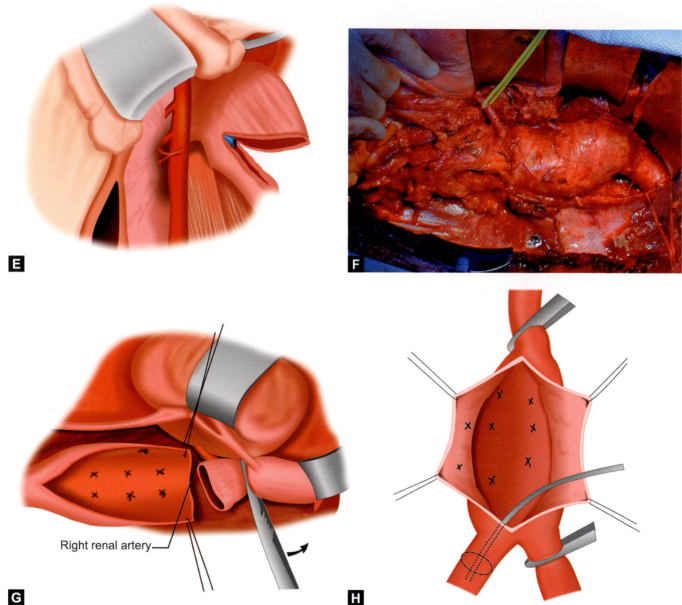

Right renal artery

Figs. 14.5E to H: (E) Exposure of visceral vessels. With superomedial mobilization of the peritoneum and viscera, division of the left crus of the diaphragm, and clearing lymphatic and connective tissue from the aorta surface the visceral vessels can be easily isolated and controlled. (F) Retroperitoneal aorta exposure. Intraoperative photograph shows the aorta exposure obtained with retroperitoneal approach and division of the diaphragmatic crus for supraceliac control. The left renal artery is isolated and controlled with a small vascular loop for later reimplantation. (G) Entering the aneurysm. Systemic heparinization (50–100 units/kg) is administered prior to clamping aorta or iliac arteries. Proximal aorta and iliac arteries free of atherosclerotic disease should be isolated for clamp placement to reduce the chance of vessel clamp injury or atheroembolization. Clamps are placed first distally to protect against embolization that may result from proximal aorta cross-clamping. The aneurysm sac is incised at the aortic bifurcation and continued to a point at least 1.0 cm below the proximal aortic cross-clamp. The incision is then carried transversely forming a "T" with division of the lateral aortic wall. Upon entering the aneurysm sac bluntly dislodge and remove mural thrombus. Back-bleeding lumbar, middle sacral, and inferior mesenteric arteries are ligated from within the aneurysm sac with figure-of-eight interrupted 2-0 silk sutures. (H) Balloon control of iliac arteries. Exposure and control of the right common iliac artery can be challenging in a retroperitoneal approach. An appropriately sized balloon catheter may be placed within the lumen of the iliac artery to provided hemostasis during aneurysm repair.

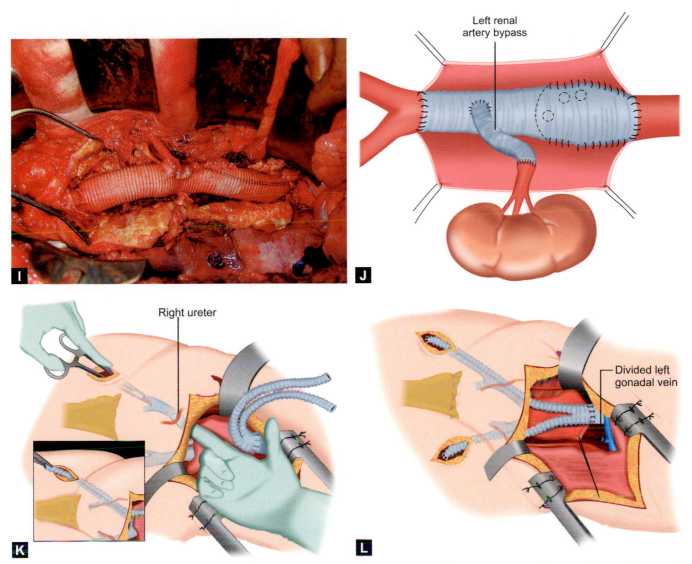

Figs. 14.5I to L: (I) Aortic tube graft. Aortic sizers are available for best measure of the appropriate diameter for prosthetic graft sizing. Stretch the graft to length prior to trimming redundant prosthetic material. Aortic replacement begins with the proximal aortic anastomosis. Avoid creation of anastomoses on aneurysmal or ectatic tissues as they are at increased risk for continued aneurysmal degeneration. Using 3-0 polypropylene suture, perform running anastomosis with double thickness of posterior aortic wall for increased strength. Teflon or Dacron pledgets may be used if aortic tissue is friable. After completing proximal anastomosis, clamp the prosthetic graft then briefly release aortic cross-clamp to test the integrity of suture line and reinforce as needed. The intraoperative photograph illustrates aortic tube graft replacement with reimplantation of the left renal artery via a Carrel-type patch of native aortic wall. (J) Left renal artery bypass. The left renal artery may also be reimplanted via an interposition bypass. The native renal artery is beveled, a graftotomy of appropriate size is created on the prosthetic graft, and an end-to-side 6 mm prosthetic interposition graft is placed. (K) Aortic bifurcated graft. Iliac anastomoses are preferred over femoral due to lower rates of infection and pseudoaneurysm formation. In the setting of severe iliac atherosclerotic occlusion or aneurysmal degeneration distal anastomoses are created at the femoral level. A plane for passage of the bifurcated limbs is created with blunt dissection anterior to the external iliac and common femoral arteries. A clamp may be placed from the dissected femoral space anterior to the external iliac to guide the bifurcated limb to the femoral artery. It is important to tunnel the iliac limbs posterior to the ureters as they cross over the iliac arteries, as extrinsic compression of the ureters can incite an inflammatory process leading to profound ureteral obstruction and hydronephrosis. (L) Distal femoral anastomoses. Femoral anastomoses are created in standard fashion using 5-0 or 6-0 polypropylene in a running continuous suture. Prior to completion of first femoral limb, release inflow clamp to flush any formed thrombus or debris from within the graft prior to restoring extremity perfusion. When anastomosis is completed, gradually remove outflow clamp to prevent hypotension from release of vasoactive substances.

3.3 Follow-Up

- Postsurgery evaluation within 1-month following discharge
- Surveillance cross-sectional imaging at 1-year post-operatively
- Lifelong best medical management of comorbidities

3.4 E-mail an Expert

- *E-mail address*: mshames@health.usf.edu

3.5 Web Resources/References

- www.vascularweb.org
- www.ncbi.nlm.nih.gov
- www.usfvascularsurgery.com

REFERENCES

1. American College of Cardiology/American Heart Association guideline update for perioperative cardiovascular evaluation for noncardiac surgery-executive summary. Circulation. 2002;105:1257.
2. Cambria RP, Brewster DC, Abbott WM. Transperitoneal versus retroperitoneal approach for aortic reconstruction: a randomized prospective study. J Vasc Surg. 1990;11(2):314.
3. Cronenwett JL, Johnston KW. Rutherford's Vascular Surgery, 7th edition. Philadelphia; Saunders; 2010.
4. Darling RC III, Shah DM, McClellan WR. Decreased morbidity associated with retroperitoneal exclusion treatment for abdominal aortic aneurysm. J Cardiovasc Surg (Torino). 1992;33(1):65.
5. Lederle FA, Wilson SE, Johnson GR, et al. for the Aneurysm detection and management (ADAM) Veterans Affairs Cooperative Study Group. Immediate repair compared with surveillance of small abdominal aortic aneurysms. N Engl J Med. 2002;346:1437.
6. Moore WS. Vascular and Endovascular Surgery, A Comprehensive Review, 7th edition. Philadelphia: Saunders; 2006.
7. Sicard GA, Reilly JM, Rubin BG, et al. Transabdominal versus retroperitoneal incision for abdominal aortic surgery: report of a prospective randomized trial. J Vasc Surg. 1995;21(2):174-81.
8. The UK Small Aneurysm Trial Participants: mortality results for randomized controlled trial of early elective surgery or ultrasonographic surveillance for small abdominal aortic aneurysms. Lancet. 1998;352:1649.
9. The United Kingdom Small Aneurysm Trial Participants: long term outcomes of immediate repair compared with surveillance of small abdominal aortic aneurysms. N Engl J Med. 2002;346:1445.

QUIZ

Question 1. Relative indications for a retroperitoneal approach to repair of an AAA include all of the following except?
a. Left-sided inferior vena cava
b. Urinary or enteric stoma
c. Inflammatory aneurysm
d. Aneurysm sac rupture

Question 2. Retroperitoneal repair of an AAA is the preferred approach for which clinical scenario?
a. Acute AAA rupture with hemodynamic instability
b. Morbidly obese patient with a midline enteric stoma
c. Patient with previous resection of a left-sided retroperitoneal sarcoma
d. 7 cm infrarenal aneurysm with an aortoenteric erosion

Question 3. In contradistinction to transabdominal approach, a retroperitoneal repair offers which advantages?
a. Shorter length of in-hospital stay
b. Reduced incidence of postoperative paralytic ileus
c. Fewer pulmonary complications
d. All of the above

Question 4. Disadvantages of the retroperitoneal approach include which of the following?
a. Potential injury to the intercostal nerve in the line of incision, resulting in a flank "bulge"
b. Contents of the peritoneal cavity not available for direct inspection
c. Inaccessible distal right common iliac artery
d. All of the above

Question 5. Which of the following maneuvers is essential in performing an aortic replacement with a bifurcated graft?
a. Trimming the redundant prosthetic material principally from the iliofemoral limbs
b. Creating the distal iliofemoral anastomoses prior to the proximal aortic
c. Tunneling the iliofemoral limbs posterior to the ureters
d. Utilizing an obturator bypass to avoid inguinal incisions

ANSWERS: 1. d 2. b 3. d 4. d 5. c

Aortobifemoral Bypass

Lindsay Gates, Jeffrey Indes

1 PREOPERATIVE

1.1 Indications

- Patients with aortoiliac occlusive disease who have TASC C/D lesions presenting with ischemic rest pain or lower extremity tissue loss.

1.2 Evidence

- Two large meta-analyses evaluated the comprehensive experience with aortobifemoral bypass grafting results indicating 30-day morbidity and mortality rates of 4%.[1]
- Several single center studies also conducted looking at 30-day mortality and found rates as low as 1%.[2,3]
- Five-year cumulative patency found to be around 96% for patient's >60, younger patients and those with small aortas are more vulnerable to late graft failure.[1,4]

1.3 Materials

- Open vascular surgery tray including assortment of vascular clamps
- Self-retaining abdominal retractor [e.g. Omnilink (Fig. 15.1A), Bookwalter (Fig. 15.1B), or Balfour]

- Major abdominal laparotomy instruments
- Knitted Dacron or PTFE bifurcated graft
- Bovie electrocautery
- Cell saver

1.4 Preoperative

Planning:
- Preoperative CT scan of Abdomen and pelvis with bilateral lower extremity run-off
- Preoperative cardiopulmonary risk evaluation and optimization

Risk assessment:
- *Low risk*:
  - Age <80
  - No, or minor, American College of Cardiology (ACC) clinical predictors of increased perioperative cardiovascular risk-abnormal EKG, arrhythmia, history of cerebrovascular accident, low functional capacity, uncontrolled hypertension
  - Age appropriate functional status
  - Non-smokers
- *Intermediate risk*:
  - Age over 80

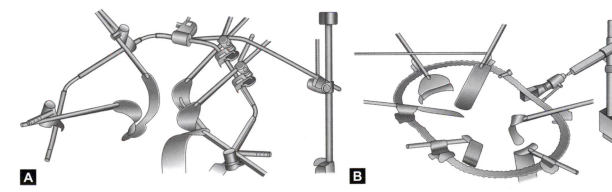

Figs. 15.1A and B: (A) Omni Retractor. (B) Bookwalter.

- Intermediate ACC clinical predictors-mild angina, previous myocardial infarction or pathological Q waves on EKG, compensated or history of heart failure, diabetes mellitus, renal insufficiency
- Chronic obstructive pulmonary disease (COPD).
- *High risk*:
  - Age over 80
  - Major ACC clinical predictors-unstable coronary syndromes (acute or recent myocardial infarction, unstable or severe angina), decompensated heart failure, significant arrhythmias (high-grade atrioventricular block, symptomatic ventricular arrhythmias, supraventricular arrhythmia with uncontrolled rate), valvular disease
  - COPD with FEV1< 1 L/s, or oxygen dependence
  - Pugh-Child's class B or C hepatic failure[5]

1.5 Preoperative Checklist

Sign-in:

- Verify patient identity, operative site, planned procedure, and consent
- Cardiopulmonary risk assessment review by anesthesiology
- Review patient allergies
- Ensure adequate intravenous access, hemodynamic monitors, availability of blood products

Time out:

- All members of operating room staff, surgery team and anesthesiology team introduce themselves and role
- Surgeon, anesthesiologist and nurse confirm correct patient, site, and procedure
- Anesthesiology review any patient specific concerns
- Equipment sterility and/or issues are confirmed
- Verify appropriate antibiotics administration within 60 minutes of incision.

Sign out:

- Nursing confirms procedure performed, correct instrument/sponge/needle counts, labeling of any surgical specimen.
- Surgeon, anesthesiologist, and nurse review tenets of postoperative management.

1.6 Decision-Making Algorithm

- *See* Flowchart 15.1.

1.7 Pearls and Pitfalls

Pearls:

- If thrombus or significant calcification limits safe cross-clamping of the aorta or iliac arteries, control may be obtained by intraluminal balloon deployment.
- If collateral veins are intact, left renal vein may be divided at the level of the vena cava for added proximal aortic exposure when needed.
- In the case of asymmetric plaque, clamp soft plaque against hard plaque to minimize risk of emboli and traumatic clamp injury.
- End-to-end proximal anastomosis: allows for more complete thromboendarterectomy of proximal stump and better in-flow with less turbulence.
- End-side anastomosis maintains antegrade flow to inferior mesenteric artery and hypogastrics, in cases of external iliac occlusion. If only aorta or CIA occlusion, end-to-end preferred.
- Do not leave diseased common femoral arteries. End-arterectomy and anastomosis to profunda origin to maintain outflow.

Pitfalls:

- Review preoperative imaging to evaluate for aberrant vascular anatomy (such as multiple renal collaterals).
- Avoid suturing aortic graft to inflamed aortic tissue when possible.
- Avoid extensive dissection anterior to the aortic bifurcation and proximal left iliac artery because the autonomic nerve plexus regulation of erection and ejaculation sweeps over this region in men.
- If proximal graft protrudes to far anteriorly or has no tissue covering it, could lead to erosion through posterior part of duodenum.

1.8 Surgical Anatomy

- *See* Figure 15.2.

1.9 Positioning

- *See* Figure 15.3.

1.10 Anesthesia

- Obtain adequate intravenous access, intra-arterial pressure monitoring, and preoperative antibiotic administration.
- Placement of epidural catheter for pain control in acceptable cases.
- Most will need to be placed under general endotracheal anesthesia.

Flowchart 15.1: Decision-making algorithm.

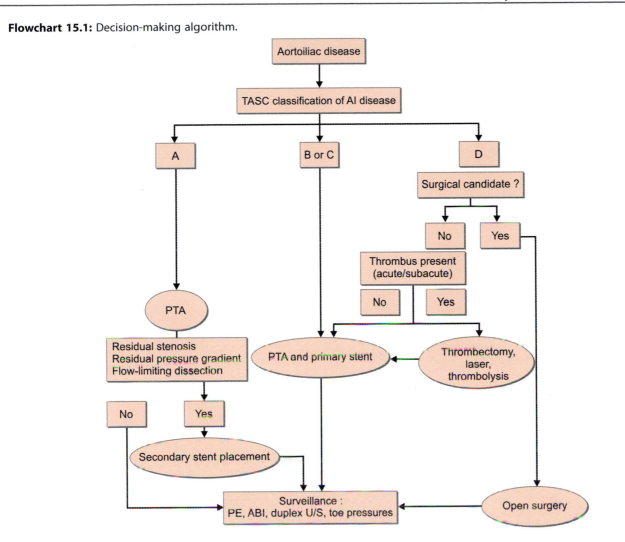

- Use of a pulmonary artery catheter may assist in the monitoring of patients with coronary atherosclerotic or valvular disease.
- Systemic heparinization (50–100 units/kg) is provided prior to aortic cross-clamping , with coagulation status monitored with frequent measures of activated clotting time.
- Avoid hypothermia, acidosis, and hypovolemia to offset potential hemodynamic compromise upon restoration of visceral or lower extremity arterial circulation.

2 PERIOPERATIVE

2.1 Incision

- *See* Figure 15.4.

2.2 Steps

- *See* Figures 15.5A to E.

2.3 Closure

- *See* Figure 15.6.

3 POSTOPERATIVE

3.1 Complications

Early:
- Cardiac complications
- Acute renal failure
- Sexual dysfunction
- Hemorrhage
- Wound infection

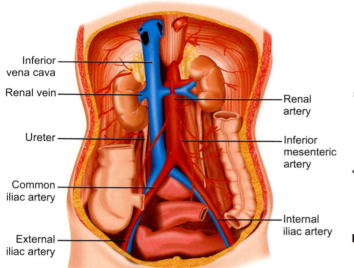

Inferior vena cava

Renal vein

Ureter

Common iliac artery

External iliac artery

Renal artery

Inferior mesenteric artery

Internal iliac artery

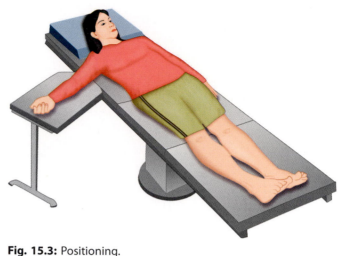

Fig. 15.3: Positioning.

Fig. 15.2: The infrarenal aorta origin is around the cephalad end of the second lumbar vertebra and continues until it bifurcates at the fourth lumbar vertebra. Paired lumbar arteries come off the posterior portion of the aorta with the inferior mesenteric artery arising off the left anterior portion of the aorta as the only visceral branch in this segment. The gonadal vessels and ureters lie along the psoas muscles in the paravertebral gutters and cross anterior to the iliac vessels in the pelvis.

Late:
- Graft thrombosis
- Graft infection
- Aortoenteric fistula
- Anastomotic pseudoaneurysm

3.2 Outcomes

- 5-year patency between 80% and 96%
- 95% of patients report initial improvement of symptoms or complete resolution of symptoms; this decreases to about 80% at 5 years.

3.3 Follow-Up

- Postoperative surgical follow-up in 2–3 weeks to assess wound
- Will need surveillance US for graft
- Life-long medical management of comorbidities

3.4 E-mail an Expert

- *E-mail address*: Jeffrey.indes@yale.edu

3.5 Web Resources/References

- www.vascularweb.org
- www.mcbi.nim.nih.gov
- Cronenwett JL, Johnston KW. Rutherford's Vascular Surgery, 7th edition. Sanders, 2010, Philidelpha, PA.
- Moore WS. Vascular and Endovascular Surgery, A Comprehensive Review, 7th edition. Saunders, 2006.

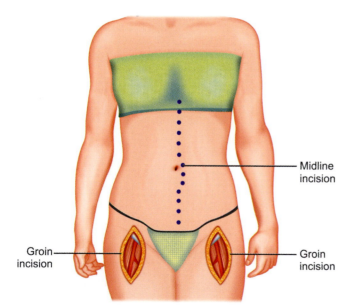

Midline incision

Groin incision

Groin incision

Fig. 15.4: Incision.

- Wound dehiscence
- Limb ischemia
- Graft thrombosis
- Bowel ischemia

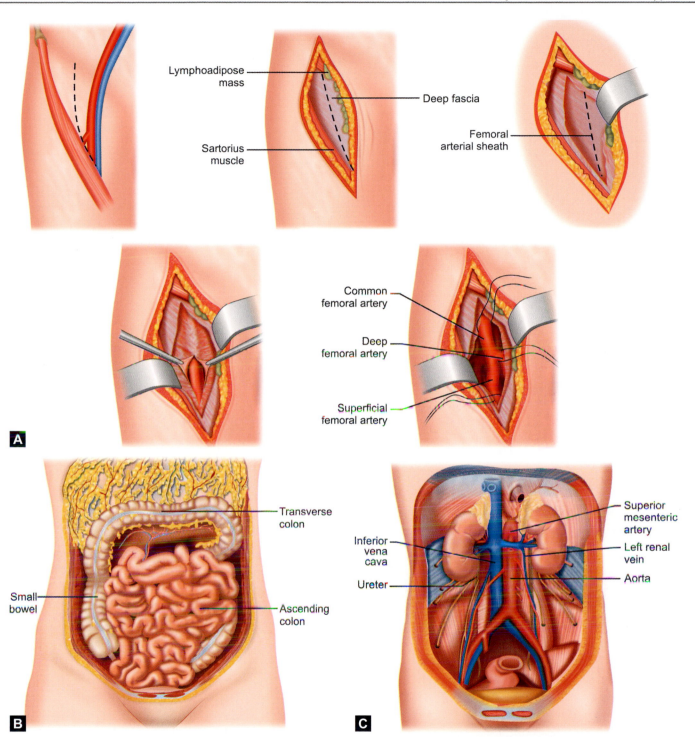

Figs. 15.5A to C: (A) Groin incision made bilaterally one third of the way between the pubic tubercle and anterior superior iliac spine. Incision deepened through skin and subcutaneous tissues. The common femoral artery, profunda femoris artery, and the superficial femoral artery need to be identified and dissected free from surrounding tissue circumferentially. (B) Via the midline incision from the subxiphoid to suprapubic region enter the abdominal cavity. Explore for any intra-abdominal abnormalities and palpate the stomach to ensure proper positioning of the nasogastric tube. Next retract transverse colon cephalad. Then divide the ligament of Treitz to mobilize the duodenum and allow for retraction of the small bowel to the right using a self-retaining abdominal retractor. (C) Incise the retroperitoneum overlaying the aorta. Continue proximally until the left renal vein is identified. Dissect the aorta just below the level of the left renal vein and prepare for clamping. Then continue dissecting the retroperitoneum distally to the level of the aortic bifurcation.

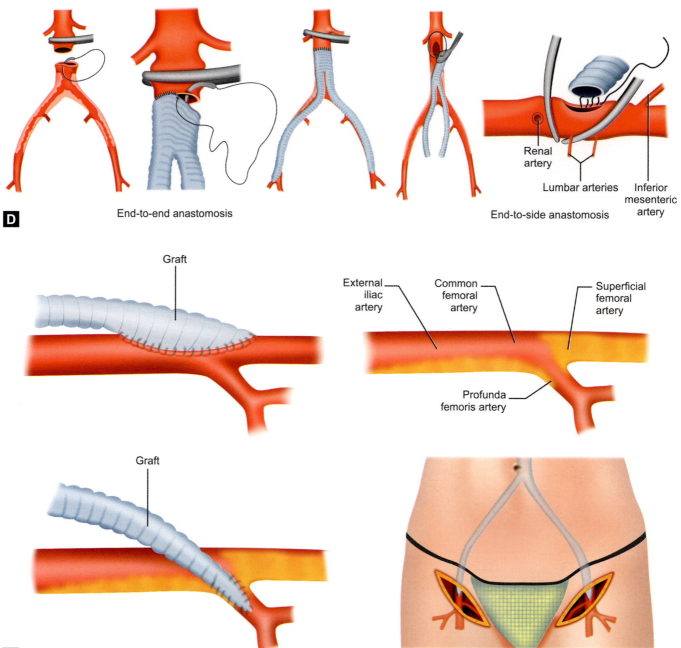

D   End-to-end anastomosis

Renal artery

Lumbar arteries   Inferior mesenteric artery

End-to-side anastomosis

Graft

External iliac artery   Common femoral artery   Superficial femoral artery

Profunda femoris artery

Graft

E

Figs. 15.5D and E: (D) Create a tunnel from each of the common femoral arteries to the aortic bifurcation. It is important to remember to stay anterior to the iliac vessels but posterior to the ureters. On the left the tunnel passes beneath the sigmoid mesentery and slightly more lateral. Moist umbilical tapes or Penrose drains are passed with a smooth aortic clamp to mark tunnels. At this point administer Heparin (or a direct thrombin inhibitor for patients with a history of HIT) for systemic anticoagulation (75–100 units/kg). After 5 minutes, apply proximal clam on the aorta just below the renal arteries. Next apply the distal clamps on the aorta at the level of the IMA. If planning on an end-to-end anastomosis, transect aorta below the proximal clamp and oversew distal aorta in two layers. If proceeding with an end-to-side anastomosis make a longitudinal arteriotomy measuring 2–3 cm. Then proceed with the proximal anastomosis. (E) Pass the right and left limb of the bifurcated graft through their respective tunnel. Clamp CFA, SFA, and profunda femoris arteries. Make a longitudinal arteriotomy in the CFA. Extend to the profunda for patients with significant SFA disease. Construct end-to-side anastomosis. Back-bleed femorals and forward flush graft.
(IMA: Inferior mesenteric artery; CFA: Common femoral artery; SFA: Superficial femoral artery).

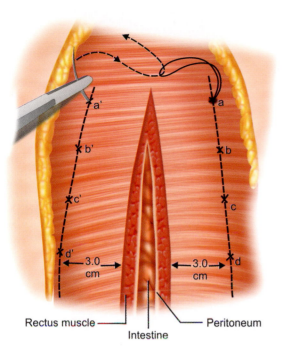

Rectus muscle —

Intestine

— Peritoneum

Fig. 15.6: Prior to closure assess distal perfusion. Reversal of systemic anticoagulation with protamine sulfate (1 mg/100 units circulating heparin); this is optional. Close retroperitoneum over proximal anastomosis and portion of aorta that will be sitting behind duodenum. If not enough retroperitoneum to cover anastomosis behind duodenum, a sleeve of omentum to separate the graft from bowel can be used. Remove retractor, close abdominal fascia then skin. Turn attention to bilateral groin incisions, close each in several layers.

REFERENCES

1. Onohara T, Komori K, Kume M, et al. Multivariate analysis of long-term results after aortobifemoral bypass in patients with aortoiliac occlusive disease. J Cardiovasc Surg. 2001; 42:381.
2. DeVries SO, Hunink MGM, et al. Results of aortic bifurcation grafts for aortoiliac occlusive disease: a meta-analysis. J Vasc Surg. 1997;26:558.
3. McDaniel MD, Macdonal PD, Haver RA, et al. Published results of surgery for AIOD. Ann Vasc Surg. 1997;11:425.
4. Reed AB, Conte MS, Donaldson MC, et al. The impact of patient age and artic size on the results of aortobifemoral bypass grafting. J Vasc Surg. 2003;37:1219-25.
5. Fleisher L, Beckman J, Brown K, et al. American College of Cardiology/American Heart Association Guideline Update for Perioperative Cardiovascular Evaluation for Noncardiac Surgery—Executive Summary. Circulation105: 1257, 2002.

QUIZ

Question 1. When performing an aortobifemoral bypass, the decision to perform an end-to-side anastomosis is primarily based on:
a. The presence of a calcified aorta
b. The presence of an occluded IMA
c. The presence of thrombus extending to the renal arteries
d. To preserve forward flow in the aorta

Question 2. When performing an aortobifemoral bypass, the decision to perform an end-to-end anastomosis is primarily based on:

a. The presence of a calcified aorta
b. The presence of an occluded IMA
c. The presence of thrombus extending to the renal arteries
d. To preserve forward flow in the aorta

Question 3. When tunneling each limb of the aortobifemoral graft the pathway should be?
a. Subcutaneous
b. Through the inguinal ligament
c. Anatomically under the ureter
d. Anatomically over the ureter

ANSWERS:

1. d   2. c   3. c

Aortoiliac Artery Angioplasty

Lindsay Gates, Jeffrey Indes

1 PREOPERATIVE

1.1 Indications

- Aortoiliac disease in patients with lifestyle-limiting claudication, rest pain, and/or tissue loss
- Trans-Atlantic Inter-Society Consensus (TASC) A and B aortoiliac lesions and some TASC C lesions in selected patients

1.2 Evidence and References

- 4-year primary patency after PTA between 58% and 86%[1]
- Complications from PTA between 3% and 7.9%[1,2]
- Aortic bifurcation disease treated with kissing iliac stents have good primary and secondary patency rates of 78% and 98%, respectively, at 3 years[2,3]

1.3 Materials Needed

- Stationary imaging system or a portable imaging system
- Micropuncture needle and wire
- 0.035 glidewire
- Lunderquist wire
- Calibrated flush catheter
- Assorted sheaths
- Assorted balloon and self-expandable stents
- Assortment of wires and catheters for difficult to transverse anatomy

1.4 Preoperative Planning and Risk Assessment

Planning:
- Duplex scan
- Computed tomography angiography, occasionally conventional angiography

- Preoperative cardiopulmonary evaluation and medical optimization of other comorbidities

Risk assessment:
- *Low risk*:
  - Age <80
  - *No or minor American College of Cardiology (ACC) clinic predictors of increased perioperative cardiovascular risk*: Abnormal electrocardiogram (EKG), arrhythmia, history of cerebrovascular accident, low functional capacity, uncontrolled hypertension
  - Life-time nonsmoker
- *Intermediate risk*:
  - Age over 80
  - *Intermediate ACC clinical predictors*: Mild angina, previous myocardial infarction or pathological Q waves on EKG, compensated or history of heart failure, diabetes mellitus, renal insufficiency
  - Chronic obstructive pulmonary disease (COPD) with FEV1 >1 L/s
  - Tortuous anatomy or heavily calcified vessels
- *High risk*:
  - Age over 80
  - *Major ACC clinical predictors*: unstable coronary syndromes (acute or recent myocardial infarction, unstable or severe angina), decompensated heart failure, significant arrhythmias (high-grade atrioventricular block, symptomatic ventricular arrhythmias, supraventricular arrhythmia with uncontrolled rate), valvular disease[4]
  - Oxygen-dependent COPD with FEV1 <1 L/s
  - Pugh-Child's class B or C hepatic failure
  - Patient comorbidities (age, smoking, coronary artery disease [CAD], COPD, chronic kidney disease [CKD], etc.)
  - Tortuous anatomy, heavily calcified vessels, areas of intra-arterial occlusion

Flowchart 16.1: Decision-making algorithm.

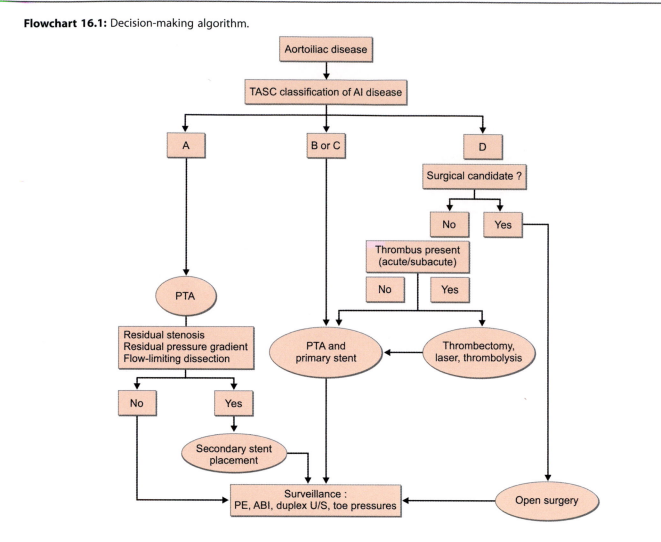

1.5 Preoperative Checklist

Sign in:
- Verified patients identity, planned procedure
- Cardiopulmonary risk assessment completed
- Review patient allergies and medications
- Review patient INR and platelet levels as well as renal function
- Ensure adequate intravenous access and hemodynamic monitors

Time out:
- Staff introduces themselves and role in surgery
- Operator and nurse reconfirms correct patient and procedure
- Any specific concerns about procedure addressed
- Perioperative antibiotics given when appropriate
- Verify equipment availability

Sign out:
- Surgeon and nurse confirm correct instrument counts, and procedure performed as well as contrast used and fluoroscopy time.

1.6 Decision-Making Algorithm

- *See* Flowchart 16.1.

1.7 Pearls and Pitfalls

Pearls:
- Geometric mismatch refers to the presence of unconformities between the native aortic lumen (both diseased and nondiseased-stented segments) and the final configuration of the stents following aortobiiliac stent reconstruction (Fig. 16.1A). Determinants of mismatch include aortic anatomy and configuration (straight vs tapered

shape), which is determined by the anatomy of the distal aorta and the pattern and extent of atherosclerotic disease.[3]

- The resulting dead-space between the stent pair and the native aortic wall can be minimized by a number of strategies, including appropriate oversizing of the stents to ensure proper filling of the dead-space. This can be better accomplished using segmental, lumen-conforming nitinol stent designs, which when appropriately oversized can allow a mirror-D configuration as opposed to a double-barrel configuration with the meshed designs such as Wallstent or with balloon-expanded stents (Fig. 16.1B).[3,4]
- Practically speaking, however, there are two main types of stent reconstructions: the abutting and crossing configurations (Fig. 16.1C). The type of aortoiliac reconstruction should be customized to the pattern of involvement in each patient. For example, in unilateral or bilateral ostial common iliac artery stenosis, an abutting stents reconstruction of the bifurcation (low neobifurcation) using either self-expanding or balloon expandable stents (when short-segment focal disease is present) was preferred.
- When disease involves the distal aorta or iliac disease extends into the distal aorta one option is to use the a unimodular aortic stent graft system which abuts the aortic bifurcation and sits low enough below the renal arteries as to not impede a possible future open surgical procedure (Fig. 16.1D).

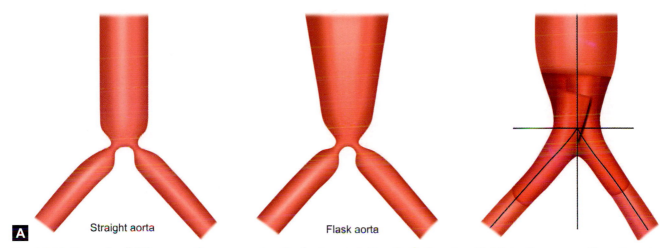

A Straight aorta Flask aorta

Fig. 16.1A: Example of different aortic anatomy showing both a straight and a flask aorta with bilateraly common iliac artery stenosis. The third diagram shows a geometric mismatch between the stents placed and the aortic wall.

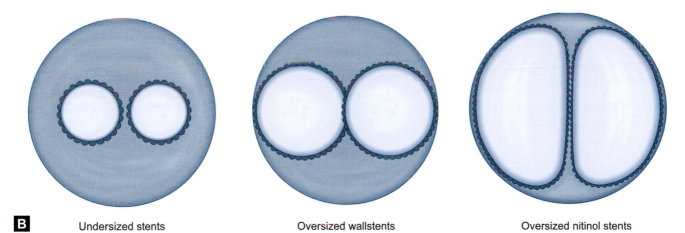

B Undersized stents Oversized wallstents Oversized nitinol stents

Fig. 16.1B: Cross-sectional view of distal aorta after iliac stent placement. First picture shows undersized stents, which leave a significant area between stent wall and aortic wall. The second picture shows double-barrel configuration with oversized wallstents or balloon-expanded stents; one still can see a significant amount of dead space between stent and aortic wall. Third illustration shows oversized lumen conforming nitinol stents, resulting in a mirror-D configuration. This reduces the amount of remaining dead space and optimized lumen diameter.

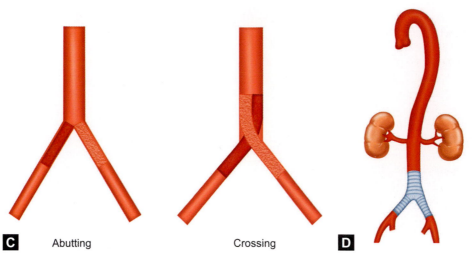

C   Abutting   Crossing   D

Figs. 16.1C and D: (C) Two major common iliac artery stent configurations abutting and crossing. (D) Example of a unimodular stent graft system, which can be used for iliac disease that extends into the distal portions of the aorta.

Pitfalls:
- When a crossing-stents configuration is used, geometric mismatch of the deployed stent pair relative to the distal aorta may be problematic because of the resulting detrimental flow disturbances, which may promote thrombosis and/or exaggerated intimal proliferation.[1–3]

1.8 Surgical Anatomy

- *See* Figure 16.2.

1.9 Positioning

- Patient is placed in the supine position.
- Bilateral groins are prepped and draped using standard sterile surgical technique.

See Figure 16.3.

1.10 Anesthesia

- Local anesthesia with intravenous sedation and intra-arterial blood pressure monitoring is used for the majority of cases.

2 PERIOPERATIVE

2.1 Incision

- Vascular access is obtained on the ipsilateral common femoral artery at the level of the femoral head in a retrograde direction using a Seldinger needle and a 0.035-in. glidewire, which is advanced under fluoroscopic guidance into the aorta.

– If the CIA is occluded, contralateral flush catheter placement should be considered so that a complete diagnostic study can be performed before any intervention (this also provides access to protect the contralateral CIA from injury during ipsilateral CIA intervention).

See Figure 16.4.

2.2 Steps

See Figure 16.5A.
- Exchange micropuncture catheter for arterial sheath.
- Advance glidewire through ipsilateral groin and cross the lesion with the use of a catheter–guidewire combination:
  – An angled tip catheter with a floppy-tipped guidewire is used to cross the lesion first, followed by the catheter.
  – In difficult cases, hydrophilic guidewires may be used.
- After advancing the catheter across the lesions, the wire is removed and aspirated. Blood return ensures that the catheter tip is intraluminal.
  – When attempting to recanalize occluded iliac artery it is possible that the wire can travel subintimal. When this occurs one can attempt an antegrade approach from the contralateral side. Once a hydrophilic wire is navigated past the lesion it is advanced into the ipsilateral EIA where it can be snared from the ipsilateral CFA and a catheter can be advanced over this wire and past the lesion.

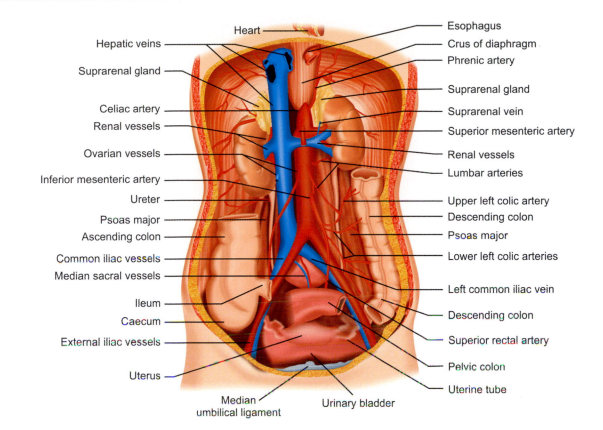

Fig. 16.2: Surgical anatomy of the abdomen and pelvis.

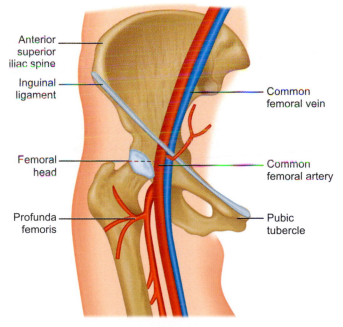

Fig. 16.4: Anatomy at the groin. The inguinal ligament runs between the anterior superior iliac spine and the pubic tubercle. The common femoral artery should be about one-third of the way along that line, lateral to the common femoral vein. The goal is to puncture at the level of the femoral head.

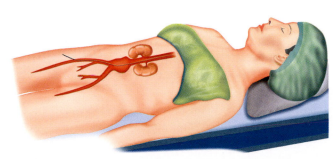

Fig. 16.3: Patient positioning in the supine position with bilateral groins prepped and draped. Allows access to bilateral common femoral arteries.

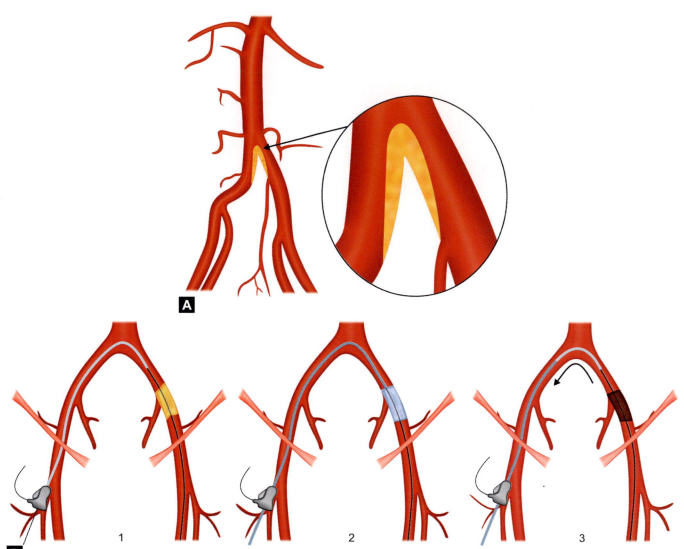

Figs. 16.5A and B: (A) Left CIA high grade stenosis. (B) Treatment from a contralateral approach. (1) Access obtained via the right CFA. A wire has been advanced up and over the bifurcation and through the left CIA lesion. Subsequently a sheath (white) has been advanced up and over into the common iliac artery. (2) A balloon or stent is advanced over the wire, through the sheath, into the area of stenosis, and inflated/deployed. (3) Removal of balloon/stent catheter. Dark red portion shows resolution of lesion.

- *At this time an angiogram can be performed*:
  - Oblique projections over the pelvis may better show the iliac artery bifurcation.
- To determine the significance of the lesion can obtain pressure measurements across lesion.
  - *Method 1*: Connect hub of the catheter and the side arm of the sheath to the intra-arterial pressure monitor (the catheter needs to be one French size smaller than the sheath).
  - *Method 2*: Using an end-hole catheter, connect to an intra-arterial pressure monitor and withdraw from proximal to distal across the lesion over a 0.014-in. wire.
  - If the pressure gradient is 10 mmHg or greater the lesion should be considered for treatment.

See Figure 16.5B and C.

- Once lesion has been assessed, proceed with passing selected angioplasty balloon over wire and centering in the lesion. Inflate until no residual waste remains.
  - Will often need to treat bilateral iliac lesions; this can be done by repeating the steps above for the contralateral side. Then would advance one angioplasty

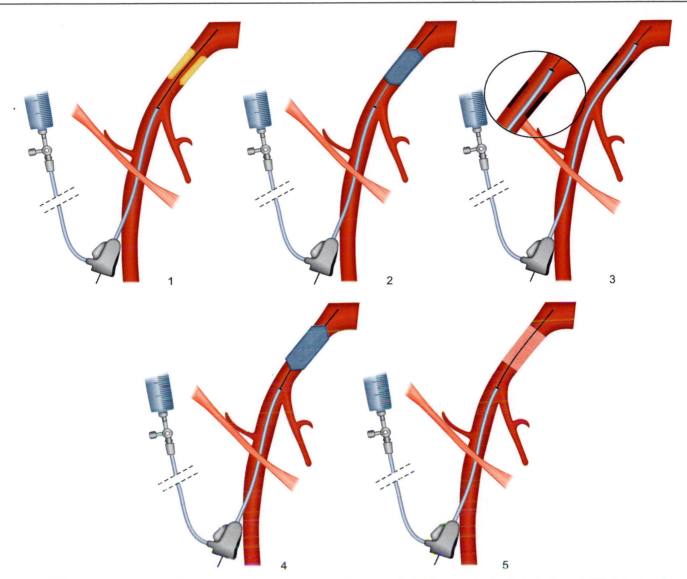

Fig. 16.5C: Treatment of CIA lesion via an ipsilateral or retrograde approach. (1) Access obtained via ipsilateral CFA. Wire has been advance accross the lesion and catheter has been placed in EIA. (2) Balloon angioplasty performed. (3) Pressures across residual stenosis can be obtained to assess for hemodynamic significance. Intravascular US also can be used to assess residual lumen diameter. (4) Stent placed across lesion. (5) Stent laced, with resolution of stenosis.

balloon into each lesion and inflate them simultaneously (Kissing Balloons). This allows the bifurcation to maintain its integrity and does not narrow either side.

– Stents should be placed for residual stenosis or in many cases as primary therapy. Stents should be sized based on the size of the patent vessel.

2.3 Closure

– Once no residual stenosis remains, wires and catheters can be removed.

– Depending on sheath size, closure device or 30-minutes manual pressure for hemostasis can be used.

3 POSTOPERATIVE

3.1 Complications

- Vessel dissection, abrupt closure, spasm and thrombus formation
- Distal embolization
- Arterial perforation

3.2 Outcomes

- 44% to 65% 4-year success rates for iliac angioplasty
- 17–21% of patients need reintervention after PTA with selective stenting.
- *For TASC A and B lesions*: Cumulative patency around 71% at 10 years, limb salvage rates are around 95% and 87% at 5 and 10 years, respectively.
- For TASC C and D lesions: Primary patency at 4 years with PTA and selective stenting is 75.5%; limb salvage rates are around 97% at 3 years.

3.3 Follow-Up

- Follow up with routine US.

3.4 E-mail an Expert

- *E-mail address*: jeffrey.indes@yale.edu

3.5 Web Resources/References

- www.vascularweb.org

- www.mcbi.nim.nih.gov
- Cronenwett JL, Johnston KW. Rutherford's Vascular Surgery, 7th edition. Sanders; 2010.
- Moore WS. Vascular and Endovascular Surgery: A Comprehensive Review, 7th edition. Saunders; 2006.

REFERENCES

1. Bosch J, Hunink M. Meta-analysis of the results of percutaneous transluminal angioplasty and stent placement for aortoiliac occlusive disease. Radiology. 1997;204:87-96.
2. Johnston KW. Iliac arteries: reanalysis of results of balloon angioplasty. Radiology. 1993;186:207-12.
3. Kudo T, Chandra FA, Ahn SS. Long-term outcomes and predictors of iliac angioplasty with selective stenting. J Vasc Surg. 2005;42(3):466-75.
4. ACC/AHA task force on practice guidelines. Eagle K, Berger P, Calkins H, et al. American College of Cardiology/American Heart Association Guideline Update for Perioperative Cardiovascular Evaluation for Noncardiac Surgery-Executive Summary. Circulation105: 1257, 2002.

QUIZ

Question 1. You have placed a common iliac stent for occlusive disease. Completion angiography shows extravasation of contrast the next step in management should be:
a. Place another bare metal stent
b. Inflate a balloon at the site
c. Open the patient and repair the artery
d. Place a covered stent

Question 2. You see a patient with a TASC D lesion that is deemed an acceptable operative candidate. The best treatment for this patient would be:

a. PTA and selective stenting
b. Open surgery
c. Primary stenting
d. Atherectomy and PTA with selective stenting

Question 3. The most accurate way of determining if a stenosis is hemodynamically significant is:
a. Duplex ultrasound
b. Angiography
c. Computed tomography angiogram (CTA)
d. A resting systolic pressure gradient of >10 mm Hg

1. d   2. b   3. d

ANSWERS:

Endovascular Aneurysm Repair

Neil Moudgill

1 PREOPERATIVE

1.1 Indications

- 5.5 cm diameter infrarenal aortoiliac aneurysm in suitable male patients
- 5.0 cm diameter infrarenal aortoiliac aneurysm in suitable female patients
- Symptomatic or ruptured infrarenal aortoiliac aneurysm in suitable patients
- *Contraindications*:
  - Inadequate proximal or distal landing zones (< 10 mm proximally)
  - Aortic neck angulation > 60°
  - Significant Iliac occlusive disease
  - Circumferential thrombus at proximal neck
  - Extensive calcification at proximal landing site

1.2 Evidence

- *Dutch Randomized Endovascular Aneurysm Management trial—randomly assigned 351 patients to open repair or endovascular aneurysm repair (EVAR):*[1]
  - All patients were candidates for EVAR.
  - All patients had aneurysms > 5 cm in maximal diameter.
  - 30-day mortality was lower in the EVAR group (1.2% EVAR vs 4.6% open).
  - There was no difference in overall survival (89.7% EVAR vs 89.6% open).
- The EVAR versus open repair in patients with abdominal aortic aneurysm (AAA) (EVAR1) trial—randomly assigned 1252 patients to AAA repair with EVAR (626) versus open repair (626)
  - 30-day mortality was significantly less for EVAR (1.8%) versus open (4.3%).
  - There was no significant difference in overall mortality.
  - Graft related complications occurred more frequently in the EVAR group.[2]

1.3 Materials Needed

- Computed tomography angiography (CTA)
- Measurement sheet
- Main body endograft and contralateral limb
- Additional proximal and distal cuffs
- Femoral artery access needle
- 5-Fr sheath[2]
- .035 guidewire (medium stiffness)
- Angled hydrophilic catheter, other catheters used to access contralateral gate
- .035 Stiff guidewire (Amplatz, Meier, Lundquist)[2]
- .035 Hydrophilic guidewire (soft)
- Large ipsilateral and contralateral sheaths appropriate for selected device introduction (no separate sheaths required for devices with included delivery system)
- Flush catheter
- Fluoroscopy table
- C-arm
- Hybrid endosuite
- Intra-arterial contrast material
- IVUS (can be used as adjunctive imaging modality)
- Aortic occlusion balloon

1.4 Preoperative Risk Assessment

Low risk:
- No prior cardiac history
- No prior femoral artery surgery
- No pulmonary disease
- No renal disease

Intermediate risk:
- Prior cardiac interventions, no ongoing cardiac ischemia
- Prior femoral artery surgery

- Moderate pulmonary disease
- Borderline renal function
- Age > 70

High risk:
- Severe cardiac disease
- Severe pulmonary disease
- Impending renal failure, however, not currently requiring dialysis
- Need for emergent repair due to rupture
- Age > 80

1.5 Preoperative Checklist

Sign in:
- Correct patient.
- Review updated history since preoperative evaluation.
- Mark surgical site.
- Evaluate groins and abdomen for abnormalities (infection, rash, injury, etc.).
- Assess lower extremity pulses and document baseline for future reference.
- Examine lower extremities.
- Review preoperative laboratory studies prior to entering operating room.

Time out:
- Verify correct patient.
- Verify correct position.
- Verify antibiotic administration.
- Verify pertinent patient comorbidities (cardiac, pulmonary, renal, etc.).
- Review patient allergies and ensure no materials to be used will elicit allergic response.
- Review critical procedural details with team members in operating room.
- Ensure necessary equipment is functional and appropriate staff available.
- Ensure endograft is available and present in the operating room.

Sign out:
- Review essential case details, any deviations from initial plan.
- Ask anesthesia for summary of care rendered from their standpoint.
- Discuss plan for immediate postoperative care specifics and patient's proposed location prior to transfer from operating room.

1.6 Decision-Making Algorithm

- *See* Flowchart 17.1.

Flowchart 17.1: Decision-making algorithm.

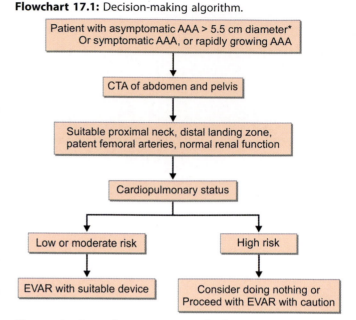

*Proper size for males > 5.5cm AAA, for females > 5.0 cm; rapid growth is > 1.0 cm/year.

- Aneurysm detected by imaging modality
- Computed tomography (CT) angiogram of abdomen and pelvis with images through femoral bifurcation
- AAA >5.5 cm for men and 5.0 cm in women
- *Assess aneurysm suitability for endovascular treatment*:
  - Proximal and distal landing zones (size, angulation, thrombus burden)
  - Access vasculature
  - Location and involvement of hypogastric arteries
- If treatment indicated—evaluate patient candidacy for surgical therapy. Discuss risks, benefits, alternatives
- Preoperative specialty evaluation (cardiac, pulmonary, renal, other).
- If suitable for endovascular treatment—obtain measurements of proximal and distal landing zones
- Select endograft and ensure availability.

1.7 Pearls and Pitfalls

Pearls:
- The left renal artery is often the lower of the two renal arteries. Its origin is typically best viewed with a slight craniocaudal (5°–10°) and right anterior oblique (5°–10°) projection of the C-arm.
- It is useful to identify (on preoperative imaging) the bony vertebral landmark most closely associated with the origin of the lowest renal artery. This allows positioning of the flush catheter and main body endograft in the pararenal aorta without contrast.

- Often the contralateral gate is oriented to deploy in an anterior or anterolateral position. This facilitates cannulation of the gate.
- Type 1A and 1B endoleaks should be corrected at the initial operation. These types of endoleaks may lead to further aneurysm expansion if left untreated.
- The final arteriographic image obtained after complete graft deployment should be continued for several seconds after the contrast bolus has passed through the distal extent of the endograft. This will allow visualization of any late endoleaks emanating from prominent branches associated with the aneurysm sac.

Pitfalls:
- Placement of an endograft in patients with anatomy that is not suitable for endovascular repair will result in graft failure, continued aneurysm expansion, or intraoperative complications.
- Posterior deployment of the contralateral gate results in challenging cannulation.
- Excessive use of iodinated contrast material or fluoroscopy can result in renal dysfunction or tissue burns.
- Acute coverage of one or both of the hypogastric arteries may lead to pelvic ischemia.
- Extensive femoral or iliac occlusive disease may preclude sheath placement or graft delivery. Additionally, graft expansion in an atherosclerotic vessel may lead to arterial rupture.

1.8 Surgical Anatomy
- *See* Figure 17.1.

1.9 Positioning
Patient is placed supine on a fluoroscopy table. The arms are secured at the patient's side (*see* Fig. 17.2).

1.10 Anesthesia
- General anesthesia, spinal anesthesia, and local anesthesia are acceptable based on surgeon/anesthesiologist preference.
- Central venous catheter placement may not be necessary for all cases; however, sufficient intravenous access for large volume resuscitation should be obtained.
- Continuous arterial pressure monitoring is required; any abrupt changes in blood pressure should be communicated to the operating team.
- Any decline in urine output should be communicated to the operating team.
- Systemic anticoagulation will be required and should be monitored at fixed intervals. Additional dosing will be prescribed by the surgical team.
- Ventilation will be held several times during the procedure.

2 PERIOPERATIVE

2.1 Incision
- *See* Figures 17.3A and B.

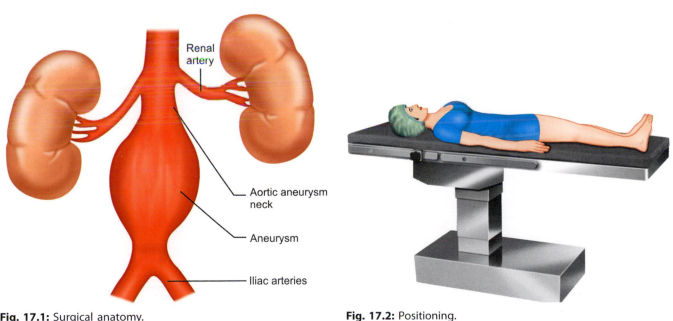

Fig. 17.1: Surgical anatomy.

Fig. 17.2: Positioning.

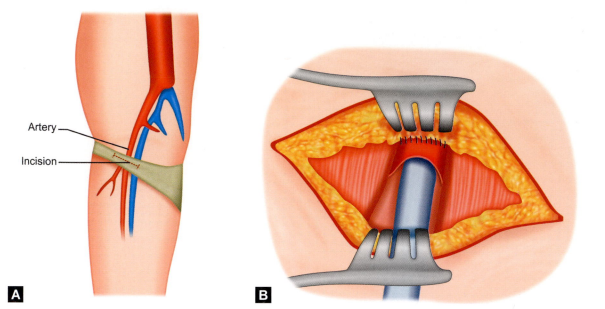

Figs. 17.3A and B: (A) An oblique incision 3 cm below the inguinal ligament is created. (B) The femoral artery is identified at the base of the dissection. It is dissected circumferentially and controlled with vessel loops proximally and distally in preparation for puncture.

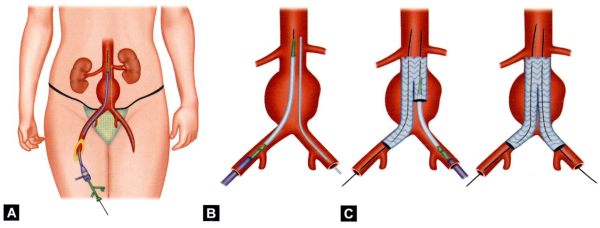

Figs. 17.4A to C: (A) Femoral access is obtained bilaterally. The main body of the endograft is positioned and a flush catheter is placed in the pararenal aorta. (B) The main body is deployed to the level of the contralateral gate; the gate is then cannulated. The ipsilateral iliac limb is then completely deployed. (C) The contralateral limb is deployed.

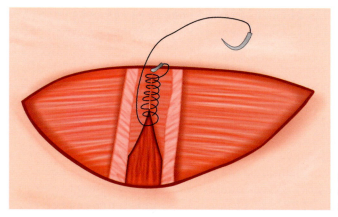

Fig. 17.5: The fascia overlying the femoral artery is closed after direct repair of the vessel. The overlying soft tissues are reapproximated in multiple layers.

2.2 Steps

- *See* Figures 17.4A to C.

2.3 Closure

- *See* Figure 17.5.

3 POSTOPERATIVE

3.1 Complications

Most common complications:
- Endoleak
- Local wound complications
- Access artery injury
- Contrast nephropathy

Least common complications:
- Spinal cord ischemia
- Bowl ischemia
- Ischemic nephropathy
- Stent graft infection

3.2 Outcomes

- Aneurysm size regression
- Maintenance of proximal and distal seal zones
- Distal pulse examination should be unchanged after EVAR
- Preserved native renal artery flow

3.3 Follow-Up

- Clinic visit 1–2 weeks after procedure to assess for local wound complications.
- CTA of abdomen and pelvis at 1, 6, and 12 months and annually thereafter to assess for fixation, endoleak, and obtain aneurysm diameter measurements post-EVAR.

3.4 E-mail an Expert

- *E-mail address*: nmoudgil@health.usf.edu

3.5 Web Resources/References

- Medline Plus http://www.nlm.nih.gov/medlineplus/ency/article/007391.htm
- Vascular Web http://www.vascularweb.org/vascularhealth/Pages/endovascular-stent-graft.aspx
- Cronenwett JL, Johnston KW. Rutherford's Vascular Surgery, 7th edition. Sanders; 2010.

REFERENCES

1. Blankensteijn JD, deJong SE, Prinssen M, et al. Two-year outcomes after conventional or endovascular repair of abdominal aortic aneurysms. N Engl J Med. 2005;352:2398.
2. EVAR trial participants. Endovascular aneurysm repair versus open repair in patients with abdominal aortic aneurysm (EVAR 1): randomized and controlled trial. Lancet. 2005;365:2179.

QUIZ

Question 1. Infrarenal aortic aneurysm repair is indicated in women when:
a. The aneurysm is >4 cm in maximal diameter
b. The aneurysm is >5 cm in maximal diameter
c. The aneurysm has thrombus lining it
d. The aneurysm is angulated >60°

Question 2. Which of the following is not a required material to perform EVAR?
a. Computed tomography angiogram (CTA)
b. Stiff .035 wire
c. Hydrophilic .018 wire
d. Flush catheter

Question 3. The origin of the left renal artery is often best viewed in which projection?
a. 75° left anterior oblique
b. 10° caudocranial and 5° right anterior oblique (RAO)
c. 10° craniocaudal
d. 5°–10° RAO and 5°–10° craniocaudal

Question 4. Deployment of the contralateral gate in which orientation may result in difficult cannulation?
a. Anterior
b. Posterior
c. Crossed
d. Anterolateral

Question 5. The ipsilateral limb of the main body endograft is deployed after which step?
a. Cannulation of the contralateral gate
b. Positioning of the main body endograft in the para-renal aorta
c. Deployment of the contralateral limb
d. Cannulation of the hypogastric artery

ANSWERS: 1. b   2. c   3. b   4. b   5. a

Hypogastric Artery Embolization

Neil Moudgill

1 PREOPERATIVE

1.1 Indications

- *Indications*:
  - Aortoiliac artery aneurysm with involvement of the hypogastric artery
  - Isolated hypogastric artery aneurysm
- *Contraindication*:
  - Prior long segment aortic repair (endovascular or open)
  - Occlusion of the contralateral hypogastric artery
  - Bilateral hypogastric artery occlusion required.

1.2 Evidence

- Preliminary embolization of the hypogastric artery to expand the applicability of endovascular aneurysm repair.[1]
  - Retrospective review of 101 patients undergoing embolization of 133 hypogastric arteries.
  - 19 hypogastric arteries embolized with coils, 114 with plugs.
  - 35% developed buttock claudication, 16% developed erectile dysfunction.
- *Buttock claudication and erectile dysfunction after internal iliac artery embolization in patients prior to endovascular aortic aneurysm repair[2]*:
  - Review of 634 patients undergoing internal iliac artery embolization.
  - Buttock claudication occurred in 31% of those with unilateral embolization and 35% with bilateral embolization.
  - Erectile dysfunction occurred in 17% overall.

1.3 Materials Needed

- CTA for planning and measurement

- Percutaneous access needle
- .035 Guidewire (medium stiffness)
- 5-Fr sheath
- Flush catheter
- Contrast material
- Hydrophilic .035 guidewire
- Sos-Omni catheter
- Angled tracking catheter
- 45-cm 5-Fr sheath
- Embolization coils or Occluding Plug (may require larger sheath) *See* Figures 18.1A and B.

1.4 Preoperative Risk Assessment

Low risk:
- Normal contralateral hypogastric artery flow with significant cross-pelvic collaterals
- Patent iliofemoral arterial system with preservation of circumflex iliac arteries.

Intermediate risk:
- Poor cross-pelvic collateralization
- Atheroscerotic femoral disease, loss of circumflex iliac arteries.

High risk:
- Prior long segment aortic repair
- Occlusion of contralateral hypogastric artery

1.5 Preoperative Checklist

Sign in:
- Correct patient
- Review updated history since preoperative evaluation
- Mark surgical site
- Evaluate groins and abdomen for abnormalities (infection, rash, injury, etc).
- Assess lower extremity pulses and document baseline for future reference.

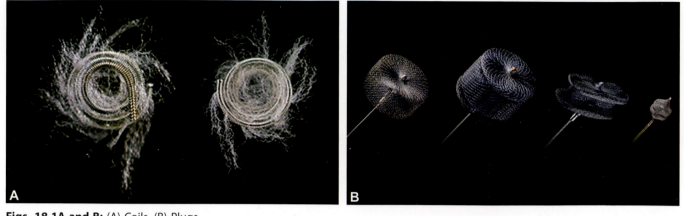

Figs. 18.1A and B: (A) Coils. (B) Plugs.

- Examine lower extremities.
- Review preoperative laboratory studies prior to entering operating room.

Time out:
- Verify correct patient
- Verify correct position
- Verify antibiotic administration
- Verify pertinent patient comorbidities (cardiac, pulmonary, renal, etc.).
- Review patient allergies and ensure no materials to be used will elicit allergic response.
- Review critical procedural details with team members in operating room.
- Ensure necessary equipment is functional and appropriate staff available.
- Ensure endograft is available and present in the operating room.

Sign out:
- Review essential case details and any deviations from initial plan.
- Ask anesthesia for summary of care rendered from their standpoint.
- Discuss plan for immediate postoperative care specifics. and patient's proposed location prior to transfer from operating room.

1.6 Decision-Making Checklist

- Aortoiliac or isolated hypogastric artery aneurysm identified:
  - Obtain CTA for evaluation and measurement:
    - Evaluate bilateral hypogastric arteries.
    - Measure aneurysm.
    - Assess options to preserve hypogastric artery flow bilaterally.

  - If deemed necessary to sacrifice flow in one or both hypogastric arteries:
    - Discuss with patient (risks, benefits, alternatives).
    - Determine best approach for hypogastric artery embolization.
    - Plan on either simultaneous or staged embolization if bilateral.
  - Select device/method of embolization:
    - Review anatomy of hypogastric artery (origin diameter, branches, collateral vessels).
    - Select device that will allow occlusion of proximal portion of hypogastric artery.

1.7 Pearls and Pitfalls

Pearls:
- Access obtained in the contralateral femoral artery often allows the best approach to the hypogastric artery for embolization. In difficult cases, access from the left brachial artery may be useful.
- Embolization of the proximal most portion of the hypogastric artery will allow continued flow through the pelvic collaterals and minimize the risk of pelvic ischemia.
- For hypogastric artery aneurysms—embolization of the individual feeding branches is necessary to minimize the risk of ongoing aneurysm expansion and rupture.
- Staged hypogastric artery embolization may be useful to prevent excessive use of contrast as well as allow development of further pelvic collaterals in the intervening time.
- Plugs can often be more specifically deployed than coils, allowing a more precise embolization if desired.

Pitfalls:
- Simultaneous bilateral hypogastric artery embolization can lead to acute pelvic ischemia.

- The proximal hypogastric artery can be challenging to embolize; care should be taken not to deploy embolization materials outside the origin of the hypogastric artery particularly when coverage of the origin is not planned.
- Rupture of the hypogastric artery can result from manipulation of catheters and wires or during attempts at embolization.
- The hypogastric artery can be challenging to catheterize, once accomplished, loss of wire access may result in an inability to recatheterize or embolize the vessel.
- Inadequate packing of coils or mis-sizing of embolization plugs may result in continued flow through the hypogastric artery.

1.8 Surgical Anatomy

- *See* Figure 18.2.

1.9 Positioning

- *See* Figure 18.3.

1.10 Anesthesia

- Ventilation will be held several times during the procedure.
- Locoregional or general anesthesia may be used.
- Continuous arterial blood pressure monitoring is required and any abrupt changes in blood pressure should be communicated to the operating team.

- Systemic anticoagulation will be required and should be monitored at fixed intervals and additional dosing will be prescribed by the surgical team.

2 PERIOPERATIVE

2.1 Incision

- *See* Figures 18.4A to C.

2.2 Steps

- *See* Figures 18.5A and B.

2.3 Closure

- *See* Figures 18.6A and B.

3 POSTOPERATIVE

3.1 Complications

Most common complications:
- Buttock claudication
- Erectile dysfunction
- Bowel ischemia

Least common complications:
- Spinal ischemia
- Perineal necrosis

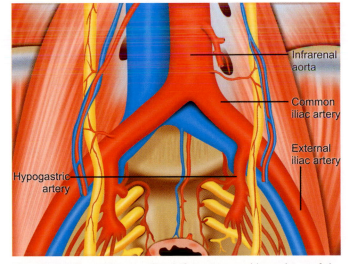

Fig. 18.2: Infrarenal aorta, Iliac bifurcation, and branching of the hypogastric artery.

Infrarenal aorta

Common iliac artery

External iliac artery

Hypogastric artery

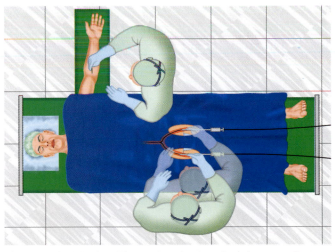

Fig. 18.3: Positioning. The patient is placed supine on a fluoroscopy table. If needed, the left arm can be placed at 90° for ease of access to the brachial artery.

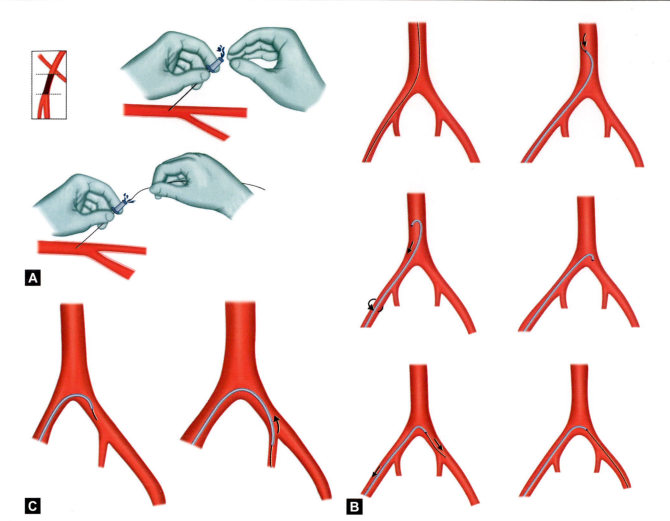

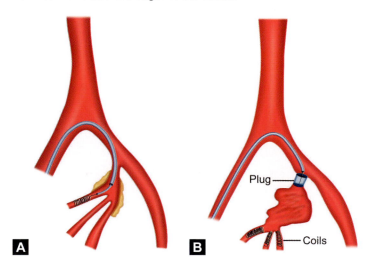

Figs. 18.4A to C: (A) Guidewire access is obtained in the femoral artery. (B) The contralateral external iliac artery is catheterized. A long sheath is then directed over the iliac bifurcation. (C) The hypogastric artery is catheterized and the long sheath is then advanced over a stiff wire into the origin of the vessel.

Figs. 18.5A and B: (A) Coils are delivered into each of the branches of the hypogastric artery to prevent retrograde filling. (B) A plug or larger coils can be used to occlude the origin of the hypogastric artery.

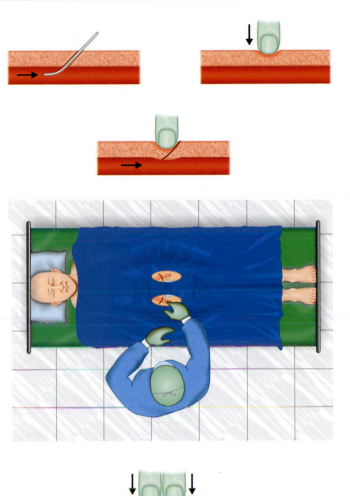

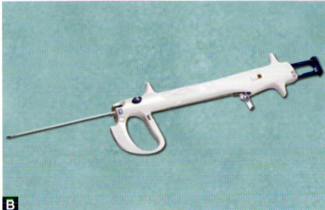

Figs. 18.6A and B: (A) Manual pressure is held over the puncture site after sheath removal. (B) In some cases, a percutaneous closure device may be useful to facilitate hemostasis (starclose, Perclose, angioseal, catalyst, etc.).

3.2 Outcomes

- Successful exclusion of the hypogastric artery origin.
- Absence of endoleak.
- Persistent cross-pelvic collateral flow.

3.3 Follow-Up

- Evaluation of the femoral artery puncture/incision site after embolization.
- History regarding symptoms related to buttock claudication and sexual dysfunction.
- Close observation for signs/symptoms related to bowel ischemia.

- Follow-up CTA to verify persistent occlusion of the embolized hypogastric artery origin.

3.4 E-mail an expert

- *E-mail address*: nmoudgil@health.usf.edu

REFERENCES

1. Wu Z, Raithel D, Ritter W, et al. Preliminary embolization of the hypogastric artery to expand the applicability of endovascular aneurysm repair. J Endovasc Ther. 2011;18(1):114-20.
2. Rayt HS, Bown MJ, Lambert KV, et al. Buttock claudication and erectile dysfunction after internal iliac artery embolization in patients prior to endovascular aortic aneurysm repair. Cardiovasc Intervent Radiol. 2008;31(4):728-34.

QUIZ

Question 1. In which instance would hypogastric artery embolization NOT be indicated?

a. Aortoiliac aneurysm involving the proximal common iliac artery
b. Isolated hypogastric artery aneurysm
c. Aortoiliac artery aneurysm with extensive occlusive disease of the external iliac artery on one side
d. Large common iliac artery aneurysm

Question 2. The hypogastric artery is most easily cannulated from the ipsilateral groin?

a. True
b. False

Question 3. Most patients will experience which clinical findings after hypogastric embolization of a single hypogastric artery:

a. Buttock claudication
b. Spinal ischemia
c. Bowel ischemia
d. None of the above

Fenestrated Endovascular Aortic Repair Cook Zenith

Susan M Shafii, F Ezequiel Parodi

1 PREOPERATIVE

1.1 Indications

- Juxtarenal or Short-neck (<4 mm) abdominal aortic aneurysm >5.5 cm or rapid growth (>5 mm in 6 months)

1.2 Intended use

- Nonaneurysmal infrarenal neck >4 mm
- Diameter outer wall to outer wall no >31 mm and no <19 mm
- Adequate iliac and femoral access
- Angle <45° relative to long axis of the aneurysm
- Angle <45° relative to the axis of the suprarenal aorta
- Ipsilateral iliac artery distal fixation site >30 mm in length and 9–21 mm in diameter
- Contralateral iliac artery distal fixation site >30 mm in length and 7–21 mm in diameter

1.3 Contraindications

- Patients with known sensitivity or allergy to stainless steel, polyester, nitinol, solder, polypropylene, or gold
- Patients with systemic or local infection that might increase risk of endovascular graft infection
- Patients that do not meet the instructions for use for the aortic neck/length landing zone

1.4 Evidence

- *See* references 1 to 3.

1.5 Planning

- High-resolution computer tomography
- Centerline imaging recommended
- Zenith fenestrated device planning and sizing worksheet (Fig. 19.1)
- Analysis of iliofemoral system for introduction of device (ideally left side)

1.6 Surgical Anatomy

- *See* Figure 19.2.

1.7 Positioning

- Supine position
- Left arm accessible in case brachial access is needed

2 PERIOPERATIVE

2.1 Incision

- Bilateral transverse or longitudinal femoral incisions

2.2 Materials

- 18-gauge/9-cm percutaneous entry needle
- 150-cc .035 Starter Wire (Boston Scientific)
- 5-Fr sheath 10 cm (Cook Medical)
- Floppy glidewire 260 cm (Terumo)
- Lunderquist wire 300 cm (Cook Medical)
- Rosen wire 260 cm (Cook Medical)
- 20 Fr Check Flo 25 cm (Cook Medical)
- 7 Fr Ansel-1 Sheath 55 cm (Cook Medical) × 2
- Pigtail catheter .035 100 cm (Cook Medical)
- KMP catheter .035 65 cm (Cook Medical)
- VS1 catheter .035 65 cm (Cook Medical)
- Van Schie 4 catheter .035 65 cm (Cook Medical)
- Curved glide catheter .035 100 cm (Terumo)
- Dilators 16 to 22 Fr 45 cm (Cook Medical)
- iCast stent (Atrium)
- 32 Coda Balloon (Cook Medical)

Zenith® Fenestrated

AAA ENDOVASCULAR GRAFT

DEVICE PLANNING AND SIZING WORKSHEET

Date: _____ Patient ID: _____

Hospital: _____

Physician Name: _____

Physician Phone #: _____

Physician E-mail: _____

Physician Signature: _____

Step 1: Locate Anatomic Positions

Use bottom of celiac axis as "0" point (reference point).

	Measurement	2D Clock Position	Centerline Distance from Reference	Inner Aortic Diameter mm
	Bottom of celiac Reference: 0 position		0	
	Middle of SMA			
	Bottom of SMA			
Highest	Middle of renal artery right◯ left◯			
Lowest	Middle of renal artery right◯ left◯			
	Accessory renal artery right◯ left◯			
	Accessory renal artery right◯ left◯			
LVR	Bottom of lowest artery			
	Start of aneurysm			
L1	Aortic bifurcation			
L2	Distal iliac fixation site (contralateral)			
L3	Distal iliac fixation site (ipsilateral)			
Access	Right external iliac (EI) (Minimum inner diameter from introduction site to aorta)			
Access	Left external iliac (EI) (Minimum inner diameter from introduction site to aorta)			
PE	Edge of proximal graft to bifurcation			

Step 2: Measure Primary Diameters (mm)

D1	Largest aortic neck diameter along 15 mm sealing zone	
D2	Largest iliac outer diameter through contralateral fixation site	
D3	Largest iliac outer diameter through ipsilateral fixation site	
Dmax	Maximum AAA diameter	
	Inner aortic diameter at chosen level	

Anatomic Measurement Key

L1 Distance from celiac (reference) to aortic bifurcation

L2 Distance from celiac (reference) to contralateral iliac fixation site

L3 Distance from celiac (reference) to ipsilateral iliac fixation site

LVR Distance of lowest vessel from celiac (reference)

PE Planned distance of proximal edge of graft to aortic bifurcation

D1 Largest aortic neck diameter along 15 mm sealing zone

D2 Largest iliac diameter through contralateral fixation site

D3 Largest iliac diameter through ipsilateral fixation site

Graft Measurement Key

PBL Proximal body graft length

PBD Proximal body graft diameter

DBL Distal body graft length

DLL Distal graft ipsilateral limb length

DD3 Distal graft ipsilateral limb diameter

Corrected Reference Drawing
(Draw visceral vessels)

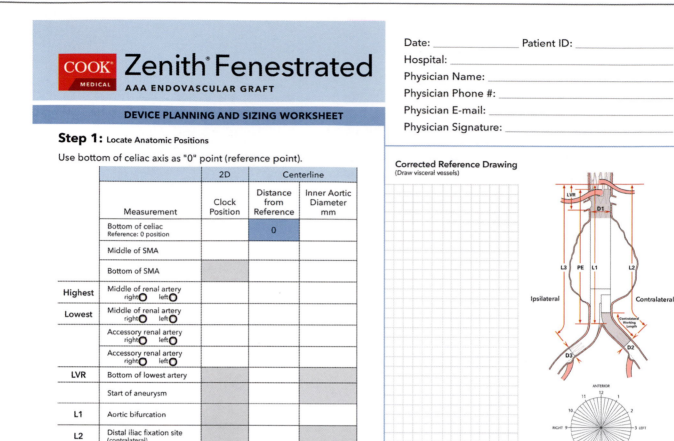

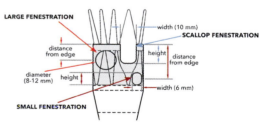

Step 3: Choose Fenestration(s)

	Vessel	#1	#2
Scallop Fenestration All scallops are 10 mm wide. Height ranges from 6 to 12 mm.	Width	10 mm	10 mm
	Height		
	Clock position		
Large Fenestration Diameters are 8, 10 or 12 mm. Stent struts may cross large fenestration. Distance from edge must be ≥ 10 mm.	Diameter		
	Clock position		
	Distance from edge		
Small Fenestration All small fenestrations are 6 mm wide. Heights are either 6 or 8 mm. Distance from proximal edge must be ≥ 15 mm.	Width	6 mm	6 mm
	Height		
	Clock position		
	Distance from edge		

Contd....

Contd....

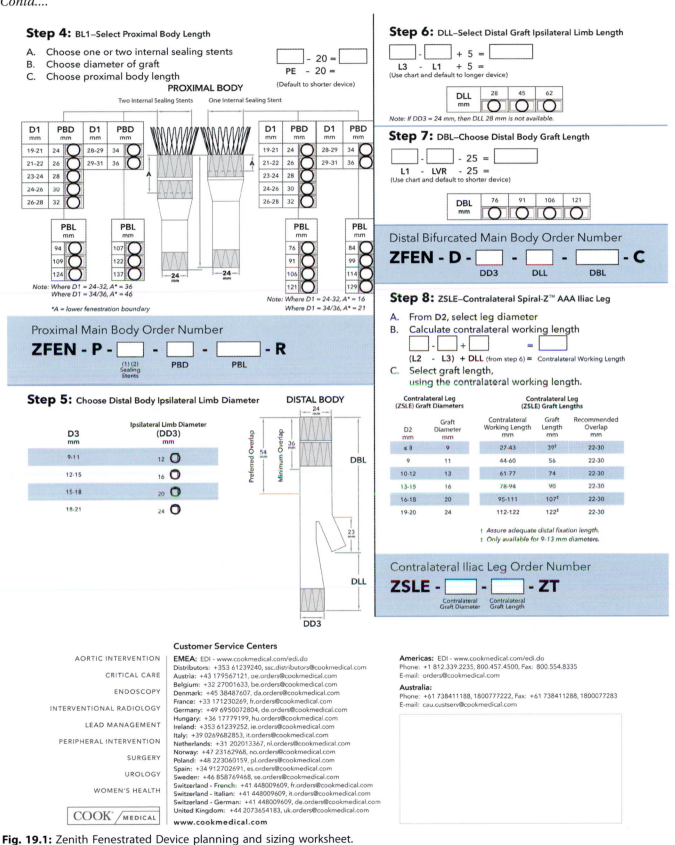

Fig. 19.1: Zenith Fenestrated Device planning and sizing worksheet.

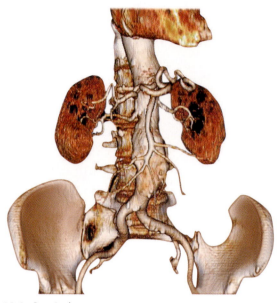

Fig. 19.2: Surgical anatomy.

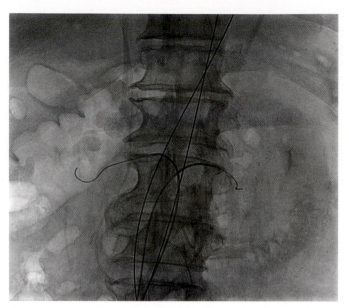

Fig. 19.3: Cannulate one renal artery via the 5-Fr sheath using KMP/VS1 or curved glide catheter of choice and glidewire.

2.3 Steps

- Obtain control of bilateral common femoral arteries via transverse or longitudinal femoral artery exposure.
- Full anticoagulation prior to access is ideal for continuous goal activated clotting time >300, with either IV heparin sulfate (100 U/kg) or direct thrombin inhibitor with bivalirudin.
- Gain endovascular access in both common femoral arteries and place a floppy system into the thoracic aorta, i.e. kumpe catheter and floppy guidewire. Proceed to exchange the floppy system for stiff system, i.e. *Lunderquist* wires, under fluoroscopic guidance.
- Select the *femoral/iliac* artery (healthiest, straightest, longest) for main device insertion.
- Insert a 20-Fr Check-Flo 25 cm (Cook) sheath into the planned contralateral side over the stiff guide wire.
- Double-puncture the 20-Fr sheath and place three 5-Fr short sheaths.
- Cannulate one renal artery via the 5-Fr sheath using KMP/VS1 or curved glide catheter of choice and glidewire. Leave the catheter and wire in place as seen in Figure 19.3.
- Repeat step 7 and cannulate the contralateral renal.
- Orient the main device prior to placing in the patient under fluoroscopy making sure check mark is anterior (Fig. 19.4)
- Introduce the main fenestrated device through the desired groin and position aligning check marks and

fenestration marks with the previously cannulated renal arteries. Make sure the anterior check mark is indeed anterior via both AP and lateral views.
- Partially deploy device by unsheathing only and aligning the renal arteries. A pigtail catheter can be placed through the third 5-Fr sheath to image before and during unsheathing. Do not release the trigger wires at this point!! You should leave the device on the delivery system.
- KMP catheter and a glidewire are introduced through the third unused 5-Fr sheath in the contralateral groin. Cannulate the bottom of the graft to get into the device and then cannulate the renal fenestration and subsequently the patient's renal artery. Once catheter is safely in the renal artery, exchange the glidewire to a Rosen wire. The catheter and 5-Fr sheath are then exchanged to a 7-Fr Ansel 1 55-cm sheath. Sheath is advanced into the renal artery and dilator is removed (Fig. 19.5).
- Repeat step 12 into the contralateral renal artery.
- Once both 7-Fr sheaths are in the renal arteries, the main device deployment is then completed by removing the trigger wires and deploys the suprarenal stents. Then remove the inner component of the main body device, leaving the sheath in place.
- Perform selective angiography of each renal artery via the respective 7-Fr Ansel sheaths and place a covered balloon-expandable stent (iCast). It is important to

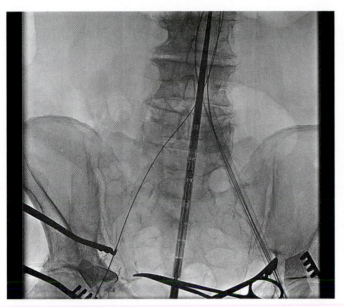

Fig. 19.4: Orient the main device prior to placing in the patient under fluoroscopy making sure check mark is anterior.

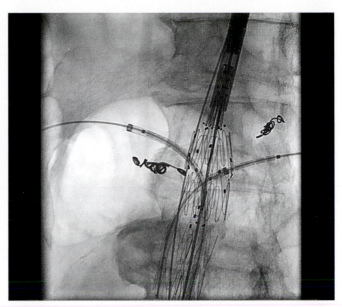

Fig. 19.5: Sheath is advanced into the renal artery and dilator is removed.

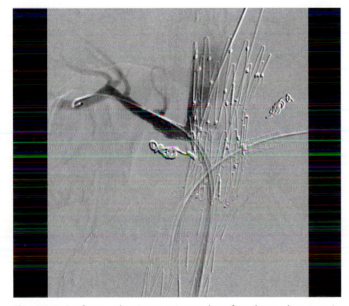

Fig. 19.6: Perform selective angiography of each renal artery via the respective 7-Fr Ansel sheaths and place a covered balloon-expandable stent (iCast).

leave approximately 5 mm of the stent into the aorta lumen. After stent deployment, flare the stent with a 10 × 2 balloon (Fig. 19.6). The flare technique seals the covered stent to the aortic stent. Recapture the balloon by advancing the sheath back into the renal stent ostia. If there is significant angulation of the renal artery (as in diving posterior), it may be necessary to place a

self-expanding stent to ease the transition of blood flow from the rigid balloon-expandable stent.

- Repeat step 15 for the contralateral renal artery.
- Perform aortogram at the level of the renals and visceral vessels to ensure patency.
- Then perform aortogram to mark aortic bifurcation and hypogastric arteries in preparation for placement of the bifurcated component.
- Remove empty main body sheath and place the bifurcated component up the same side as the main body fenestrated component was delivered. Take care as the bifurcated device is delivered to not crush the renal stents. To avoid renal stent crush, leave the Ansel sheaths in place until the device is introduced. Prior to deployment of the bifurcated component, the Ansel sheaths will need to be pulled back into the iliac artery.
- Deploy bifurcated device making sure there is at least a two stent overlap, cannulate contralateral limb, and deploy limb extension (Fig. 19.7).
- Inflate a 32-Coda balloon on overlap segment of the fenestrated and bifurcated components.
- Perform completion aortogram (Fig. 19.8).

3 POSTOPERATIVE

3.1 Complications

- Endoleak

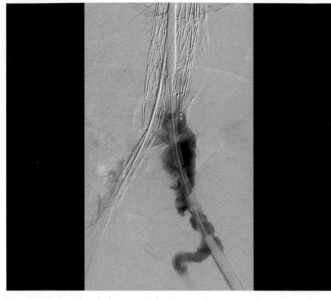

Fig. 19.7: Deploy bifurcated device making sure there is at least a two stent overlap, cannulate contralateral limb and deploy limb extension.

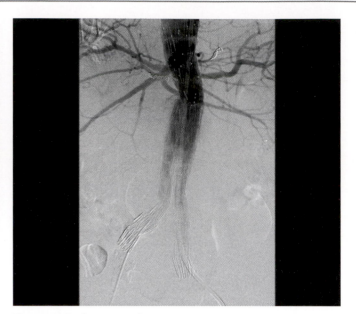

Fig. 19.8: Perform completion aortogram.

- Renal artery dissection
- Groin access injury

3.2 Follow-up

- Mesenteric ultrasound/Renal duplex
- CTA of aorta
- Monitor for aneurysm growth/endoleak
- Surgical follow-up of groin incisions

REFERENCES

1. The Zenith Fenestrated (Cook Medical) AAA Endovascular Graft US clinical study. Non-randomized, multi-center study. Available from Clinicaltrials.gov/show/NCT00875563. [Accessed August 23, 2014].
2. Scurr JRH, Brennan JA, Gilling-Smith GL, et al. Fenestrated EVAR repair for juxtarenal aortic aneurysm. Br J Surg. 2008;95:326-32.
3. Kakra H, Michael W. Endovascular repair of juxtarenal aneurysms. Circulation. 2012;125:2684-5.

chapter 20

Obturator Bypass

J Westley Ohman, Patrick J Geraghty

1 PREOPERATIVE

1.1 Indications

- Need for circumventing the femoral triangle:
  - Localized infection of vascular prosthetic graft
  - Infected femoral pseudoaneurysm
  - Limb ischemia in the presence of irradiated groin
  - Extensive prior groin dissection/complex wound healing/flap coverage
  - Contraindications
- Extensive retroperitoneal infection and/or diffuse infection of aortofemoral graft

1.2 Evidence

- In a meta-analysis, patency rates at 1 and 5 years were 72.7% ± 5.0% and 56.9% ± 7.0%, respectively; and survival rates at 1 and 5 years were 80.5% ± 4.0% and 53.3% ± 7.0%.[1,2]
- The most recent case series demonstrates 5-year graft patency of 80% and limb salvage of 60%.

1.3 Materials Needed

- Standard instrument set for aortic and femoropopliteal bypass procedures
- Kelly-Wick (or similar) prosthetic graft tunnelers
- Omni-Tract (or similar) fixed retractor
- Externally supported expanded polytetrafluoroethylene (e-PTFE) graft

1.4 Preoperative Risk Assessment

Planning:
- Computed tomography angiography or standard arteriography to define anatomy

Low risk:
- Radiation-induced tissue changes without evidence of infection
- Infection secondary to percutaneous access without sepsis

Intermediate risk:
- Complex atherosclerotic disease of inflow and/or outflow arteries
- Infected aortofemoral prosthetic graft

High risk:
- Active femoral hemorrhage
- Systemic sepsis
- High medial risk due to medical comorbidities

1.5 Preoperative Checklist

Sign in:
- No special precautions

Time out:
- Preoperative pulse examination and marking
- Administration of broad-spectrum intravenous antibiotics (including coverage of methicillin-resistant Staphylococcus aureus and any previously identified pathogens)
- Review CT imaging and mark expected extent of infectious process.
- Communicate details of two-stage prep to operating team (prep infected groin wound, isolate with Ioban drape, and then prep in proximal and distal fields with additional Ioban draping).

Sign out:
- Postoperative pulse examination

1.6 Decision-Making Algorithm

- *See* Flowchart 20.1.

Flowchart 20.1: Decision–making alogrithm.

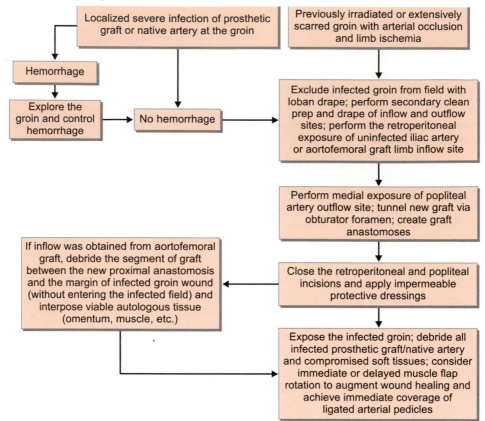

1.7 Pearls and Pitfalls

Pearls:

- As a fallback option, prep in the ipsilateral infraclavicular axillary artery. If the retroperitoneum is found to be contaminated, this alternate inflow site can be used for performance of axillopopliteal grafting through clean tissue planes.
- Placement of ipsilateral ureteral stent after anesthetic induction may help the surgeon identify and protect this structure, particularly when scarring is expected due to prior pelvic irradiation or aortofemoral graft placement.
- When preparing to tunnel the graft, palpate the margins of the obturator foramen, and locate the small fascial hiatus (the obturator canal) through which the obturator vessels pass. From the proximal (retroperitoneal) wound, use a long Kelly or tonsil clamp to penetrate the foramen at a site distinct from the canal, thus avoiding incidental trauma to these vessels. With a fingertip, guide the tip of the Kelly-Wick tunneler to the aperture you have created, and smoothly advance the tunneler to the popliteal exposure.
- At the time of groin debridement, autologous vein patching of the distal common femoral artery can be utilized to maintain retrograde flow from the popliteal outflow site to the profunda femoris artery.

Pitfalls:

- When the obturator bypass is originated from a clean proximal portion of an aortofemoral or iliofemoral graft limb, it is critically important for the surgeon to remove the segment of the old graft from the new proximal anastomosis to the margin of the groin infection, and interpose viable autologous tissue in that intervening space prior to closure. At the subsequent removal of infected graft from the groin, all gross contamination should be carefully removed before retrieving the ligated distal stump of the graft from under the inguinal ligament—this will minimize the likelihood of cross-contamination of the proximal clean field.

1.8 Surgical Anatomy

- *See* Figures 20.1A and B.

1.9 Positioning

- *See* Figure 20.2.

1.10 Anesthesia

- Muscle relaxants necessary to manipulate ipsilateral lower extremity for tunneling
- Central venous catheters preferentially placed in contralateral internal jugular vein
- Arterial lines restricted to contralateral upper extremity
- Type and cross-match a minimum of 2 units packed red blood cells

2 PERIOPERATIVE

2.1 Incision

- *See* Figures 20.3A and B.

2.2 Steps

- *See* Figures 20.4A to D.

2.3 Closure

Both the abdominal and popliteal exposures are closed in standard fashion with running layered absorbable suture. After closure of these clean wounds is complete, impermeable dressings are applied. The groin wound is then exposed for debridement and possible flap rotation.

3 POSTOPERATIVE

3.1 Complications

Most common complications:
- Recurrent hemorrhage from groin site
- Persistent soft tissue infection at groin site
- Obturator nerve injury
- Pelvic organ injury (ureter, bladder, rectum)

Least common complications:
- Isolated thigh tissue necrosis (interval necrosis) from hypoperfusion of profunda femoris

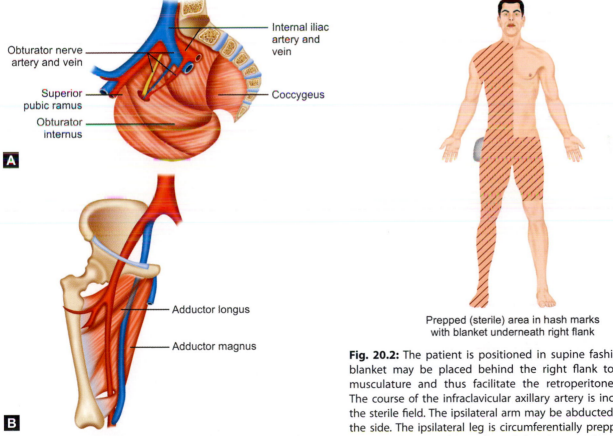

Figs. 20.1A and B: (A) Image of hemipelvis with identification of vital structures. (B) Completed obturator bypass.

Prepped (sterile) area in hash marks with blanket underneath right flank

Fig. 20.2: The patient is positioned in supine fashion. A folded blanket may be placed behind the right flank to extend the musculature and thus facilitate the retroperitoneal exposure. The course of the infraclavicular axillary artery is included within the sterile field. The ipsilateral arm may be abducted or tucked at the side. The ipsilateral leg is circumferentially prepped. Popliteal artery exposure and tunneling of the obturator bypass are aided by external rotation at the hip and partial flexion of the knee joint.

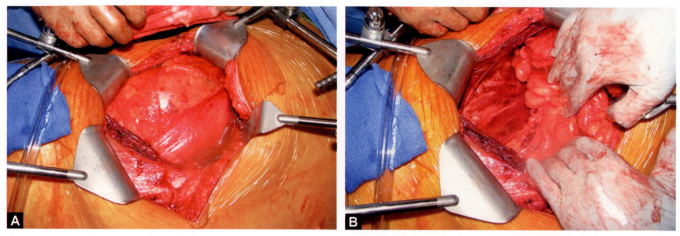

Figs. 20.3A and B: (A) Oblique abdominal incision used for retroperitoneal approach (the near end of the incision extends close to the patient's midline; cephalad direction is to the right). This incision is similar to that used for kidney transplantation. The usual medial incision for popliteal exposure is also made (not shown). (B) The peritoneum is then swept medially. The psoas is visualized and the ureter is identified and protected. Ureteral stents may assist in the latter process.

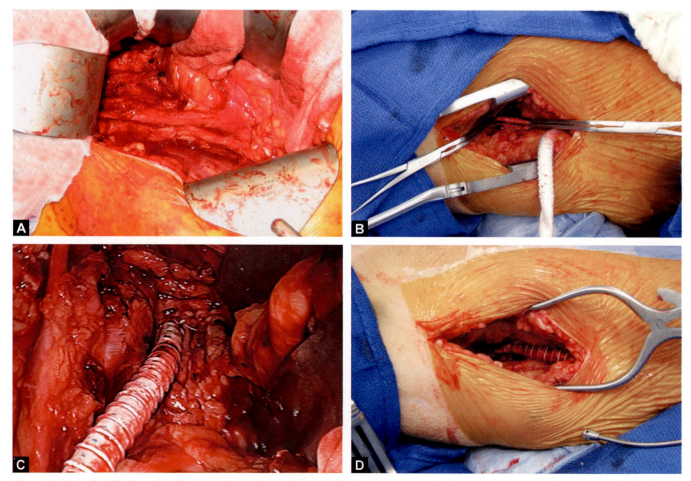

Figs. 20.4A to D: (A) Completed retroperitoneal exposure of distal aorta and right iliac artery (viewed from patient's flank, with cephalad direction to the left). (B) Medial exposure of right popliteal artery for distal anastomosis. (C) PTFE graft has been tunneled via obturator foramen (viewed from pelvic brim—bladder and rectum swept medially to the left). (D) Completed distal anastomosis to popliteal artery. (PTFE: Polytetrafluoroethylene).

- Graft occlusion from sitting upright for prolonged periods of time
- Infection of new PTFE graft or proximal aspect of aortofemoral graft

3.2 Outcomes

Expected outcomes:
- Maintenance of lower extremity circulation
- 5-year graft patency of >75%
- Eradication of infection
- Successful (albeit often delayed) healing of complex groin wound

3.3 Follow-Up

- Wound care, possible muscle flap, for groin coverage
- Postoperative ankle-brachial index
- Physical therapy evaluation for lower extremity neuromuscular deficits

- Goal is for patient to return to preoperative function within 30 days of surgery.
- 4-week follow-up visit for surgical site inspection with repeat ankle-brachial index.
- Follow-up yearly (or as needed) thereafter.
- Daily antiplatelet therapy for prosthetic graft patency.

3.4 E-mail an Expert

- *E-mail address*: geraghtyp@wustl.edu

REFERENCES

1. Patel A, Taylor SM, Langan EM 3rd, et al. Obturator bypass: a classic approach for the treatment of contemporary groin infection. Am Surg. 2002;68(8):653-8; discussion 658-9.
2. Sautner T, Niederle B, Herbst F, et al. The value of obturator canal bypass. A review. Arch Surg. 1994;129(7):718-22.

QUIZ

Question 1: Obturator bypass can be utilized for diffuse aortofemoral graft infection:
a. True
b. False

Question 2: Which of the following necessitates addressing the groin prior to completion of the obturator bypass?
a. Groin skin necrosis with active purulent drainage
b. Active hemorrhage from femoral vessels
c. Severely diminished (<0.3) ipsilateral ankle-brachial index on preoperative evaluation.
d. History of prior irradiation to ipsilateral groin.

Question 3: All of the following are true except:
a. Contamination of the retroperitoneal space is not a contraindication for obturator bypass.

b. Infected groins can be safely bypassed prior to debridement.
c. Lesions due to radiation are generally lower risk than those due to infection of prior prosthetic material.
d. Ureteral stent placement may facilitate identification and protection of this structure.

Question 4: After adequate groin debridement, the soft tissues cannot be closed over the ligated vascular pedicles. An appropriate next step would be:
a. Hip disarticulation.
b. Close the groin wound with Prolene mesh.
c. Rotation of a muscle flap to provide coverage of the vascular pedicles.
d. Cover the pedicles with Silvadene ointment.

ANSWERS: 1. b   2. b   3. a   4. c

Iliac Aneurysm Open Repair

Lindsay Gates, Jeffrey Indes

1 PREOPERATIVE

1.1. Indications

- Isolated iliac artery aneurysm 3.5 cm or larger
- Symptomatic aneurysm, regardless of size, that cannot otherwise be treated with an endovascular approach.

1.2. Evidence

- Aneurysm <3 cm per year expand more slowly than larger (3–5 cm) ones (11 26 mm/year).[1]
- Isolated iliac artery aneurysms constitute 0.6–2.0% of abdominal aortoiliac aneurysms. Typically involves the common iliac artery (CIA) 70–90% of the time.[1,2]
- For emergent open surgical repair, mortality averaged 28% compared to elective operations that averaged 5%.[3,4]

1.3. Materials Needed

- Open vascular surgery tray
- Major abdominal laparotomy instruments
- Self retaining retractor (Bookwalter Fig. 21.1A, Omni Fig. 21.1B, etc.)
- Headlamps (optional) (Figs. 21.1C and D)
- Dacron or polytetrafluoroethylene graft
- Bovie electrocautery
- Cellsaver

1.4. Preoperative Planning and Risk Assessment

- *Planning*:
  - Computed tomography angiography (CTA) of abdomen and pelvis (look for associated abdominal aortic aneurysm [AAA])
  - Bilateral lower extremity arterial duplex or CTA to assess for femoral-popliteal aneurysms or disease
  - Preoperative cardiopulmonary risk assessment
- *Risk assessment*:
  - *Low risk*:
    - Age <80
    - No, or minor, American College of Cardiology (ACC) clinical predictors of increased perioperative cardiovascular risk: abnormal EKG, arrhythmia, history of cerebrovascular accident, low functional capacity, uncontrolled hypertension[5]
  - *Intermediate risk*:
    - Age over 80
    - *Intermediate ACC clinical predictors: Mild angina,* previous myocardial infarction or pathological Q waves on EKG, compensated or history of heart failure, diabetes mellitus, renal insufficiency
    - Chronic obstructive pulmonary disease (COPD) with FEV1 >1 L/s
    - Asymptomatic, small (3.5) aneurysm
  - *High risk*:
    - Age over 80
    - *Major ACC clinical predictors*: Unstable coronary syndromes (acute or recent myocardial infarction, unstable or severe angina), decompensated heart failure, significant arrhythmias (high-grade atrioventricular block, symptomatic ventricular arrhythmias, supraventricular arrhythmia with uncontrolled rate), valvular disease
    - Oxygen-dependent COPD with FEV1 <1 L/s
    - Smoker
    - Infected/inflammatory aneurysm

1.5 Preoperative Checklist

- Preoperative administration of β-blockers for risk reduction of cardiovascular events.

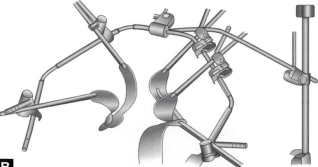

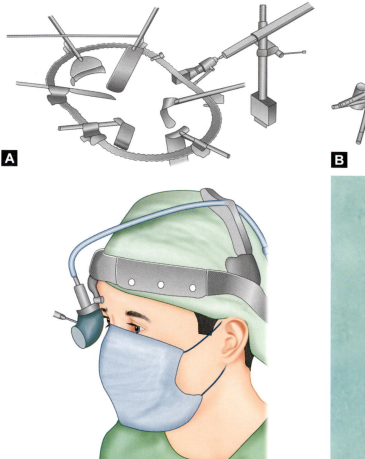

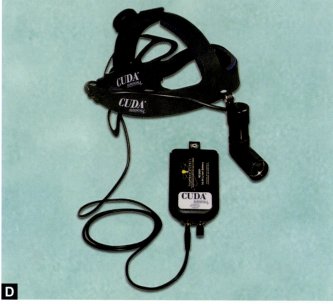

Figs. 21.1A to D: (A) Bookwalter; (B) Omni retractor; (C and D) Headlamps.

Sign in:
- Verified patient identity, operative site, planned procedure and consent
- Cardiopulmonary risk assessment reviewed by anesthesiology
- Review patient allergies and use of β-blockers
- Ensure adequate intravenous access, hemodynamic monitors, availability of blood products.

Time out:
- Team members introduce themselves and role
- Surgeon, anesthesiologist, and nurse reconfirm correct patient, site, and procedure
- Surgeon reviews critical steps, operative duration, and estimated blood loss
- Anesthesiology reviews any patient-specific concerns
- Equipment sterility and/or issues are confirmed
- Verify appropriate antibiotic administration within 60 minutes of incision.

Sign out:
- Nursing confirms procedure performed, correct instrument/sponge/needle counts, labeling of any surgical specimen.
- Surgeon, anesthesiologist, and nurse review tenets of postoperative management.

1.6. Decision-Making Algorithm

- *See* Flowchart 21.1.

1.7. Pearls and Pitfalls

Pearls:
- Avoid iatrogenic injuries by using minimal dissection and balloon arterial occlusion.
- If aneurysmorrhaphy with interposition prosthetic graft is not feasible, ligation proximal and distal to aneurysm can be combined with a crossover ilio- or femorofemoral

Flowchart 21.1: Decision-making algorithm.

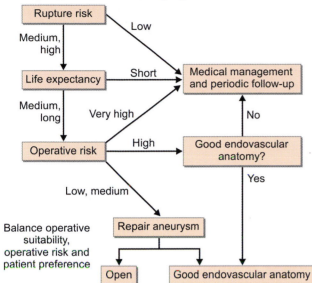

bypass (treatment of choice for mycotic aneurysm or contaminated field).
- Often useful to reflect the cecum and/or the sigmoid colon medially to gain control of the right and left external iliac artery, then trace this back to the origin of the internal iliac artery to avoid ureter injury.

Pitfalls:
- Not identifying ureter as crossed bifurcation.
- Can have significant venous bleeding and bleeding from side branches that can be difficult to control deep in pelvis. Adequate exposure is essential.
- Interruption of internal iliac artery with diseased or occluded contralateral iliac artery aneurysm. Can lead to hip claudication, ischemic colitis, neurologic deficits, bowel or bladder dysfunction, and impotence.

1.8. Surgical Anatomy

Common iliac artery starts at the aortic bifurcation and continues distally along the medial border of the ipsilateral psoas major muscle. It then divides into an external and internal iliac artery at level of sacroiliac joint. The right CIA crosses anterior to the left common iliac vein. The common iliac veins lie on the posteromedial side of the common iliac arteries. The ureter on each side crosses in front of the CIA bifurcation. The internal iliac artery branches off the CIA on the posteromedial side. The internal iliac artery then runs posterior to and parallel with the ureter then dives into medial pelvis where it divides into anterior and posterior divisions. The external

iliac arteries continue laterally until it crosses beneath the inguinal ligament, becoming the common femoral artery (Fig. 21.2).

1.9. Positioning (Figs. 21.3A and B)

- Supine
- Prep from nipples to knees

1.10. Anesthesia

- Obtain adequate intravenous access, with intra-arterial pressure monitoring and preoperative antibiotic administration.
- Up to date type and screen with at least 4 units crossed blood available.
- Foley catheter placement
- Endotracheal anesthesia
- Epidural catheter for pain control when appropriate. This will aid with postoperative pain control and reduce the surgical stress response as well as cardiovascular demands.

2 PERIOPERATIVE

2.1 Incision

- Patient should be supine on the operating table.
- The abdomen is prepped and draped using standard sterile surgical technique.
- A curvilinear incision is made in the left or right lower quadrant (depending on lesion location) extending from 1 cm above the pubic symphysis to 2–4 cm lateral to the anterior superior iliac spine (Fig. 21.4).

2.2 Steps

The incision is carried down through the subcutaneous tissue. Then divide the muscle with electrocautery and mobilize the peritoneum medially to expose the retroperitoneum. The retroperitoneum is entered and the external iliac artery and vein are mobilized free from the surrounding connective tissue, taking care to ligate all lymphatics to prevent lymphocele formation. It is important to identify the spermatic cord in men. It can be secured with a vessel loop and retracted away from the operative field. In women the round ligament can be ligated and divided (Figs. 21.5A1 and A2).

Continue the dissection proximally and distally along the iliac artery. An adequate proximal length is needed

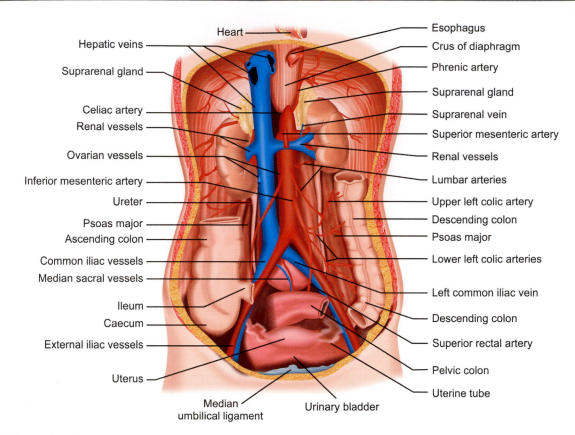

Heart
Esophagus
Hepatic veins
Crus of diaphragm
Suprarenal gland
Phrenic artery
Celiac artery
Suprarenal gland
Renal vessels
Suprarenal vein
Ovarian vessels
Superior mesenteric artery
Inferior mesenteric artery
Renal vessels
Ureter
Lumbar arteries
Psoas major
Upper left colic artery
Ascending colon
Descending colon
Common iliac vessels
Psoas major
Median sacral vessels
Lower left colic arteries
Ileum
Left common iliac vein
Caecum
Descending colon
External iliac vessels
Superior rectal artery
Uterus
Pelvic colon
Uterine tube
Median
umbilical ligament
Urinary bladder

Figs. 21.2: Surgical anatomy.

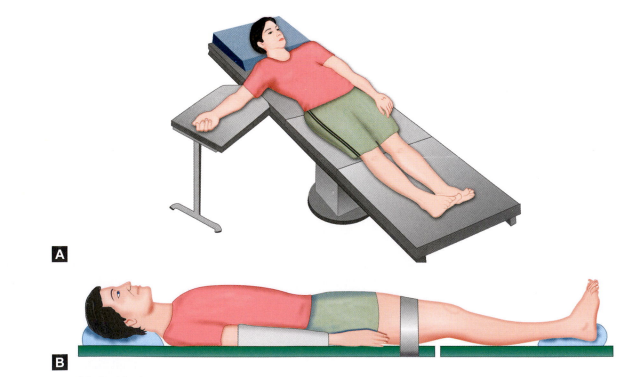

A

B

Figs. 21.3A and B: Positioning.

on the CIA to cross-clamp; also, an adequate length is needed along both the internal and external iliac artery to clamp distal. During dissection make sure to be aware of the location of the ureter at all times.

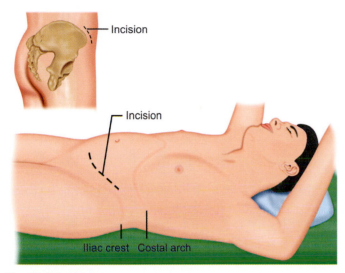

Fig. 21.4: Incision.

Once dissection is complete give the patient heparin (usually between 75-100 units/kg) and check ACT during the surgery, with a goal of 200–300. Once patient heparinized and an appropriate amount of time has passed, proceed with placing proximal clamp on the CIA as proximal as possible (best if just distal to the bifurcation). If unable to place cross-clamp due to significant disease, one will need to use occlusion balloons. This can be done by making a longitudinal arteriotomy and passing an occlusion balloon proximal and inflate just past its origin off the distal aorta (care taken not to occlude circulation to the contralateral iliac limb) (Fig. 21.5B).

Next one will need to place the distal clamp on the external iliac artery as well as place the clamp on the internal iliac artery. Again if unable to get control on these vessels one can also place occlusion balloons (Fig. 21.5B).

Once all vessels are controlled perform aneurysmorrhaphy and proceed with inlay of the prosthetic graft. Proceed with an end-to-end anastomosis on normal segment of the proximal CIA. Once completed with the proximal anastomosis next proceed with the distal

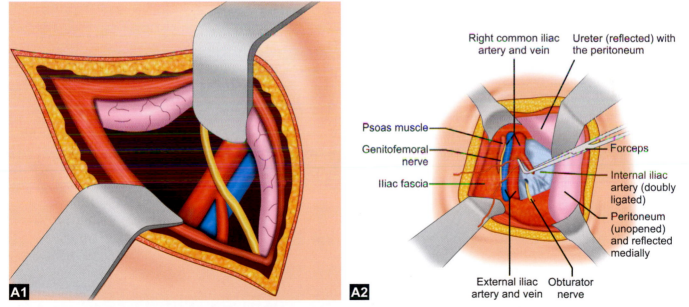

Figs. 21.5A1 and A2: (A1) Exposure of the iliac vessels carried through a curvilinear incision in the left or right lower quadrant. Entry through the retroperitoneum will expose the external iliac artery and vein. These are mobilized from surrounding subcutaneous tissue. When dissecting around the iliac bifurcation care must be taken to evaluate the ureter crossing over in this location towards the bladder. (A2) Another view of dissection to the iliac vessels. The peritoneum and ureter will be reflected medially as dissection carried down to iliac vessels in pelvis. Both the genito-femoral nerve and obturator nerve are in close proximity to iliac vessels in this location and care should be taken during dissection to prevent nerve injuries.

The retroperitoneum is entered and the external iliac artery and vein are mobilized free from the surrounding connective tissue, taking care to ligate all lymphatics to prevent lymphocele formation. It is important to identify the spermatic cord in men. It can be secured with a vessel loop and retracted away from the operative field. In women the round ligament can be ligated and divided.

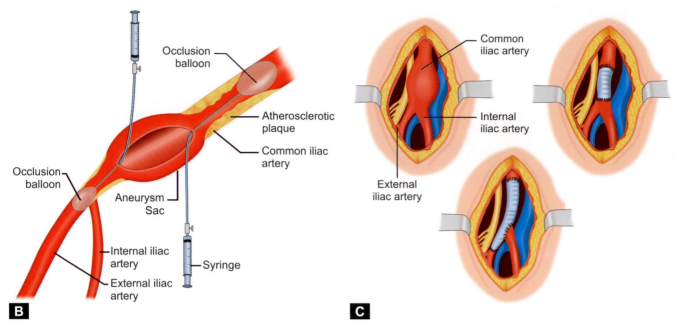

Figs. 21.5B and C: (B) For patients with significantly calcified proximal and distal disease, vascular control can be accomplished with occlusion balloons as shown. (C) Common iliac artery aneurysm shown can be repaired with either an interposition graft with an end to end anastomosis proximal to the origin of the internal iliac artery or an end to end interposition graft between the common iliac artery and external iliac artery with re-implantation of the internal iliac artery to perfuse the pelvis.

anastomosis. Depending on the anatomy of the aneurysm, one can perform distal anastomosis: (1) end-to-end to disease-free CIA, (2) end-to-end to the external iliac artery (this will exclude the internal iliac artery so need to make sure the contralateral side is patent), and (3) end-to-side to the external iliac artery to perfuse the internal iliac artery with over sewing of the CIA just proximal to the bifurcation. Once completed the distal anastomosis release clamps and ensure adequate flow distal to the graft (Fig. 21.5C).

2.3 Closure

- Abdominal wound is irrigated and closed in layers.

3 POSTOPERATIVE

3.1 Complications

- Artheroembolization
- Buttock claudication
- Ureteral injury
- Postoperative hemorrhage
- Anastomotic leak
- Anastomotic aneurysm formation

3.2 Outcomes

- 30-day mortality 6%–8%[3]
- Mortality for ruptured iliac artery aneurysms ranges from 30% to 50%.[2,4]

3.3 Follow-Up

- Follow up postoperative visit for 2–4 weeks
- Will need surveillance US at 6 months and 1 year, then yearly after
- Additional imaging required for new symptoms or concerns.

3.4 E-mail an Expert

- *E-mail address*: jeffrey.indes@yale.edu

3.5 Web Resources/References

- www.vascularweb.org
- www.mcbi.nim.nih.gov
- Cronenwett JL, Johnston KW. Rutherford's Vascular Surgery, 7th edition. Philidelphia, PA, Sanders; 2010
- Moore WS. Vascular and Endovascular Surgery, A Comprehensive Review, 7th edition. Philidelphia, PA Saunders; 2006.

REFERENCES

1. Levi N, Schroeder. Isolated iliac artery aneurysms. Eur J Vasc Endovasc Surg. 1998;16:342-4.
2. Sandhu R, Pipinos I. Isolated iliac artery aneurysms. Semin Vasc Surg. 2005;18 (4):209-15.
3. Kasirajan V, Hertzer R, Beven EG, et al. Management of isolated common iliac artery aneurysms. Cardiovasc Surg. 1998;6(2):171-7.
4. Patel NV, Long GW, Cheema ZF, et al. Open vs endovascular repair of isolated iliac artery aneurysms: a 12-year experience. J Vasc Surg. 2009:49(5):1147-53.
5. Fleisher L, Beckman J, Brown K, et al. American College of Cardiology/American Heart Association Guideline Update for Perioperative Cardiovascular Evaluation for Noncardiac Surgery—Executive Summary. Circulation. 2002;105: 1257.

QUIZ

Question 1. Which patient would benefit most from an open repair of an iliac artery aneurysm?
a. 90-year-old-man with COPD on home oxygen and an ejection fraction of 20%
b. 54-year-old man with hypertension
c. 70-year-old woman who is also an endovascular candidate
d. 75-year-old man who is also an endovascular candidate

Question 2. When is the most appropriate time to administer heparin to a patient during open iliac aneurysm repair?
a. Immediately after the artery is exposed
b. After clamping the artery
c. If using a graft after the graft is tunneled and prior to clamping
d. Prior to exposing the artery

Question 3. With regards to open repair of iliac aneurysms which of the following is true?
a. A Foley catheter is usually never needed
b. Arterial access does not aid in monitoring during repair
c. Epidural anesthesia will aid in postoperative pain control
d. A large self-retaining retractor is usually not needed

ANSWERS:

1. b   2. c   3. c

Endovascular Iliac Artery Aneurysm Repair

Lindsay Gates, Jeffrey Indes

1 PREOPERATIVE

1.1. Indications

- Isolated iliac artery aneurysm 3.5 cm or larger
- Symptomatic aneurysm (pain, rupture, embolus), regardless of size

1.2. Evidence

- Expansion rates are relatively slow, 11 mm/year for aneurysms <3 cm in diameter and 25–30 mm/year for larger aneurysms.[1]
- Rupture rates reported from 15% to 70%, but there have been no reported ruptures in aneurysms
- <30 mm in diameter.[1,2]
- Mostly asymptomatic and found incidentally. Some can present with symptoms related to acute expansion, rupture, iliac vein compression, ureteral obstruction, or erosion into adjacent structures.[3]
- Endovascular repair has been associated with a reduced length of stay, reduced operative blood loss, reduced need for invasive monitoring/intensive care unit care postoperatively, and reduced perioperative complications.[3,4]

1.3. Materials Needed

- Stationary imaging system or a portable imaging system
- Micropuncture needle and wire
- 0.035 glidewire
- Lunderquist wire
- Calibrated flush catheter
- Sheath
- Balloon or self expandable covered stent grafts (10–20% oversized compared with target vessel)
- Embolization coils
- Intravascular ultrasound (IVUS) (optional)
- Bifurcated AAA endograft (optional for short proximal necks that do not have an adequate seal zone)

1.4. Preoperative Planning and Risk Assessment

Planning:
- Computed tomography angiography, occasionally conventional angiography
- Preoperative cardiopulmonary evaluation and medical optimization of other comorbidities
- Bilateral lower extremity arterial duplex to assess for femoral-popliteal aneurysms

Risk assessment:
- *Low risks*:
  - Age <80
  - No, or minor, American College of Cardiology (ACC) clinical predictors of increased perioperative cardiovascular risk: abnormal electrocardiogram (EKG), arrhythmia, history of cerebrovascular accident, low functional capacity, uncontrolled hypertension[5]
- *Intermediate risk*:
  - Age over 80
  - *Intermediate ACC clinical predictors*: Mild angina, previous myocardial infarction or pathological Q waves on EKG, compensated or history of heart failure, diabetes mellitus, renal insufficiency
  - Chronic obstructive pulmonary disease (COPD) with FEV1 >1 L/s
  - Asymptomatic, small (3.5) aneurysm
- *High risk*:
  - Age over 80
  - Major ACC clinical predictors—unstable coronary syndromes (acute or recent myocardial infarction, unstable or severe angina), decompensated heart

failure, significant arrhythmias (high-grade atrioventricular block, symptomatic ventricular arrhythmias, supraventricular arrhythmia with uncontrolled rate), valvular disease
- Oxygen-dependent COPD with FEV1 <1 L/s
- Smoker
- Infected/inflammatory aneurysm

1.5 Preoperative Checklist

- Completion of cardiac evaluation and medically optimized
- Up to date laboratories, including type and screen

1.6 Decision-Making Algorithm

- *See* Flowchart 22.1.

1.7. Pearls and Pitfalls

Pearls:
- In extremely tortuous arteries a "buddy wire" system can be used to straighten the arterial pathway. Place two 0.035-in. glidewires through the sheath and position in the infrarenal aorta. Exchange catheters passed over each wire and then one is replaced with and Amplatz stiff wire and the other for a Lunderquist wire. Once in position sheath removed and exchanged for a larger sheath only over the Amplatz wire with the Lunderquist buddy wire outside the sheath providing structural support.
- If a suitable proximal common iliac seal zone is not available or if there is associated significant aneurysm disease

of the infrarenal aorta or contralateral common iliac artery (CIA), an aortobiiliac endograft should be considered.
- If there is not an adequate proximal landing zone, will need to use a bifurcated endograft graft that will provide an excellent seal at the bifurcation.
- There are data to support covering a hypogastric artery that is not aneurysmal and not having to embolize it.

Pitfalls:
- Not obtaining an adequate proximal or distal sealing zone. Will result in a type 1 endoleak.
- Failing to embolize vessels that feed the aneurysm sac. Will result in a type 2 endoleak.

1.8. Surgical Anatomy

- *See* Figure 22.1.

1.9. Positioning

- Patient is placed in the supine position.
- Bilateral groins are prepped and draped using standard sterile surgical technique.

1.10. Anesthesia

- Local anesthesia with intravenous sedation and intra-arterial blood pressure monitoring is used for the majority of cases.

2 PERIOPERATIVE

2.1 Incision

- Vascular access is obtained on the ipsilateral common femoral artery in a retrograde direction using a Seldinger needle and a 0.035-in. glidewire, which is advanced under fluoroscopic guidance into the aorta.

2.2 Steps

See Figure 22.2A.
- An introducer sheath is then passed over the wire and positioned in the ipsilateral external iliac artery (sheath size often depends on the stent that will be used).
- Advance a short calibrated flush catheter with 1-cm markers (such as a pigtail or omni-flush catheter) over the wire into the distal aorta.
  - Patient is told to hold breath (or anesthesia informed to hold respirations) and digital subtraction angiography (DSA) is obtained.

Flowchart 22.1: Decision-making algorithm.

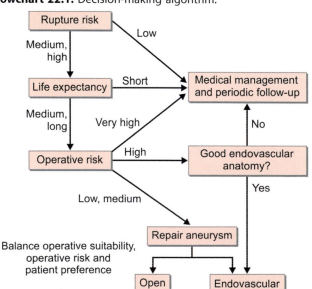

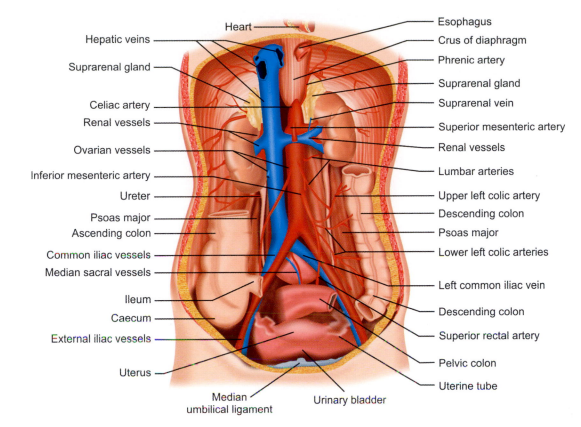

Fig. 22.1: Anatomy of abdomen and pelvis.

- A 30° contralateral oblique projection may also be performed to provide additional anatomic detail and further evaluate the internal iliac artery.
- Use calibrations on the catheter to measure length of stent needed and wall diameter.

See Figure 22.2B.

- (Alternatively) IVUS is used next to measure diameters of the external and common iliac arteries, length of the common iliac artery, and localization of the orifice of the hypogastric artery. It is also used to identify other pathology of the arterial wall, e.g. calcification, thrombus, etc. (optional- measurements can be made based on preoperative CTA with conformation by intra-operative angiogram).

See Figure 22.2C.

- *If there is 10–25 mm of normal arterial wall "neck" available on the CIA (proximal to the bifurcation), can proceed with advancing a Lunderquist wire into the abdominal aorta:*
  - Next advance stent over wire and deploy per packaging instructions.

- After deployment remove devise and advance flush catheter back into abdominal aorta and take final angiogram to insure exclusion of aneurysm.

See Figure 22.2D.

- *If there is not an adequate distal neck and the aneurysm extends to the iliac bifurcation the hypogastric artery should be coiled or plugged:*
  - Using a glide catheter and glide wire maneuver wire into the internal iliac artery.
  - Deploy coil/plug into the proximal portion of the internal iliac artery to exclude circulation.
  - Important to maintain anterior and posterior branches to avoid pelvic ischemia.
  - Through the sheath shoot an angiogram to confirm exclusion from circulation.
  - Next advance Lunderquist wire through sheath into the intra-abdominal aorta. Over wire advance selected stent into place with landing zone in the proximal CIA and distally in external iliac artery (EIA).
  - Once stent deployed remove device and replace Flush catheter for completion angiogram.

- If final angiogram satisfactory the sheath and wire can be removed.

See Figure 22.2E.

- If unable to land stent proximal or distal may need to use aortic stent graft either modular or a bifurcated unibody device to seal iliac aneurysm for a more advanced and complex procedure. Possible configurations shown.

2.3 Closure

- Usually need closure device for closure due to larger sheath size.

3 POSTOPERATIVE

3.1 Complications

- Can have symptoms of ischemia after coil of IIA (buttock claudication, impotence, colonic ischemia)

- Stent thrombosis
- Distal embolization or occlusion requiring intervention or thrombolysis

3.2 Outcomes

- Reintervention rates relatively high 11–28%[2,4]
- Higher reintervention rates seen with increased diameter and decreased length of proximal landing zone[4]
- Distal landing zone diameter >24 mm also had higher reintervention rates[4]
- Increased rate of limb occlusion with extension into the external iliac artery.[3]

3.3 Follow-up

- Patient will need to follow up at 2–4 weeks after initial procedure for US.
- Will need routine US surveillance at 6 months, 1 year and yearly after procedure.

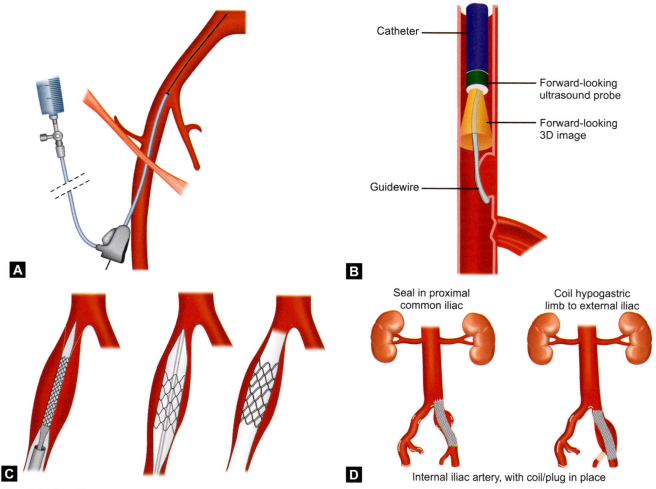

Figs. 22.2A to D

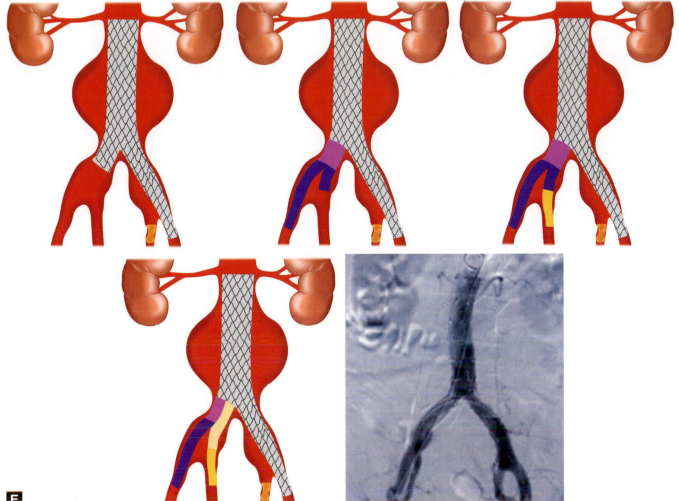

Figs. 22.2A to E: (A) Access via the ipsilateral common femoral artery (CFA) with wire across the aneurysm in the CIA. Sheath advanced into the external iliac artery. (B) IVUS catheter in the iliac artery, for measurement of diameter and assessment of suspected stenosis. (C) Balloon expandable stent placed across aneurysm. Stent placed so that proximal and distal end against adequate length of normal arterial wall to exclude aneurysm from circulation. (D) Image of adequate distal seal zone. In second image the aneurysm extends to the iliac bifurcation. Stent has been extended to cover the internal iliac artery with a coil place to prevent endoleak. (E) Multiple configurations of aortic stent grafts with modular limbs to revascularize patients with inadequate distal necks (aneurysms that extend to the iliac bifurcation). Last image shows angiogram after modular stent graft placed excluding bilateral common iliac aneurysm.

3.4 E-mail an Expert

- *E-mail address*: jeffrey.indes@yale.edu

3.5 Web Resources/References

- www.vascularweb.org
- www.mcbi.nim.nih.gov
- Cronenwett JL, Johnston KW. Rutherford's Vascular Surgery, 7th edition. Sanders, 2010.
- Moore WS. Vascular and Endovascular Surgery: A Comprehensive Review, 7th edition. Saunders, 2006.

REFERENCES

1. Richardson JW, Greenfield LJ. Natural history and management of iliac artery aneurysms. J Vasc Surg. 1998;8:165-71.
2. Zayed H, Attia R, Modarai B, et al. Predictors of reintervention after endovascular repair of isolated iliac artery aneurysm. Cardiovasc Intervent Radiol. 2011;34:61-6.
3. Buckley C, Buckley S. Technical tips for endovascular repair of common iliac artery aneurysms. Semin Vasc Surg. 2008;21:31-4.
4. Esposito G, Franzone A, Cassese S, et al. Endovascular repair for isolated iliac artery aneurysms: case report and review of the current literature. J Cardiovasc Med. 2009;10:861-5.

5. ACC/AHA task force on practice guidelines. Eagle K, Berger P, Calkins H, et al. American College of Cardiology/American Heart Association Guideline Update for Perioperative Cardiovascular Evaluation for Noncardiac Surgery-Executive Summary. Circulation. 2002;105:1257

QUIZ

Question 1. Which of the following is correct regarding the repair of internal iliac aneurysms?
a. They can be safely covered with a stent graft originating in the common iliac artery extending into the external iliac artery.
b. Coil embolization is required.
c. Open repair is technically simple.
d. The ipsilateral approach is preferable to the contralateral approach.

Question 2. What is the cause of a Type II endoleak?
a. Porosity of the graft fabric
b. Flow around the graft proximally
c. Retrograde flow from a patent branch vessel
d. Flow between to overlapping stent grafts

Question 3. What is the most common side effect associated with embolization of an internal iliac artery aneurysm?
a. Thigh necrosis
b. Buttock claudication
c. Sexual dysfunction
d. Toe gangrene

ANSWERS: 1. b   2. c   3. b

Endoleak Management: Translumbar

Kamal Massis

1 PREOPERATIVE

1.1 Indications/Contraindications

- *Indication*:
  - Type II endoleak with enlarging aneurysm sac
  - Failed attempt at transarterial embolization
- *Contraindication*:
  - Uncorrectable coagulopathy
  - Active infection
  - Renal insufficiency
  - Type I or III endoleak

1.2 Evidence

- The natural history of type II endoleaks is not benign and there is a higher association with continued sac expansion, sac rupture, conversion to open repair, and reintervention compared to those without endoleaks.[1]
- Translumbar sac embolization has a 71–92% success rate in controlling type II endoleaks. This is compared to much lower success rates in transarterial embolization of 20% to 38%.[2,3]

1.3 Materials Needed

- 21-gauge styletted needle (Fig. 23.1)
- 4–5 Fr vascular sheath (Fig. 23.2)
- 4–5 Fr catheter
- Microcatheter
- Coils
- Liquid embolic agent, ethylene vinyl alcohol copolymer (Onyx) or N-butyl cyanoacrylate (NBCA) glue

1.4 Preoperative Risk Assessment

Planning:
- Preoperative computed tomography (CT) of the abdomen
  - Assess safe entry into aneurysm sac and direct pathway to endoleak nidus.
- Preoperative angiogram
  - Assess flow pattern of endoleak:
    - Inflow and outflow vessels involved

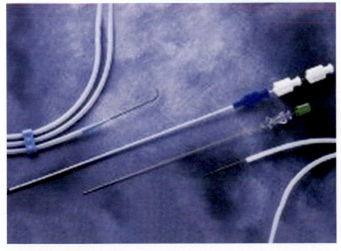

Fig. 23.1: Stylet needle.

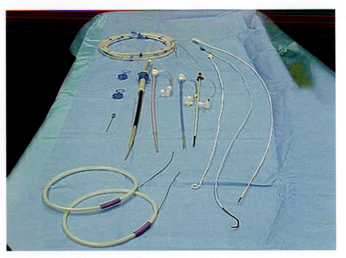

Fig. 23.2: Catheters sheaths wires.

Risk assessment:
- *Low risk*:
  - Large endoleak nidus
  - Small body habitus with short and direct tract to endoleak nidus.
  - No nearby organs or vessels that could be damaged
- *Intermediate risk*:
  - Small endoleak nidus
  - Large body habitus with longer tract to endoleak nidus
  - Close proximity to kidney, IVC, bowel, crossing vessel
- *High risk*:
  - Poorly visualized endoleak nidus
  - IVC or kidney in direct path of needle tract
  - Very large body habitus with >20 cm tract to endoleak nidus

1.5 Preoperative Checklist

Sign in:
- ___Has the patient confirmed his/her identity, procedure, and consent?
- ___Is the site marked?
- ___Is the anesthesia machine and medication check complete?
- *Does the patient have a*:
  - Y/N—Known allergy?
  - Y/N—Difficult airway?
  - Y/N—Uncorrected coagulopathy?

Time out:
- ___Confirm patient's name, procedure, and where incision will be made.
- Y /N—Has antibiotic prophylaxis been given within last 60 minutes?
- *Anticipated critical events*:
  - *To surgeon*:
    - ___How long will case take?
    - ___What is the anticipated blood loss?
  - *To anesthetist*:
    - ___Are there any patient-specific concerns?
  - *To nursing/technologist team*:
    - ___Has sterility been confirmed?
    - ___Are there any equipment issues or concerns?
  - Y/N—Is the essential imaging displayed?

Sign out:
- *Nurse verbally confirms*:
  - ___Name of the procedure
  - ___Were there any equipment problems that need to be addressed?

- *To surgeon, anesthetist, and nurse*:
  - ___What are the key concerns for recovery and management of this patient?

1.6 Decision-Making Algorithm

- *See* Flowchart 23.1.

1.7 Pearls and Pitfalls

Pearls:
- Carefully review the preoperative imaging to understand the exact level of the endoleak nidus and the vessels involved, along with the flow pattern.
  - *Measure on the preoperative CT (Figs. 23.3 and 23.4)*:
  - *The level of entry using fluoroscopic landmarks, usually spine anatomy*
  - *The distance from the spinous process of the entry point*
  - *The angle of entry relative to vertical axis*
  - *The depth of the tract from skin entry to aortic wall and to endoleak nidus*
- The vast majority of cases will involve a left paraspinal approach, with few cases requiring a right-sided paraspinal approach or transvena caval approach.

Pitfalls:
- Embolization without coil protection of a patent inferior mesenteric artery increases the risk of nontarget embolization of colonic arteries and bowel ischemia.
- Avoid tracts that are in close proximity to adjacent vessels or organs. Stay as near to midline as possible, as more lateral approaches have a higher likelihood of hitting kidneys or colon.

1.8 Surgical (Radiographic) Anatomy

- Axial and coronal enhanced CT images through abdomimal aortic aneurysm (AAA) sac showing the endoleak and relevant anatomy (Figs. 23.5 and 23.6).

1.9 Positioning

- Prone positioning is required to gain access into the AAA sac.
- Arms must be clear of the abdomen to allow for imaging in the lateral position. The best position of the arms is abducted above shoulders and secured to a long-arm board.
- There must be adequate clearance for the C-arm to travel over the patient and leave space for the access needle.
- Attention to the monitoring cables and tubes must be given if angiographic/C-arm CT imaging is to be performed.

Flowchart 23.1: Endoleak flowchart.

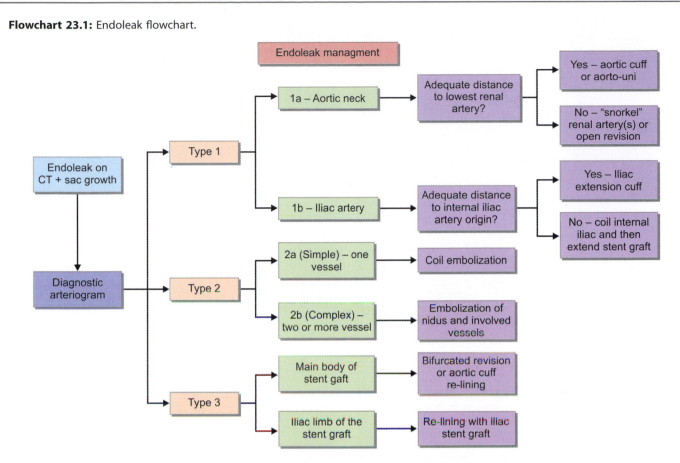

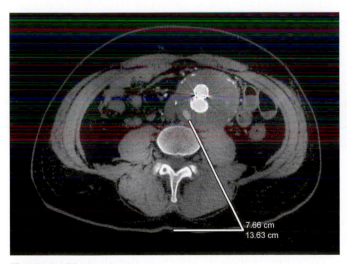

Fig. 23.3: CT measurements.

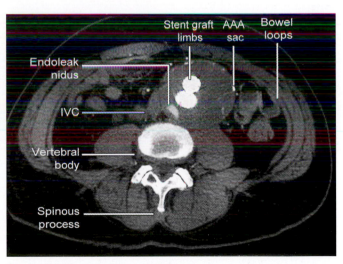

Fig. 23.4: CT axial with annotations.

1.10 Anesthesia

- General endotracheal anesthesia is preferred to conscious sedation because of airway protection and patient cooperation in the prone position.

- Deep anesthesia is not necessary as the pain level is very low with sac puncture.
- Paralysis is preferred so as to have proper breath-holds during digital subtraction angiography.

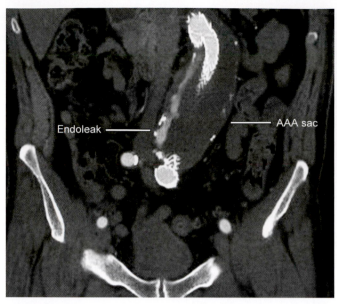

Fig. 23.5: CT coronal.

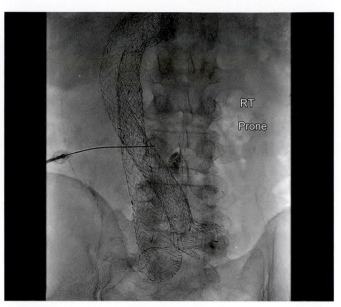

Fig. 23.6: Fluoroscopic image of needle entry.

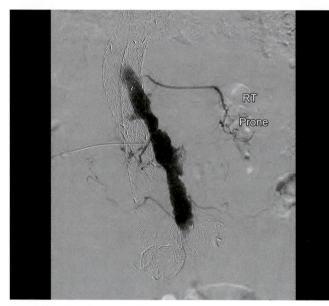

Fig. 23.7: DSA from needle.

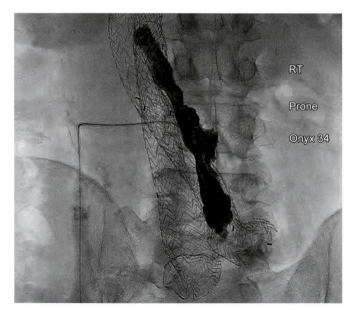

Fig. 23.8: Onyx embolization.

2. PERIOPERATIVE

2.1 Incision

- Stab incision with 11 blade at the needle entry site to allow passage of the sheath.

2.2 Steps

- Using fluoroscopic guidance, locate the skin entry site and place 21-gauge needle in a "gunsight" position.

- Enter in same angle as the C-arm projection toward the endoleak nidus.
- Once tract is secured, oblique C-arm in lateral position to assess depth of needle.
- Remove needle stylet and assess for pulsatile blood return (Fig. 23.7).
- Perform digital subtraction angiogram to evaluate endoleak nidus and contiguity with feeding and outflow arteries (Fig. 23.8).
- Place guide sheath and catheter into endoleak nidus.

- Occlude the nidus with coils/liquid embolic. If possible, occlude feeding and outflow vessels to decrease likelihood of recurrent or persistent endoleak (*See* Flowchart 23.1).

2.3 Closure

- Once hemostasis is achieved and confirmed with the cessation of pulsatile flow, the guiding catheter/sheath can be withdrawn.

3 POSTOPERATIVE

3.1 Complications

- *Most common*:
  – Hematoma, small
  – Extravasation of embolic material into retroperitoneum
  – Nontarget embolization of lumbar arteries or inferior mesenteric artery
- *Least common*:
  – Colonic ischemia
  – Hematoma, large
  – Spinal ischemia
  – Aneurysm rupture

3.2 Outcomes

- Complete occlusion of the endoleak nidus in 70% to 90% of patients

3.3 Follow-Up

- 23-hour observation to assess for evidence of retroperitoneal bleeding or ischemic complications
- 1-month follow-up computed tomography angiography (CTA) to assess for residual endoleak
- 6-month follow-up CT to assess for change in aneurysm sac dimensions and assure sac stabilization or involution

3.4 E-mail an Expert

- *E-mail addresses*: massis.kamal@gmail.com

REFERENCES

1. Jones JE, Atkins MD, Brewster DC, et al. Persistent type 2 endoleak after endovascular repair of abdominal aortic aneurysm is associated with adverse late outcomes. J Vasc Surg. 2007;46:1-8.
2. Baum RA, Carpenter JP, Golden MA, et al. Translumbar embolization of type 2 endoleaks after endovascular repair of abdominal aortic aneurysms. J Vasc Interv Radiol. 2001; 12:111-6.
3. Timaran CH, Ohki T, Rhee SJ, et al. Predicting aneurysm enlargement in patients with persistent type II endoleaks. J Vasc Surg. 2004;39:1157-62.

chapter 24

Endoleak Management: Transarterial

Kamal Massis

1 PREOPERATIVE

1.1 Indications/Contraindications

- *Indication*:
  - Endoleak with enlarging aneurysm sac
- *Contraindication*:
  - Uncorrectable coagulopathy
  - Active infection
  - Renal insufficiency

1.2 Evidence

- *Introduction*:
  - *Endoleak types*:
    - *See* Figures 24.1 and 24.2.
- The natural history of type 2 endoleaks is not benign and there is a higher association with continued sac expansion, sac rupture, conversion to open repair, and reintervention compared to those without endoleaks.[1]
- Open conversion post-EVAR has a high morbidity/ mortality.
  - Recent series showed a morbidity of 55% and mortality of 18%.[2]
  - EUROSTAR study had mortality of 24%, with main indication for open repair being endoleak with sac expansion.
- Endovascular management of endoleaks is needed and proper characterization of the endoleak is needed prior to attempt at treatment.
- Exhaustive diagnostic arteriogram is needed to determine the type of endoleak. At the time of diagnostic angiography, use of transarterial routes is less invasive and can be attempted before proceeding with direct sac puncture. If complete occlusion of the endoleak

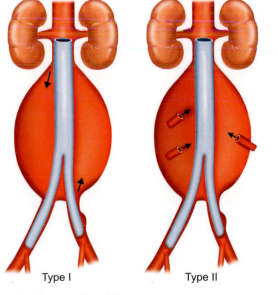

Fig. 24.1: Leak types 1 and 2.

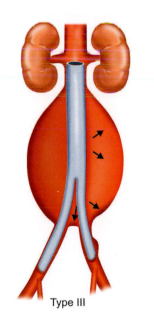

Fig. 24.2: Leak types 3 and 4.

cannot be achieved via femoral access, at least some of the culprit vessels can be occluded to minimize the risk of nontarget embolization prior to direct sac puncture.

1.3 Materials Needed

- 5–6 Fr vascular sheath (Fig. 24.3)
- 4–5 Fr catheter
- Microcatheters and wires
- Coils, pushable, and detachable
- Liquid embolic agent, ethylene vinyl alcohol copolymer (Onyx, Fig. 24.4) or N-butyl cyanoacrylate (NBCA) glue

1.4 Preoperative Risk Assessment

Planning:
- *Preoperative Computed tomography angiography (CTA) of the abdomen*:
  - Assess possible vessels involved in endoleak
  - Assess the abdominal aortic aneurysm (AAA) sac dimensions and confirm growth over prior studies
- *Diagnostic arteriogram*:
  - Exclude type 1 or 3 endoleak
  - Assess source and flow pattern of endoleak
  - Identify most favorable collateral pathway to access endoleak nidus

Risk assessment:
- *Low risk*:
  - Direct collateral pathway to endoleak nidus
  - Well circumscribed endoleak nidus
  - Few vessels involved in endoleak

- *Intermediate risk*:
  - Long tortuous collateral pathway to endoleak nidus
  - Occluded hypogastric arteries
- *High risk*:
  - Poorly visualized or poorly circumscribed endoleak nidus
  - Many vessels involved in endoleak, >5
  - Renal insufficiency
  - Very tortuous iliacs

1.5 Preoperative Checklist

Sign in:
- ___Has the patient confirmed his/her identity, procedure, and consent?
- ___Is the site marked?
- ___Is the anesthesia machine and medication check complete?
- *Does the patient have a*:
  - Y/N—Known allergy?
  - Y/N—Difficult airway?
  - Y/N—Uncorrected coagulopathy?

Time out:
- ___Confirm patient's name, procedure, and where incision will be made.
- Y/N—Has antibiotic prophylaxis been given within last 60 minutes?
- *Anticipated critical events*:
  - *To surgeon*:
    - ___How long will case take?
    - ___What is the anticipated blood loss?
  - *To anesthetist*:
    - ___Are there any patient-specific concerns?

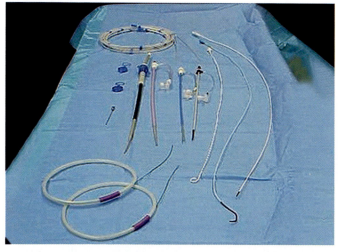

Fig. 24.3: Catheters sheaths wires.

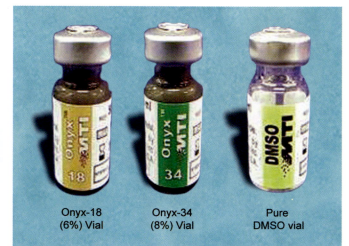

Fig. 24.4: Onyx vials.

Flowchart 24.1: Endoleak flowchart.

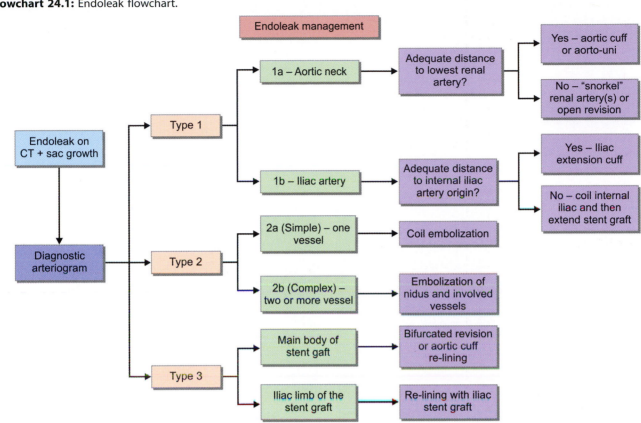

- To nursing/technologist team:
  - ___Has sterility been confirmed?
  - ___Are there any equipment issues or concerns?
- Y/N—Is the essential imaging displayed?

Sign out:
- *Nurse verbally confirms*:
  - ___Name of the procedure
  - ___Were there any equipment problems that need to be addressed?
- *To surgeon, anesthetist, and nurse*:
  - ___What are the key concerns for recovery and management of this patient?

1.6 Decision-Making Algorithm

- *See* Flowchart 24.1.

1.7 Pearls and Pitfalls

Pearls:
- Carefully review the preoperative CTA and assess the possible source of the endoleak.
- Vessels adjacent to the endoleak nidus are more likely culprits.

- Assess the proximal and distal seal zones and if there is incomplete apposition between the stent graft and the aortic neck or iliac arteries, suspicion should be raised over a possible type 1a or 1b. If the endoleak appears on the early/arterial phase of the study adjacent to the seal zones, also consider type 1 endoleak.
- If there is a large endoleak adjacent to the stent graft and not in direct contiguity with the aortic sac wall and/or a vessel, consider a type 3. Then, carefully assess the stent struts and look for fracture.
- The goal of the embolization of type 2a (simple) endoleaks is to occlude the culprit vessel, and this is best done with coils.
- The goal of embolization of type 2b (complex) endoleaks is obliteration of the endoleak nidus and involved vessels.
- If a type 3 endoleak is identified, stent graft relining is an effective technique of treatment.
- If a type 1a or 1b endoleak is identified, stent graft extension cuff placement is an effective technique of treatment, if possible based on devices available and landing zones relative to adjacent branch vessels (Renal, SMA, Internal iliacs).

Pitfalls:
- Embolization of the inferior mesenteric artery carries the highest procedural risk if attention is not made to

preserve the colonic branches and the collateral pathways. Nontarget embolization will lead to colonic ischemia.
- Use of liquid embolic agents (NBCA, Onyx) carries a risk of nontarget damage to adjacent structures, especially when done via IMA access to the endoleak nidus.
  - There is also a risk of adhering the catheter in place to the liquid embolic, if the embolic is not deployed in the recommended fashion.
- The use of large catheters in small collateral vessels will cause vasospasm and may prevent advancement of the device into the target vessel and endoleak nidus.

- Occlusion of those collateral pathways, especially the SMA-IMA, may cause arterial thrombosis and ischemia.
- Coaxial (macrocatheter, microcatheter) and triaxial guiding sheath (macrocatheter, microcatheter) systems are preferred for obtaining stable access via small and tortuous vessels.

1.8 Surgical (Radiographic) Anatomy

- *See* Figures 24.5 to 24.9.

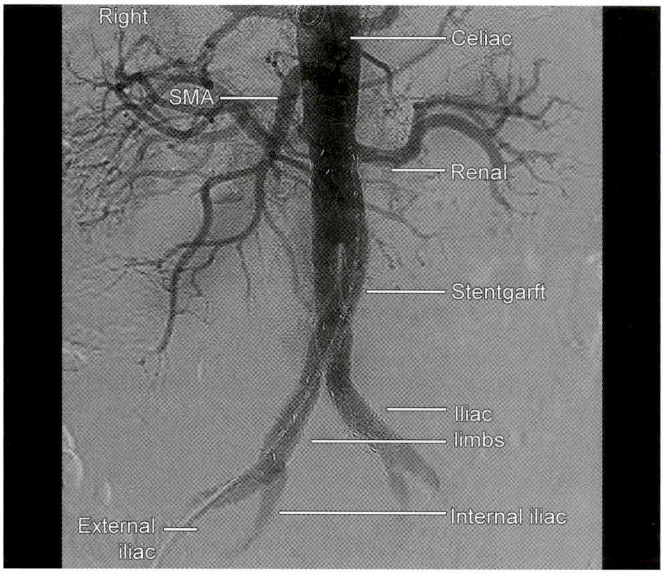

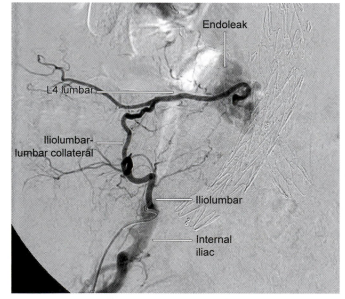

Fig. 24.5: Aortogram, flush.

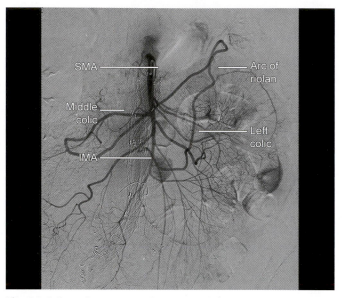

Fig. 24.6: Superior mesenteric artery to inferior mesenteric artery (SMA-IMA) collateral pathway (Arc of Riolan).

Fig. 24.7: Iliolumbar–lumbar collateral pathway.

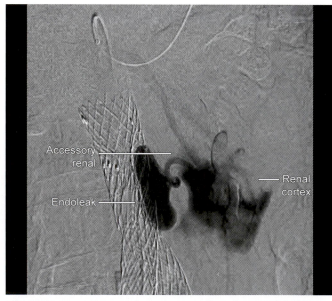

Fig. 24.8: Accessory renal artery as outflow from IMA inflow.

1.9 Positioning

- Supine position in an angiography suite.
- Bilateral groins prepped and draped for common femoral arterial access.

1.10 Anesthesia

- Conscious sedation preferred method of anesthesia, unless patient is not a candidate and then local anesthesia alone is preferred. Cooperation with breath-holds is critical for proper angiographic evaluation and treatment.

2 PERIOPERATIVE

2.1 Incision

- Common femoral arterial access with 5-Fr or 6-Fr vascular sheath

2.2 Steps

Diagnostic arteriogram:

- Perform flush aortogram for overview of the anatomy and for initial localization of the possible branch vessels involved in the endoleak, or to diagnose a type 1 or 3 endoleak.
- Obtain magnified views of the aortic neck in at least two projections (AP and lateral) to exclude proximal type 1 endoleak.

- Obtain flush angiograms within the stent graft to better assess for a type 3 endoleak and isolate limbs to localize the exact defect.
- Perform selective arteriograms of the possible culprit vessels:
  - *Superior mesenteric artery*:
    - Middle colic artery
  - Bilateral common and Internal iliac arteries
  - L1 Lumbar arteries
  - *Internal iliac arteries*:
    - Iliolumbar arteries
- Embolization (refer to Section 1.6)
- *Type 1a*:
  - Evaluate distance between lowest renal artery and top of divider of the bifurcated stent graft:
    - If enough distance according to manufacturer specifications, place aortic extension cuff.
    - If not enough distance, consider advanced maneuver such as stenting the renal artery and landing the aortic cuff higher, a.k.a "Snorkel" technique.
- *Type 1b*:
  - Evaluate distance to origin of internal iliac artery:
    - If adequate distance to obtain distal seal, >1.0 cm, then place iliac extension cuff stent graft.
    - If inadequate, coil embolization of internal iliac artery, and then place iliac extension cuff stent graft (Figs. 24.10 and 24.11).
- *Type 2a*:
  - Obtain access into culprit vessel

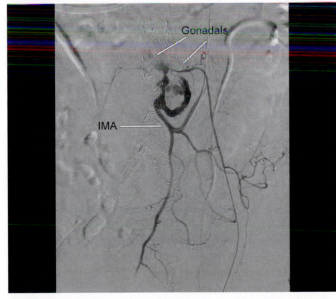

Fig. 24.9: Gonadal arteries as outflow from IMA inflow.

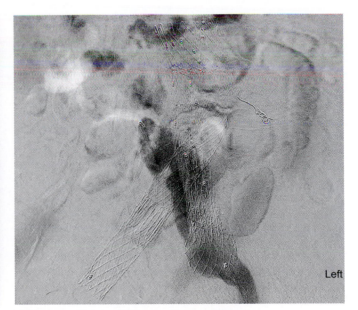

Fig. 24.10: Coil embolization of internal iliac.

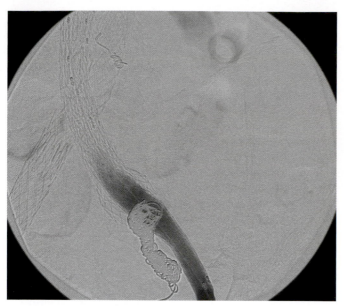

Fig. 24.11: Iliac extension cuff.

- Coil embolization (Fig. 24.12; IMA endoleak s/p coil embolization)
- *Type 2b*:
  - Obtain access into endoleak nidus
  - Fill nidus and ideally also fill the culprit arteries with liquid embolic and/or coils (Figs. 24.13 and 24.14)
- *Type 3*:
  - If located in main body of stent graft, place aortic cuff to re-line the defect or bifurcated stent graft revision
  - If located in one of the iliac stent graft limbs, reline with iliac extension cuff (Figs. 24.15 and 24.16)

2.3 Closure

- Remove sheath and use manual compression to obtain hemostasis:
  - Arterial closure devices may also be used.
- If larger access is needed (>10 Fr) for placement of extension cuffs or revision, consider "preclose" with suture mediated devices versus open surgical arterial closure.

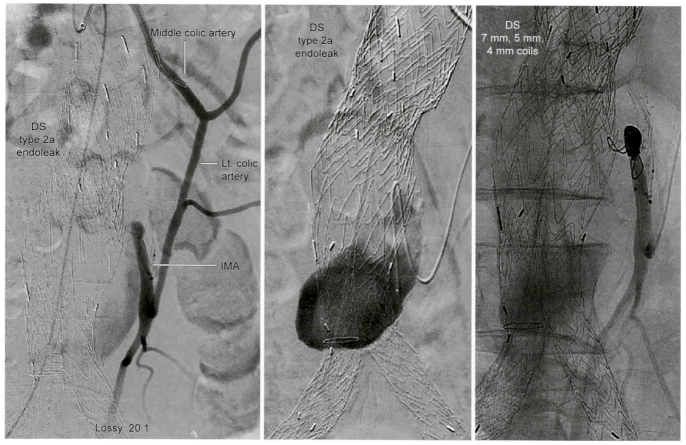

Fig. 24.12: IMA endoleak s/p coil embolization.

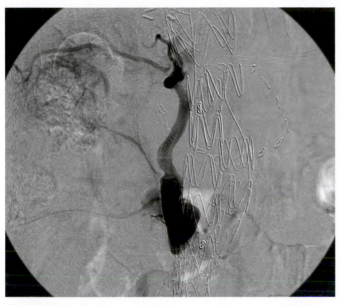

Fig. 24.13: Iliolumbar to lumbar access with microcatheter.

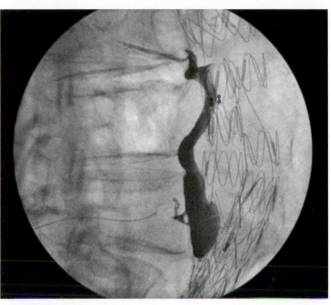

Fig. 24.14: Embolization with Onyx.

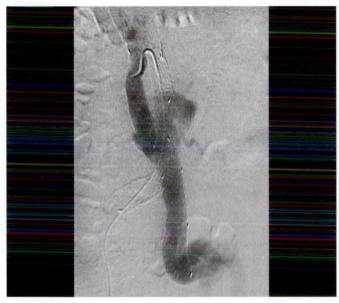

Fig. 24.15: Limb isolated and angio shows type 3 leak from crossed left iliac limb.

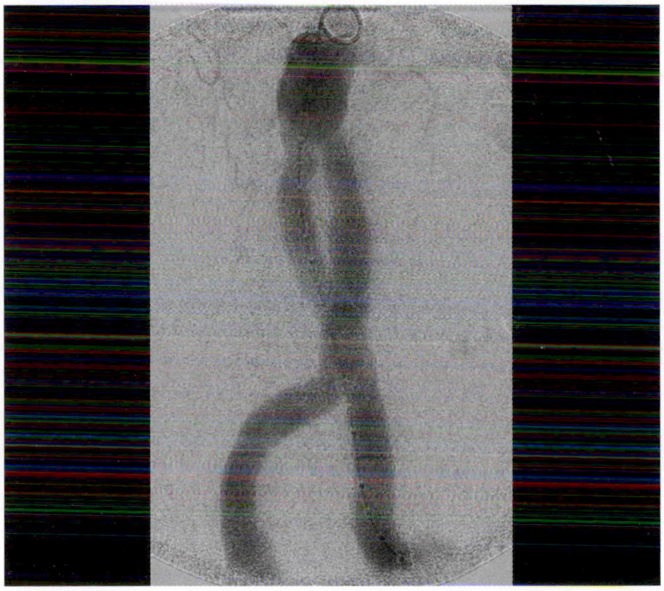

Fig. 24.16: Treated successfully with iliac extension cuff relining.

3 POSTOPERATIVE

3.1 Complications

Most common:
- Hematoma, small
- Pseudoaneurysm at the arteriotomy

- Extravasation of embolic material into retroperitoneum
- Nontarget embolization of lumbar arteries or inferior mesenteric artery

Least common:
- Arterial dissection
- Colonic ischemia

- Hematoma, large or retroperitoneal hemorrhage
- Spinal ischemia
- Aneurysm rupture

3.2 Outcomes

- Earlier studies with coil embolization alone had poor success at endoleak resolution at about 20–38%.[3,4]
- Later studies using a combination of embolic materials including coils, Onyx, and NBCA via transarterial route had an overall success rate of endoleak resolution of 59–60%.[1,5]
- More evidence is needed to determine the threshold for treatment and the long-term success rates of endoleak embolization techniques, especially type 2 endoleaks.

3.3 Follow-Up

- 6-hour observation and bed rest after sheath removed, less if closure device used
  - Assessment of groin site(s) and peripheral pulses
  - Abdominal examination and vitals to assess for bleeding or bowel ischemia
- 1-month follow-up CTA to assess for residual endoleak
- 6-month follow-up CTA to assess for change in aneurysm sac dimensions and assure sac stabilization or involution

3.4 E-mail an Expert

- *E-mail address*: massis.kamal@gmail.com

REFERENCES

1. Jones JE, Atkins MD, Brewster DC, et al. Persistent type 2 endoleak after endovascular repair of abdominal aortic aneurysm is associated with adverse late outcomes. J Vasc Surg. 2007;46:1-8.
2. Chaar CI, Eid R, Park T, et al. Delayed open conversions after endovascular abdominal aortic aneurysm repair. J Vasc Surg. 2012;55(6):1562-9.e1.
3. Baum RA, Carpenter JP, Golden MA, et al. Translumbar embolization of type 2 endoleaks after endovascular repair of abdominal aortic aneurysms. J Vasc Interv Radiol. 2001;12:111-6.
4. Timaran CH, Ohki T, Rhee SJ, et al. Predicting aneurysm enlargement in patients with persistent type II endoleaks. J Vasc Surg 2004; 39: 1157-62.
5. Massis K, Carson W, Rozas A, et al. Treatment of type II AAA endoleaks with ethylene-vinyl-alcohol copolymer (Onyx). J Vasc Endovasc Surg. 2012;46(3):251-7.

QUIZ

Question 1. The endoleak type associated with reversed flow to the aneurysm sac via a branch vessel with outflow to another branch vessel is:

a. Type Ib
b. Type IIa
c. Type IIb
d. Type III
e. Type IV

Question 2. Possible collateral pathways for the development of type II endoleaks are:

a. Superior mesenteric artery to inferior mesenteric artery
b. Internal iliac artery to iliolumbar artery to lumbar artery
c. L1 lumbar artery to L2 or L3 lumbar artery
d. Accessory renal arteries
e. All of the above

Question 3. Treatment options for repair of a Type III endoleak include:

a. Endovascular revision with stent-graft "re-lining"
b. Open surgical revision
c. Coil embolization
d. A and B
e. A and C

ANSWERS: 1. c   2. e   3. d

Explant Aortic Endograft

Paul Armstrong

1 PREOPERATIVE

1.1 Indications

- Ruptured aortic aneurysm after endovascular aneurysm repair (EVAR)
- Infected EVAR
- Persistent aneurysm growth after EVAR; suspected endoleak not amenable to secondary percutaneous intervention

1.2 Evidence

- When there is no safe endovascular solution for a failed EVAR, explantation is the only option left to solve the problem.[1,2]

1.3 Materials Needed

- Dacron or polytetrafluoroethylene tube or bifurcated aortic graft
- Deep vein or cadaver homograft

Planning:
- Cardiology consultation and risk assessment
- Preoperative CT scan (chest/abdomen/pelvis) with and without intravenous contrast of the affected aorta
  - *Graft endoleak*: Arterial sizing for new graft implant including assessment of proximal and distal "sewing rings"
  - *Graft infection*: Define degree of soft tissue and arterial infection/inflammation including
- Duplex ultrasonography of bilateral lower extremities with ankle brachial index and toe pressure

1.4 Preoperative Planning and Risk Assessment

Low risk:
- American Society of Anesthesiologists (ASA) physical status classification 1 or 2

Intermediate risk:
- ASA 3
- History of percutaneous or surgical coronary revascularization
- Creatinine >2.5 mg/dL

High risk: ASA 4 or 5:
- Class III or IV angina with unreconstructable coronary disease
- Class III or IV congestive heart failure with unreconstructable coronary disease
- Oxygen- or steroid-dependent chronic obstructive pulmonary disease (COPD)
- COPD with a forced expiratory volume in one second <30%

1.5 Preoperative Checklist

- Cardiac risk assessment
- CT-angiography of aorta and iliofemoral circulation
- Duplex ultrasonography of lower extremities with ankle brachial indices/toe pressures
- Optimize nutrition
- Optimize renal function
- Type and cross-match blood products

1.6 Decision-Making Algorithms

- *See* Flowcharts 25.1A and B.

Flowcharts 25.1A and B: Decision-making algorithm.

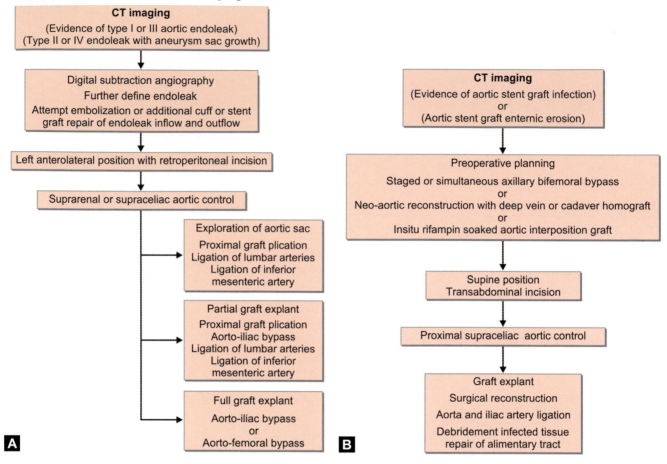

1.7 Pearls and Pitfalls

Pearls:

- Supraceliac control facilitates suprarenal stent implant removal.
- Plication of suprarenal stent grafts and partial graft removal preserve aortic integrity and are useful for endoleaks related to lumbar and iliac arteries.
- Staged reconstructions (e.g. axillary bifemoral bypass and endograft explant) within 24–48 hours offer shorter overall operative times and provide lower extremity perfusion.
- Two surgical teams are helpful, allowing for simultaneous bilateral deep vein harvests and arterial reconstructions.

Pitfalls:

- 360° of graft plication is difficult to obtain without good aortic neck dissection.
- Simultaneous explants with prosthetic explants should be limited to patients with hemodynamic instability (e.g. active gastrointestinal bleeding).
- Deep veins need detailed preparation including inversion for valve lysis and detailed monofilament suture ligation of all side branches.

1.8 Surgical Anatomy

- *Visceral aorta*:
  - Celiac and superior mesenteric arteries
  - Renal arteries
- *Iliac arteries*:
  - Common
  - Internal
  - External
- Inferior mesenteric artery
- Lumbar arteries
- Ureter
- Duodenum

1.9 Positioning

- Left anterolateral positioning with a thoracoabdominal incision provides definitive exposure for control of the aorta is optimum for suprarenal, fenestrated, or descending thoracic endografts.
- Supine midline abdominal incision is an alternative for infrarenal endovascular grafts.

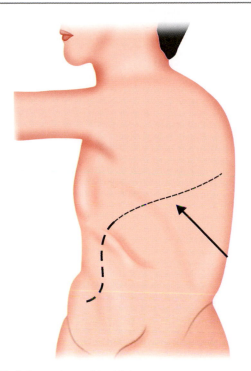

Fig. 25.1: Retroperitoneal Incision.

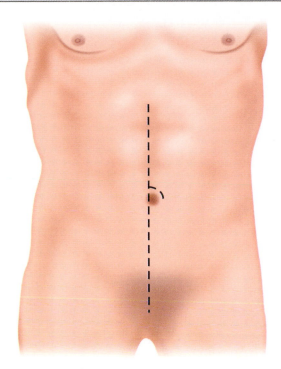

Fig. 25.2: Transabdominal Incision.

1.10 Anesthesia

- General endotracheal anesthesia
- Radial arterial line
- Large bore central venous access with consideration for Swan-Ganz monitoring
- Autotransfusion "Cell Saver"

2 PERIOPERATIVE

2.1 Incision

- Retroperitoneal (Fig. 25.1)
- Transabdominal (Fig. 25.2)

2.2 Steps

- Retroperitoneal exposure from diaphragm to the iliac bifurcation:
  - Oblique incision from the ribs to the abdominal midline. The level of rib exposure is determined by preoperative planning for controlling the proximal abdominal or thoracic aorta. In general, ribs 11 and 12 can be used to clamp below the diaphragm, while ribs 6–10 usually are associated with descending thoracic aortic control. The incision is carried toward the midline 4–5 cm inferior to the umbilicus to expose the iliac bifurcation.

- The subcutaneous tissue is divided, followed by the external oblique, internal oblique, and transversus abdominus muscles. The anterior and posterior rectus sheaths are carefully divided and the peritoneal is swept away medially to expose the psoas muscle. The blunt and sharp dissection is continued superiorly as the peritoneum is swept medially away from the diaphragm until the crus muscles are exposed.
  - The aorta is identified to include the visceral vessels. Large retroperitoneal venous drainage is just inferior to the aorta at the level of the visceral vessels and presents annoying bleeding if not properly preserved or judiciously ligated.
  - A decision is made to retract the left kidney to the right or dissect Gerota's fascia to allow for the kidney to be left in the retroperitoneal position.
  - The course of the left ureter is marked with a vessel loop and generally retracted to the right along with the peritoneum.
  - Control of the visceral vessels with vessel loops is dictated by the reconstruction plan. Balloon catheter occlusion is another option for visceral vessel control once the aortic sac is entered.
  - The common iliac arteries and the left external iliac artery are readily exposed from this position. Since the right external iliac is difficult to reach from this

exposure, it may be necessary to extend the midline incision further to the right or the graft may need to be extended to the right femoral artery.

- After heparin, the inflow and outflow arteries are clamped and the aortic sac is explored. Based on intraoperative findings, decisions are made for full or partial graft explant. Serial release of inflow aortic and outflow iliac clamps can help define the endoleak.

- *Transabdominal exposure from lesser sac to iliac bifurcation*:
    - Midline incision from the xiphoid process of the sternum to the superior pubic rami.
    - Peritoneum is opened and the transverse colon and omentum are eviscerated superiorly in a moist towel. The small intestine is wrapped in a bowel bag or moist towel and eviscerated to the right side exposing the ligament of Treitz. The duodenum and small intestine are retracted further to the right with the dissection.
    - The retroperitoneum is opened in a longitudinal manner to expose the left renal vein and arteries proximally and the external iliac arteries distally. Control can be obtained with standard vascular clamping techniques.
    - The inferior mesenteric artery is identified and ligated. Visible lumbar arteries are controlled with ligation clips or suture material
    - After heparin, the inflow and outflow arteries are clamped and the aortic sac is explored. Based on intraoperative findings, decisions are made for full or partial graft explant. Serial release of inflow aortic and outflow iliac clamps can help define the endoleak.

2.3 Closure

Retroperitoneal explant aortic endoleak:
- Closure of residual aortic sac with 2-0 absorbable suture
- Closure 3 layers (posterior sheath, anterior sheath, and transversus abdominis muscles) with #1 looped polydiaxanone (PDS)
- Subcutaneous tissue closure with 2-0 absorbable suture
- Skin closure with absorbable subcuticular stitch or skin staples

Transabdominal explant infected endograft:
- Closure retroperitoneum with 2-0 absorbable suture
- Omental flap if infected tissue planes present
- Closure midline fascia # 1 looped PDS
- Skin with absorbable subcuticular stitch or skin staples

3 POSTOPERATIVE

3.1 Complications

Most common complications:
- Renal failure
- Myocardial ischemia
- Anemia related to blood loss

Least common complications:
- Lower extremity ischemia/thrombo-embolus
- Graft infection

3.2 Outcomes

Stent graft endoleak:
- Definitive treatment for any aortic endoleak

Stent graft infection:
- Removal of contaminated graft implant and debridement of infected retroperitoneal tissue planes is a key component to therapy to treat what is frequently a lethal infectious condition

3.3 Follow-Up

Explant for endoleak:
- *2 weeks*: Clinic appointment for evaluation of incision
- *12 months*: Duplex ultrasound surveillance lower extremities for peripheral artery disease

Explant for infection:
- *2 weeks*: Clinic appointment to evaluate incision and antibiotic course
- *6 weeks*: CT scan of abdomen/pelvis to evaluate for findings of residual infection, clinical examination to determine need for additional antibiotics
- *4–6 months*: CT evaluation to exclude residual infection
- *12 months*: CT evaluation to exclude residual infection

3.4 E-mail an Expert

- *E-mail address*: parmstro@health.usf.edu

REFERENCES

1. Kelso RL, Lyden SP, Butler B, et al. Late conversion of aortic stent grafts J Vasc Surg. 2009;49:589-95.
2. Brinster CJ, Fairman RM, Woo EY, et al. Late open conversion and explantation of abdominal aortic stent grafts. J Vasc Surg. 2011;54:42-6.

· QUIZ

Question 1: The most critical element in planning the removal of an aortic endograft with a type 2 leak and possibly a type 1 endoleak includes:
a. Details contained with the original implant operative note
b. Current cardiac risk assessment and serum creatinine and glomerular filtration rate
c. Most recent aortogram with iliofemoral runoff
d. Preoperative triple phase (arterial, venous, noncontrast) CT scan abdomen and pelvis

Question 2: Treatment of a juxtarenal aortic stent graft with hooks for fixation and a type 2 endoleak may include all of the following *except*. (Choose best answer)
a. Ligation of bleeding lumbar and inferior mesenteric arteries with aortic sac exploration and closure
b. Ligation of bleeding lumbar and inferior mesenteric arteries with proximal graft plication and sac closure
c. Arteriogram with inferior mesenteric artery embolization and sac puncture with sac injection of gelfoam and ethylene vinyl alcohol
d. Laparoscopic clipping of lumbar branch vessels and inferior mesenteric artery

Question 3: Aortic reconstruction for a type I leak with a 1.2 cm proximal graft migration and type 2. Endoleak associated with the inferior mesenteric artery may include all of the following *except*:
a. Conversion of graft utilizing a suprarenal unibody graft that extends into the right iliac limb. Creation of a femorofemoral bypass and with contralateral iliac limb occlusion

b. Exploration of the aortic sac with proximal graft plication and ligation of the inferior mesenteric artery
c. Transection of the proximal stent graft body with interposition Dacron graft to iliac stent graft limbs
d. Aortic sac exploration with full graft body explant, ligation of aorta at the renal arteries, transection of lilac stent limbs at bifurcation with ligation of aortic bifurcation of common iliac artery origin, and axillary bifemoral bypass

Question 4: The surgical follow-up and surveillance protocol after explant of aortic stent graft includes. (Choose best answer)
a. Lifelong antiplatelet therapy in all patients with aspirin and clopidogrel
b. Six weeks of intravenous antibiotics
c. Duplex ultrasonography of the iliofemoral reconstruction 4–6 weeks after explant surgery
d. Serial CT scanning every 3 months for the first year then annually thereafter

Question 5: Potential solutions for treating an unstable patient actively bleeding from an aortoenteric erosion in a patient with a previous EVAR include:
a. Axillary bifemoral bypass with explant of aortic graft and ligation of distal aorta and iliac vessels
b. Explant of aortic stent graft and aortoiliac reconstruction using deep femoral veins
c. In situ replacement of endograft with rifampin soaked interposition graft and full explant of aortic endograft
d. All the above

ANSWERS:
1. d   2. d   3. a   4. c   5. d

Iliac Artery Conduit

Paul Armstrong

1 PREOPERATIVE

1.1 Indications

- Inadequate (small or occluded) native iliac artery conduit suitable for establishing sheath access to deliver aortic stent graft

1.2 Evidence

- Forcing a large sheath through a small vessel (femoral-external iliac) will lead to a tear.[1,2]

1.3 Materials Needed

- Dacron or polytetrafluoroethylene (PTFE) 10–12 mm graft limb

1.4 Preoperative Planning and Risk Assessment

Planning:
- Cardiology consultation and risk assessment
- Preoperative CT scan abdomen and pelvis with and without intravenous contrast to characterized the terminal aorta and bilateral iliofemoral arteries
- Duplex ultrasonography of bilateral lower extremities with ankle brachial index and toe pressures

Risk assessment:
- *Low risk:* ASA 1 or 2
- *Intermediate risk:* ASA 3
  - Previous lower abdominal surgery
  - Reoperative iliofemoral artery surgery
- *High risk:* ASA 4 or 5
  - Class III or IV angina with unreconstructable coronary disease
  - Class III or IV congestive heart failure with unreconstructable coronary disease

- Oxygen- or steroid-dependent chronic obstructive pulmonary disease (COPD)
- COPD with a forced expiratory volume in one second <30%

1.5 Preoperative Checklist

- Cardiac risk assessment
- CT angiography of aorta and iliofemoral circulation
- Duplex ultrasonography of lower extremities with ankle brachial indices/toe pressures
- Optimize nutrition
- Optimize renal function
- Type and cross-match blood products

1.6 Decision-Making Algorithm

- *See* Flowchart 26.1.

Flowchart 26.1: Decision-making algorithm.

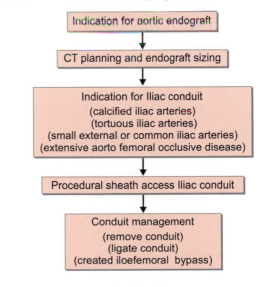

1.7 Pearls and Pitfalls

Pearls:
- The conduit should be stretched to length after creation. This can be accomplished by tunneling it to the groin or by using a sheet of Ioban to secure it to the lower extremity.
- Iliac artery calcification may determine the level of the conduit anastomosis. Conduit construction should be completed in the most normal appearing artery segment possible. If iliac arteries are to be calcified, then aortic conduit may be required.
- After conduit use should the distal external iliac artery be diseased then the conduit can be used as a bypass to the femoral vessel.

Pitfalls:
- The most difficult time to place an iliac conduit is after the artery has ruptured.
- Make as few large sheath exchanges as possible since the new suture line of the iliac anastomosis can tear or disrupt.
- Polytetrafluoroethylene grafts allow for smooth wire and catheter traversal and provides a better seal with the sheath as compared to Dacron. However, PTFE adheres to larger sheaths and does not allow for frequent smooth sheath exchanges. Dacron does allow for a smoother exchange of large sheaths but the corrugations of Dacron material can hinder smooth wire and sheath traversal.
- Large covered stents (9–12 mm) and balloon angioplasty can be used to create an iliac conduit; however, these "internal" iliac conduits are at risk for disruption or migration as delivery sheaths are exchanged. This technique should be used with caution.
- Technology demands have resulted in the first generation of balloon expandable sheaths. These sheaths have insertion profiles of 11–14 Fr and increase to sizes up to 20 Fr. They offer stability to delivery but generally require relining of the entire iliac artery upon removal, resulting in compromise of the internal iliac artery origin.

1.8 Surgical Anatomy

- *Pelvic retroperitoneum:*
  - Aortic bifurcation
  - Inferior vena cava bifurcation
  - Ureter
  - *Iliac arteries:*
    - Common
    - Internal
    - External
- *Common femoral artery:*
  - Femoral arteries

1.9 Positioning

- Supine

1.10 Anesthesia

- General endotracheal anesthesia
- Radial arterial line
- Large bore central venous access
- Autotransfusion "Cell Saver"

2 PERIOPERATIVE

2.1 Incision

- *Lower abdominal retroperitoneal exposure right or left side:*
  - Medial border rectus abdominis sheath
  - *Lateral border:* 5–7 cm medial to anterior superior iliac spine
  - *Inferior border:* 3–5 cm superior and parallel to inguinal ligament
  - *See* Figure 26.1.

2.2 Steps

- *Retroperitoneal right or left lower quadrant exposure from inguinal ligament to the iliac bifurcation:*
  - Subcutaneous tissue and muscles of anterior abdominal wall divided
  - External oblique is split in direction of its fibers
    - Internal oblique, transversus abdominus, and transversalis fascia are divided to the edge of the rectus sheath

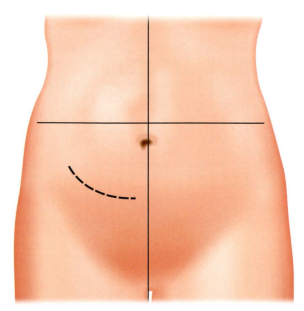

Fig. 26.1: Incision.

– Blunt dissection is used to retract the peritoneum and ureter medially
- End-to-side anastomosis of conduit with 4-0 monofilament suture to common or external iliac artery
- Tunnel conduit in subcutaneous plane to femoral incision or apply 3m Ioban drape to extend and stabilize conduit to skin. Proceed with endovascular portion of case.
- When endovascular procedure complete either transect of conduit close to anastomosis with suture ligation of conduit stump or tunnel the conduit in the retroperitoneal plane posterior to the ureter and beneath inguinal ligament and perform an end-to-side anastomosis to common femoral artery with a monofilament suture

See Figures 26.2 to 26.5.

2.3 Closure

- Closure of retroperitoneum over

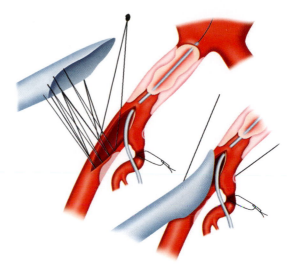

Fig. 26.2: Retroperitoneal right or left lower quadrant exposure from inguinal ligament to the iliac bifurcation.

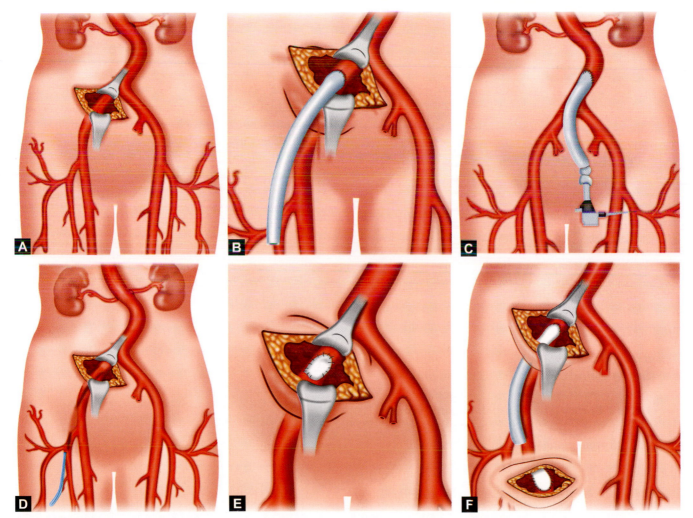

Figs. 26.3A to F: End-to-side anastomosis of conduit with 4-0 monofilament suture to common or external iliac artery.

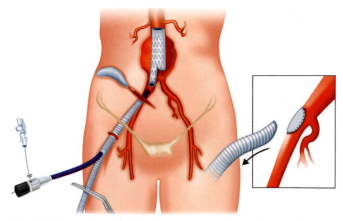

Fig. 26.4: Tunnel conduit in subcutaneous plane to femoral incision or apply 3 m loban drape to extend and stabilize conduit to skin.

- Closure transversus abdominus muscle with 2-0 absorbable suture
- Closure internal/external oblique muscles with 2-0 absorbable suture
- Closure of Scarpa's and Camper's fascia with 2-0 absorbable suture
- Skin Closure with 3-0 absorbable subcuticular stitch or skin staples

3 POSTOPERATIVE

3.1 Complications

Most common complications:
- Iliac artery or graft thrombosis
- Ureter injury

Least common complications:
- Conduit thrombosis
- Lower extremity ischemia/thrombo-embolus
- Conduit infection

3.2 Outcomes

- *Stent graft endoleak*:
  - Definitive treatment for any aortic endoleak
- *Stent graft infection*:
  - Removal of contaminated graft implant essential to treat what is often a lethal infectious condition. in order to treat infection

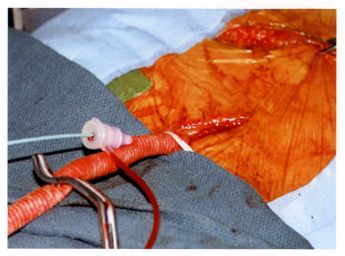

Fig. 26.5: When endovascular procedure complete either transect of conduit close to anastomosis with suture ligation of conduit stump or tunnel the conduit in the retroperitoneal plane posterior to the ureter and beneath inguinal ligament and perform an end-to-side anastomosis to common femoral artery with a monofilament suture.

3.3 Follow-Up

- *Ligation iliac conduit*:
  - *2 weeks*: Clinic appointment for evaluation of incision
  - Standard surveillance of aortic stent graft
- *Conversion conduit to iliofemoral bypass*:
  - *2 weeks*: Clinic appointment to evaluate incision and vascular examination
  - *4–6 weeks*: Duplex ultrasound examination of bypass and lower extremities
  - Annual duplex surveillance of iliofemoral bypass with clinical examination for of peripheral artery disease

3.4 E-mail an Expert

- *E-mail address*: parmstro@health.usf.edu

REFERENCES

1. Abu-Ghaida AM, Clair DG, Greenberg RK, et al. Broadening the applicability of endovascular aneurysm repair: the use of iliac conduits. J Vasc Surg. 2002;36:111-7.
2. Frank J. Criado iliac arterial conduits for endovascular access: technical considerations. J Endovasc Ther. 2007;14:347-51.

QUIZ

Question 1: Safe alternatives to sheath access for aortic endovascular stent graft deployment include all except. (Choose best answer.)
a. End-to-side anastomosis of common iliac artery conduit
b. End-to-end anastomosis of external iliac artery conduit
c. Percutaneous profunda femoris artery
d. Percutaneous femoral artery access

Question 2: If confronted with a 7-mm calcified external right iliac and 8-mm right common iliac artery with severe tortuosity and some calcification, a safe alternative to aorta access for infrarenal aortic endograft placement includes:
a. Distal aorta and common iliac artery endarterectomy.
b. Occlusion of right iliac artery occlusion and left aorta-unilateral endograft with femoral bypass.
c. Right common iliac artery conduit with attempt place aortic endograft.
d. B and C

Question 3: The most common complication associated with a left iliac arterial conduit is:
a. Conduit infection
b. Distal limb ischemia
c. Ischemia to the sigmoid colon or rectal mucosa

d. Disruption of conduit anastomosis during sheath exchange

Question 4: Indications for an external or common iliac conduit include all the following except. (Choose best answer)
a. 7-mm bilateral common iliac arteries with extensive calcification to aortic bifurcation.
b. 8 mm right tortuous iliac artery with left common iliac artery occlusion
c. Occluded right external iliac artery with 9-mm common bilateral iliac arteries.
d. 8-mm right external iliac artery with severe calcification and tortuous 9-mm common iliac artery with 3-cm aneurysm. The left external iliac artery is occluded

Question 5: After successful endograft deployment the iliac conduit can be managed by:
a. Ligation close to the anastomosis
b. Creation of a iliofemoral bypass from the right-to-left side
c. Removal of the conduit with primary artery repair
d. All of the above

ANSWERS:

1. c   2. d   3. d   4. c   5. d

SECTION

4

Visceral

Visceral Artery Bypass

Jason Jundt, Erica Mitchell

1 PREOPERATIVE

1.1 Indications

- *Acute mesenteric ischemia*:
  - Atrial fibrillation
  - Acute thrombosis of diseased artery
  - Embolization
- *Chronic mesenteric ischemia*:
  - Abdominal pain
  - Weight loss
  - Postprandial pain (abdominal angina)
  - Diarrhea
  - Food fear
  - Two of three visceral vessel occlusions

1.2 Evidence

- Open revascularization is preferred for low-risk patients, nonhostile abdomen, occlusion, severe calcification, and longer lesions.[1]
- Open surgery also has important role in the treatment of patients with extensive disease, long segment or flush occlusions, small vessel size, multiple tandem lesions, and severe calcification.[2]

1.3 Materials Needed

- Headlight
- Loupe magnification
- Self-retaining retractor set (Bookwalter or Omni retractors and various size Weitlaner retractors)
- Vascular clamp set (Debakey aortic clamp, Cherry clamp, Cooley subclavian clamp, Reverse-S aortic clamp, Profunda clamp, Satinsky clamp, Wiley hypogastric clamp)
- Vascular instrument set (various lengths and sizes of needle drivers)
- Major abdominal instrument set
- Conduit [saphenous vein graft, femoral vein graft, 6–8 mm × 40 mm or 12 mm × 6–8 mm bifurcated Dacron or polytetrafluoroethylene (PTFE) grafts]
- Polypropylene and/or PTFE suture
- Heparin saline solution (at least 10 U/mL)
- Cell saver

1.4 Preoperative Planning and Risk Assessment

Planning:
- Complete history and physical examination
- Electrocardiogram
- Echocardiogram
- Cardiac stress test
- Pulmonary function testing
- Nutritional assessment (albumin, prealbumin, preoperative parenteral nutrition)
- Laboratory testing (complete blood count, complete metabolic profile, and coagulation profile)
- Preoperative CT angiogram protocol of the chest, abdomen, and pelvis
- Preoperative visceral angiogram
- Duplex ultrasound (mesenteric duplex)
  - Superior mesenteric artery peak systolic velocity ≥ 275 cm/s[3]
  - Celiac artery peak systolic velocity ≥ 200 cm/s[3]

Risk assessment:
- Low-to-intermediate risk
  - Absence of high-risk factors
- High risk
  - Age >80
  - Severe pulmonary dysfunction
    - FEV1 <800 mL or DLCO <50% predicted
    - Resting pCO_2 >50 mm Hg or PO_2 <60 mm Hg
    - Home oxygen therapy

– Severe cardiac dysfunction
  ▪ Left ventricular ejection fraction < 25%
  ▪ New York Heart Association (NYHA) class III or IV
  ▪ Angina pectoris
  ▪ Cardiac stress test positive for myocardial ischemia
  ▪ Myocardial infarction <90 days prior to surgery
– Severe renal insufficiency (baseline Cr > 3.0 mg/dL) or dialysis dependent[4]

1.5 Preoperative Checklist

Preinduction of anesthesia (nurse and anesthetist):
- Has the patient confirmed identity, site, procedure, and consent?
- Is the site marked?
- Is the anesthesia machine and medication check complete?
- Is the pulse oximeter on the patient and functioning?
- *Does the patient have a*:
  – Known allergy?
  – Difficult airway or aspiration risk?
  – Risk of greater than 500 mL blood loss?

Before skin incision (nurse, anesthetist, and surgeon):
- Confirm all team members have introduced themselves by name and role.
- Confirm the patient's name, procedure, and where the incision will be made.
- Has antibiotics prophylaxis been given within the last 60 minutes? (Unless necrotic or perforated bowel is expected and the patient is not allergic, cefazolin is given in weight-based fashion. If allergic, then 800 mg clindamycin is the drug of choice).
- Anticipated critical events?
- *Surgeon*:
  – What are the critical or nonroutine steps?
    ▪ Administration of heparin (80–100 U/kg initial dose then 1000 U dosed on the hour)
    ▪ Mannitol administration (12.5 g/70 kg) prior to reperfusion of the intestines
    ▪ Clamping of the aorta
    ▪ Release of the aortic clamp and/or selective organ reperfusion
  – How long will the case take?
    ▪ Mesenteric bypass (3–6 hours)
  – What is the anticipated blood loss?
    ▪ Variable depending on length and difficulty (< 500 mL)
- *Anesthetist*:
  – Are there patient-specific concerns?

- *Nursing team*:
  – Has sterility been confirmed?
  – Are there equipment issues or concerns?
    ▪ Is essential imaging displayed?

Before patient leaves the operating room (nurse, anesthetist, and surgeon):
- *Nurse to confirm*:
  – Name of procedure
  – Completion of instrument, sponge and needle counts
  – Specimen labeling (read aloud, including patient name)
  – Equipment problems to be addressed
- Surgeon, anesthetist, and nurse:
  – What are the key concerns for recovery and management of this patient?[5]
    ▪ Admission to ICU
    ▪ Cardiac, respiratory and neurological monitoring
    ▪ Monitoring for bowel ischemia and urine output

1.6 Pearls and Pitfalls

Pearls:
- Infrarenal or iliac graft origin can avoid suprarenal clamp and can be combined with aortoiliac reconstruction. This is especially useful in a heavily calcified aorta.
- Antegrade bypass allows for inline flow and requires minimal dissection.

Pitfalls:
- Infrarenal or iliac graft origin can result in kinking if not oriented properly and usually requires prosthetic graft.
- Antegrade bypass requires tunneling to the SMA in a retropancreatic tunnel as well as supraceliac clamp predisposing the patient to renal ischemia and possible embolization.

1.7 Surgical Anatomy

The superior mesenteric artery is found at the root of the small bowel mesentery. When using the transperitoneal approach the SMA is exposed by releasing the ligament of Treitz and retracting the small bowel inferiorly and to the right. The celiac artery above is pictured on the other side of the transverse mesocolon. Access to the celiac artery generally requires dissection through the hepatogastric ligament (Fig. 27.1).

1.8 Positioning

The patient is placed in the supine position with arms extended. The side-rail is cleared to allow for retractor

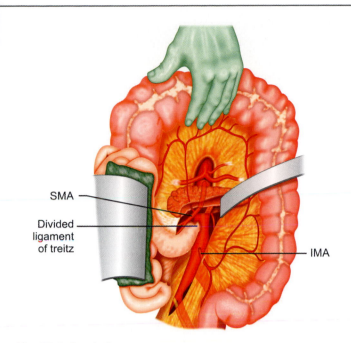

SMA

Divided ligament of treitz

IMA

Fig. 27.1: Surgical anatomy.

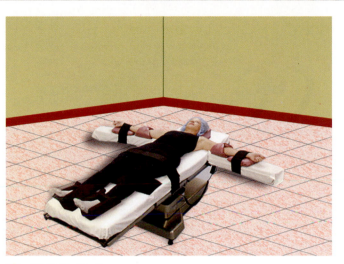

Fig. 27.2: Positioning.

placement. Anesthesia monitoring equipment is cleared from the entire chest wall and abdomen. A warming drape may be placed above the level of the nipples (Fig. 27.2).

1.9 Anesthesia

- Acute mesenteric ischemia and chronic mesenteric ischemia patients are often compensating for their underlying illness. Induction of anesthesia without proper monitoring equipment and vascular access can result in acute and rapid decompensation.
- *Aortic cross clamping*:
  - Increased afterload with proximal arterial hypertension and increased contractility, end-systolic, and end-diastolic volumes
  - Increased preload due to blood volume redistribution in supraceliac clamping but not in infraceliac clamping
  - Increased preload and afterload results in increased myocardial oxygen demand
  - Blood flow distal to the clamp is maintained by perfusion pressure and is not dependent on preload or cardiac output.[6]
- *Aortic unclamping*:
  - Unclamping hypotension
    - Central hypovolemia caused by pooling of blood into reperfused tissue distal to clamp location

- Hypoxia-mediated vasodilatation with increase in venous capacity in the extremities below the occlusion
- Accumulation of myocardial-depressant metabolites
  - Treatment of unclamping hypotension
    - Clamp for shortest period of time possible
    - Gradually release the aortic clamp
    - Careful titration of volume and vasoactive drugs[6]

2 PERIOPERATIVE

2.1 Incision

The patient is placed in the supine position with arms extended. Incision is made from the xiphoid process to below the umbilicus. If exposure is difficult, the incision and be lengthened to the pubic symphysis, although this is rarely necessary. This incision is used for antegrade and retrograde bypass techniques (Fig. 27.3).

2.2 Steps

Antegrade bypass:
- Gentle traction is applied to the transverse colon in the direction of the pubic symphysis. The gastrohepatic ligament is divided and the left lobe of the liver freed of its attachments, allowing it to be safely retracted to the right and placed beneath a retractor blade (Fig. 27.4).
- Using the intubated esophagus for guidance, the diaphragmatic crus is incised for a length of approximately

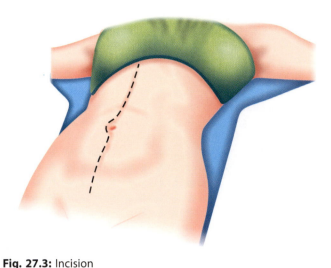

Fig. 27.3: Incision

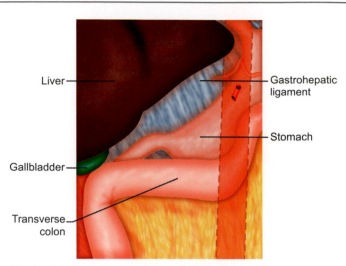

Fig. 27.4: Entry to the less sac for celiac artery exposure.

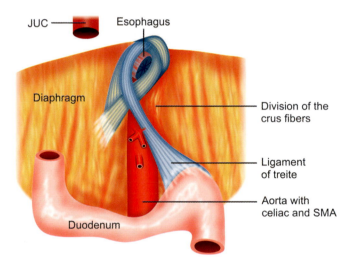

Fig. 27.5: The right and left crus of the diaphragm must be divided to expose the aorta and celiac artery.

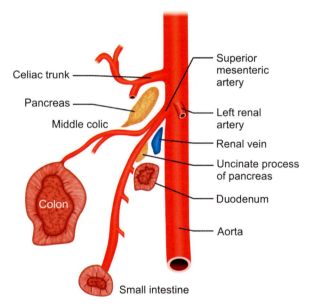

Fig. 27.6: Relationship of vessels and viscera: tunneling is along the aorta behind the pancreas.

4 cm exposing the anterior surface of the supraceliac aorta. The neural tissue overlying the celiac artery is dissected and the hepatic as well as splenic arteries are controlled with vessel loops (Fig. 27.5).

- Occasionally there is adequate superior mesenteric artery exposed above the pancreas; however, in most cases exposure is necessary at the root of the mesentery with a retropancreatic tunnel (Fig. 27.6).
- If there is no intestinal necrosis or perforation then 7 mm woven bifurcated polyester or PTFE graft may be used for antegrade bypass, especially if two vessel bypass is planned. In cases with contamination, vein graft will be necessary and most commonly the greater saphenous vein or superficial femoral vein is adequate (Fig. 27.7).

- After administration of heparin and cross-clamping of the supraceliac aorta, the proximal anastomosis is sewn to the supraceliac aorta in an end-graft to side-aorta fashion. Revascularization of the celiac axis then requires end-graft to side-common hepatic artery anastomosis. If using a bifurcated graft, the blood flow can then be restored to the celiac artery and the descending aorta with Fogarty mush clamps placed upon the limb of the graft intended for superior mesenteric artery revascularization and release of the proximal and distal clamps used for celiac revascularization (Fig. 27.8).

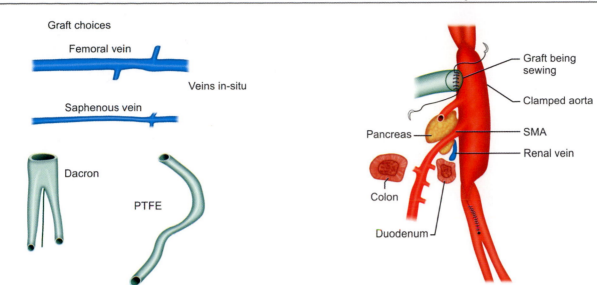

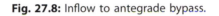

Fig. 27.7: Conduits for bypass.

Fig. 27.8: Inflow to antegrade bypass.

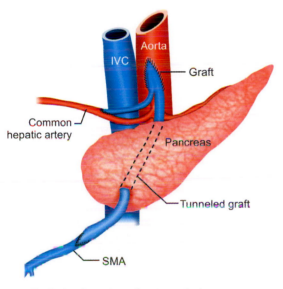

Fig. 27.9: Typical orientation of antegrade bypass.

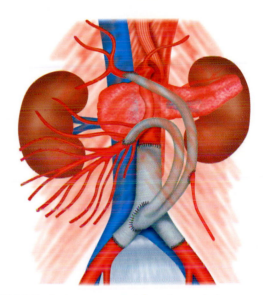

Fig. 27.10: Typical arrangement for retrograde bypass.

- The superior mesenteric artery revascularization often requires creation of a retropancreatic tunnel to bring the graft in opposition with the super mesenteric artery at an acceptable revascularization site. In cases where this is too risky due to previous pancreatic pathology, then a prepancreatic position is chosen for the graft. This positioning will place the graft in contact with the stomach and thus autologous conduit is typically used (Fig. 27.9).

Retrograde bypass:[7]

- Retrograde bypass requires inflow from the distal infrarenal aorta or common iliac artery. The operation is typically used for superior mesenteric artery revascularization (Fig. 27.10).
- Move the small bowel to the right lower quadrant and elevate the transverse colon cephalad. This will expose the duodenum. Gentle traction downward and to the right lower quadrant will expose the suspensory ligament of Treitz. The ligament of Treitz is released exposing the root of the mesentery. The superior mesenteric artery and typically be palpated in the mesentery as it emerges from under the pancreas (Fig. 27.11).
- Incise the peritoneum overlying the superior mesenteric artery at the root of the mesentery. Dissect

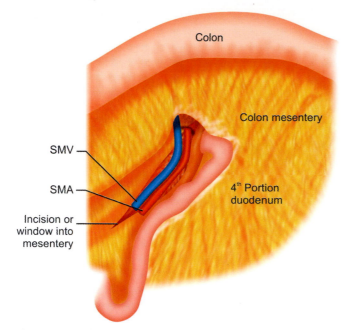

Fig. 27.11: Relationship of superior mesenteric artery and vein of the mesentery.

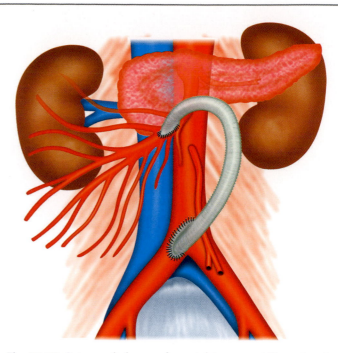

Fig. 27.12: Retrograde bypass from right common iliac artery to the superior mesenteric artery.

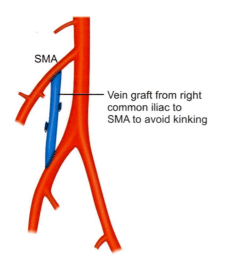

Fig. 27.13: Vein graft orientation in the setting of a bowel perforation for retrograde bypass.

proximally toward the aorta and distally to indentify jejunal branches. The superior mesenteric artery and jejunal branches are controlled with vessel loops (Fig. 27.14).

- If no intestinal necrosis or perforation then prosthetic graft is used; typically 7-mm crimped woven Dacron. The proximal anastomosis is performed to the left common iliac artery just beyond the bifurcation. The graft is passed first cephalad toward the left shoulder then turned anteriorly and inferior to be anastomosed to the anterior wall of the superior mesenteric artery. This method results in a gentle reversed "C" configuration (Fig. 27.12).

- In the presence of intestinal necrosis or perforation autologous graft is used. Greater saphenous or femoral vein is the preferred conduit but can be prone to kinking in the retrograde bypass configuration. In this situation the bypass originates on the right common iliac artery and requires a more direct route to the superior mesenteric artery with anastomosis to the posteromedial wall of the artery (Fig. 27.13).

2.3 Closure

- The retroperitoneum and ligament of Treitz are approximated with absorbable suture in both bypass situations to attempt and isolate the graft from the peritoneal cavity.

- The fascia is closed with running absorbable suture and the skin approximated with staples. If there is concern regarding the viability of bowel, the abdomen is occasionally left open with vacuum dressing in place (Fig. 27.14).[6]

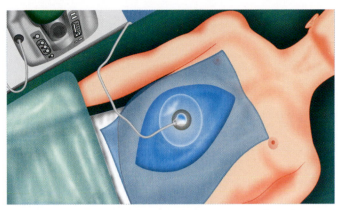

Fig. 27.14: Temporary abdominal closure can allow for rapid return to operating room for "second look" when bowel viability is questionable.

3 POSTOPERATIVE

3.1 Complications

- *Most common complications*:
  - *Systemic complications*:
    - Myocardial infarction
    - Pulmonary compromise
    - Renal failure
- *Less common complications*:
  - *Intestinal reperfusion syndrome*:
    - Rare but serious complication manifested by acidosis, pulmonary compromise, and coagulopathy
    - Treatment is given prior to restoring intestinal perfusion with administration of sodium bicarbonate and mannitol to minimize effects of metabolic acidosis and scavenge free radicals, respectively.
  - *Acute graft thrombosis*:
    - Technical error due to kinking or compression

3.2 Outcomes

- Visceral bypass has excellent patency and technical success, with reported rates of 93% at 36 months and 89% at 72 months.[8]
- Highly effective and durable therapy for chronic and acute mesenteric ischemia with 89% resolution of symptoms at 72 months.[1]

3.3 Follow-up

- *Surveillance imaging*[9]:
  - *Duplex ultrasound imaging*:
    - No guidelines regarding velocity criteria

- Recommend baseline study for patients following the operation and prior to leaving the hospital and every 6 months thereafter.
  - *Angiogram if*:
    - Markedly elevated peak systolic velocities
    - Rising peak systolic velocities on serial examinations
    - Recurrence of symptoms regardless of ultrasound evaluation
- Follow-up in 2 weeks after discharge to inspect incisions and document improvement in symptoms including nutrition
- Return to regular diet with weight gain by postoperative weeks 6–8 depending on postoperative course and complications.

3.4 E-mail an Expert

- *E-mail address*: monetag@ohsu.edu

REFERENCES

1. van Petersen A, Kolkman J, Beuk R, Open or percutaneous revascularization for chronic splanchnic syndrome. J Vasc Surg. 2010;51:1309-16.
2. Oderich G, Gloviczki P, Bower TE. Open surgical treatment for chronic mesenteric ischemia in the endovascular ear: when it is necessary and what is the preferred technique? Semin Vasc Surg. 2010;23:36-46.
3. Moneta G, Yeager R, Dalman R, et al. Duplex ultrasound criteria for diagnosis of splanchnic artery stenosis or occlusion. J Vasc Surg. 1991;14:511-20.
4. Oderich G, Bower T, Sullivan T, et al. Open versus endovascular revascularization for chronic mesenteric ischemia: risk-stratified outcomes. J Vasc Surg. 2009;49:1472-9.
5. Implementation manual WHO surgical safety checklist 2009 Safe surgery saves lives. World Health Organization publications. 2009. Available from http://whqlibdoc.who.int/publications/2009/9789241598590_eng.pdf.[Accessed August 20, 2014].
6. Gelman S. The pathophysiology of aortic cross-clamping and unclamping. Anesthesiology. 1995;82:1026-60.
7. Moneta GL. Exposure of the visceral vessels for surgical mesenteric revascularization. In: Antonino Cavallaro, Antonio V. Sterpetti, Fabrizio Barberini, Luca di Marzo (Eds). Atlas of Arterial Surgery: Basics of Anatomy and Technique. Padova: Piccin; 2012;455.
8. McMillan W, McCarthy W, Bresticker M, et al. Mesenteric artery bypass: Objective patency determination. J Vasc Surg. 1995;21:729-41.
9. Moneta GL. Screening for mesenteric vascular insufficiency and follow-up of mesenteric artery bypass procedures. Semin Vasc Surg. 2001;14:186-92.

QUIZ

Question 1. Which of the following is not a common symptom of chronic mesenteric ischemia?
a. Diarrhea
b. Nausea and vomiting
c. Weight loss
d. Abdominal angina

Question 2. Which of the following is an indication for open mesenteric bypass surgery?
a. Elderly patient with numerous comorbid conditions
b. Long segment occlusion
c. Minimal calcifications of the aorta
d. Short segment stenosis at the origin

Question 3. Please select the high risk patient from the following list:
a. 67-year-old male; EF 40%; FEV1 80% predicted
b. 79-year-old female; myocardial infarction 10 months ago; creatinine 1.1
c. 81-year-old male; no previous cardiac history, DLCO 60% predicted
d. 55-year-old female; EF 30%; FEV1 750 mL

Question 4. The WHO Surgical Safety Checklist includes all of the following except?
a. Check the pulse oximeter
b. Introduce yourself
c. State critical portions of procedure
d. The surgeon must be present for the pre-induction check

Question 5. Which of the following is true about performing a retrograde SMA revascularization with prosthetic graft?
a. The orientation of the graft is simpler
b. Dissection around the iliac arteries is avoided
c. The operation is relatively easier to perform using a familiar dissection and cross-clamping of the aorta is not necessary
d. Heavy aortic calcification is a contraindication to this procedure

Question 6. Which of the following peak systolic velocities obtained from venous duplex evaluation indicates >70% stenosis of the superior mesenteric artery?
a. 270 cm/s
b. 280 cm/s
c. 190 cm/s
d. 260 cm/s

Question 7. Aortic cross clamping causes all the following changes in cardiac function except the following?
a. Increased myocardial oxygen demand
b. Decreased afterload
c. Blood volume redistribution to the head, upper extremities, and lungs
d. Increased preload in the supraceliac clamp position

Question 8. A 55-year-old female with history of 60 packs-years of smoking, 20 pound weight loss and severe postprandial pain presents with sudden onset of severe midepigastric abdominal pain. CT angiogram demonstrates occluded SMA and celiac artery origins with a patent IMA. Following the CT angiogram the patient is found to have peritoneal signs. You take her to the operation room and are preparing to perform a retrograde SMA revascularization when you notice full thickness necrosis and perforation in the midjejunum. What is the next step?
a. Perform bypass with Dacron graft and close the abdomen
b. Abort the bypass procedure and resection the necrotic bowel
c. Staple off the bowel leaving the patient in discontinuity, perform the revascularization with vein and leave the abdomen open for second-look laparotomy
d. Resection the necrotic bowel and perform the anastomosis with Dacron graft

Question 9. The most common complication following mesenteric revascularization is which of the following?
a. Systemic complication (MI, pneumonia, or renal failure)
b. Restenosis
c. Acute thrombosis
d. Graft infection

Renal Artery Bypass with Vein

Marcus R Kret, Greg Moneta

1 PREOPERATIVE

1.1 Potential Indications

- Severe hypertension not adequately controlled with multiple medications and a hemodynamically significant renal artery lesion
- *Ischemic nephropathy*: Rapid decline in renal function and an associated hemodynamically significant renal artery lesion
- Young patients with moderate hypertension, few associated comorbidities, and a correctable lesion of the main renal artery due to atherosclerosis or fibromuscular dysplasia
- Recurrent stenosis following prior endovascular treatment
- Correction of a renal artery stenosis in conjunction with an open aortic operation to treat aortic aneurysm or aortoiliac occlusive disease
- Flash pulmonary edema
- *Contraindication:* "Prophylactic" repair of renal artery lesion in the absence of significant hypertension and/or progressive decline in renal function

1.2 Evidence

- Renal artery bypass for severe hypertension or renal salvage remains controversial.
- Two large series demonstrated improved blood pressure control in 79–85% of patients and improvement/stabilization of renal function in 76–90%[1,2]:
  - Only 8–12% of these patients were cured of hypertension (i.e. normotensive with no antihypertensive medications).
- Currently percutaneous transluminal renal artery angioplasty/stenting (PTRA/S) is generally recommended when possible as initial treatment for renal artery stenosis. In a small, single-center, prospective comparison of open revascularization versus PTRA/S[3], similar results were observed in terms of blood pressure, renal function response, as well as in overall morbidity and long-term mortality:
  - A nonsignificant trend toward improved overall primary patency at 4 years was observed in the open surgery group (88% vs 68%; *P* = .097).
- The benefit of intervention over optimal medical therapy has been challenged by the multicenter, randomized Angioplasty and STenting for Renal Artery Lesions (ASTRAL)[4] trial. The study demonstrated no clinically relevant improvements in blood pressure or renal function, nor any decrease in renal events, cardiac events or improvements in mortality attributable to percutaneous revascularization:
  - This trial included only patients whose physicians felt there was uncertainty regarding the benefit of renal artery revascularization. Therefore, patients with poorly controlled hypertension or rapidly declining renal function believed to benefit from revascularization were potentially not included in the study or included in insufficient numbers to achieve statistical benefit.
  - The Cardiovascular Outcomes with Renal Atherosclerotic Lesions (CORAL) study has also examined the efficacy of intervention for renal artery stenosis, with similar results demonstrating renal artery stenting did not add anything additional when added to comprehensive medical management in the treatment of atherosclerotic renal artery stenosis.[5]

1.3 Materials Needed

- Self-retaining retractor system
- Vascular clamps suitable for the aorta and renal arteries
- Instruments available for vein graft harvest/preparation
- 5-0, 6-0, and 7-0 polypropylene suture

1.4 Preoperative Planning and Risk Assessment

Preoperative planning:
- *Preoperative testing*:
  - *Laboratory tests*: CBC, electrolytes:
    - Consider serum and/or urinary catecholamines and cortisol levels to rule out other metabolic causes of hypertension (pheochromocytoma, Cushing's syndrome)
  - *Imaging*:
    - Duplex ultrasonography—preferred initial modality
    - Magnetic resonance angiography, computed tomography arteriography, or conventional angiography
- Required for planning a bypass procedure
- Potential for worsening renal dysfunction with indiscriminant use of contrast material
  - Conventional angiography if duplex ultrasonography suggests >60% stenosis
- Typically wait >24 hours after angiography and ensure adequate preoperative IV hydration prior to surgery.
  - *Cardiopulmonary testing*:
  - Chest X-ray
  - EKG and echocardiogram
    - Consider nuclear medicine or treadmill stress test

Low risk:
- Nonatherosclerotic renal artery disease (fibromuscular disease, Takayasu's arteritis)

Intermediate risk:
- Older age (>65)
- History of heart attack or stroke

Higher risk:
- Congestive heart failure
- Severe aortic occlusive disease
- Chronic lung disease
- Diabetes mellitus
- Chronic renal insufficiency
- Renal artery occlusion

1.5 Preoperative Checklist

Sign in:
- Radial arterial line for continuous blood pressure monitoring
- Central venous catheter for fluid/medication administration and central venous blood pressure monitoring
- Foley catheter to monitor urine output

Time out:
- *Preoperative antibiotics*: First-generation cephalosporin within 60 minutes of skin incision
- IV Heparin 50–100 units/kg IV prior to application of aortic clamp
- 25–50 g mannitol infusion prior to renal artery clamping

Sign out:
- Invasive blood pressure monitoring 24–48 hours postoperatively
- Maintain adequate postoperative hydration.

1.6 Pearls and Pitfalls

Pearls:
- The right renal artery runs posterior to the vena cava.
- Access to the distal right renal artery is facilitated by mobilization of the right colon to the left.
- Access to the proximal right renal artery can be gained between the aorta and vena cava and is more difficult, but certainly possible, from a retroperitoneal approach.
- Access to the distal left renal artery is most easily accomplished through a left retroperitoneal approach with the "left kidney up".
- Access to the distal left renal artery using a midline or transverse transabdominal approach is best achieved by mobilizing the left colon inferiorly and to the right.
- Using the right iliac artery as the inflow site for a right "aorto" renal bypass obviates the need to deal with the IVC in routing the graft to the distal right renal artery.
- Vein grafts can more readily kink when placed on the proximal aorta. A smoother course to the left renal artery is facilitated by anastomosis to the aorta several centimeters below the origin of the native renal artery.
- Incorporating a side branch into the heel of the vein graft anastomosis to the aorta or iliac artery will help prevent kinking of the vein graft at its origin.
- Spatulated end-to-end anastomosis of a vein graft to the renal artery is often technically easier for the distal anastomosis than a side-to-side anastomosis.

Pitfalls:
- Accessory right renal arteries may be encountered inferior to the main renal artery traveling anterior to the vena cava.
- Avoid using small caliber veins for conduit. A 6-mm prosthetic graft is perfectly acceptable conduit for a renal artery bypass in an adult.
- Routing vein grafts underneath the vena cava to the right renal artery induces unnecessary complexity to the operation.

1.7 Surgical Anatomy

- Depiction of renal arterial and venous supply with shaded depiction of overlying abdominal organs (Figs. 28.2 to 28.7).

1.8 Positioning

- *Midline transperitoneal approach*:
  - Supine with arms extended bilaterally
  - Pillow or roll beneath knees with subtle "frog-leg" to facilitate vein graft harvest
  - Preoperative vein mapping to select the best saphenous vein and mark the course of the vein on the skin
- *Left retroperitoneal approach*:
  - Left side up at 30–45° angle (facilitated by bean bag)
  - Hips rotated to provide groin exposure/leg access for vein graft harvest.
  - Pillow or roll placed beneath knees with subtle "frog-leg" to facilitate vein graft harvest.
  - Preoperative vein mapping to select the best saphenous vein and mark the course of the vein on the skin

1.9 Anesthesia

- General endotracheal anesthesia

2 PERIOPERATIVE

2.1 Incision

- *Midline transperitoneal approach*:
  - Midline incision from xiphoid to several centimeters below the umbilicus

  - Alternatively, a transverse infraumbilical incision from the tip of the 12th rib bilaterally also provides good transperitoneal exposure of the renal arteries.
- *Left retroperitoneal approach*:
  - Beginning over the 11th rib at the midaxillary line, the incision extends inferomedially toward the lateral border of the rectus abdominus muscle inferior to the umbilicus (Fig. 28.1)
  - After the abdominal wall muscles are divided, the peritoneum is separated from the inner surface of the abdominal wall.

2.2 Steps

- *Midline transperitoneal approach*:
  - Exposure of the proximal left renal artery is begun by retracting the small bowel to the right side of the abdomen and the transverse colon cephalad. The left renal vein is mobilized and retracted using a vessel loop. Usually cephalad retraction works best:
    - The posterior peritoneum overlying the aorta is incised, and the distal duodenum is retracted to the right. This may require division of the ligament of Treitz. The peritoneal incision is extended laterally to expose the plane posterior to the tail of the pancreas (Fig. 28.2).
    - The left renal artery typically lies posterior to the left renal vein. The vein is retracted either superiorly or inferiorly, depending on which provides better access to the artery. Full exposure of the

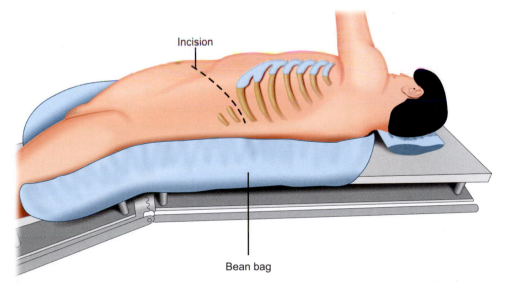

Fig. 28.1: Positioning for retroperitoneal exposure to the abdominal aorta and left renal artery.

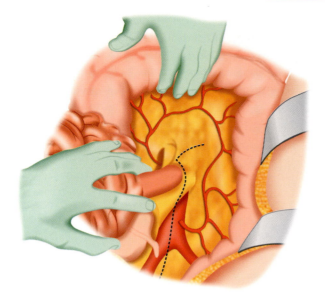

Fig. 28.2: Transperitoneal exposure of the abdominal infrarenal aorta and left renal artery begins with mobilization of the transverse colon superiorly and the small bowel to the right.

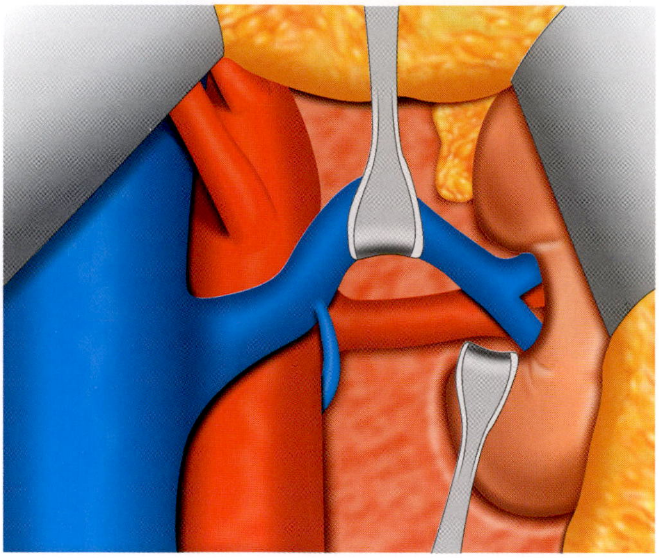

Fig. 28.3: Superior retraction of the left renal vein to expose the left renal artery.

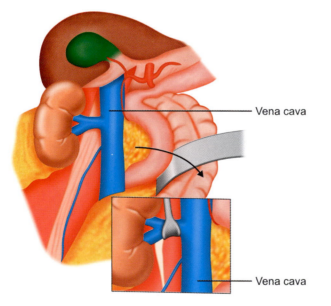

Fig. 28.4: The right colon and duodenum are mobilized medially and the right renal vein is mobilized superiorly to expose the midial and distal right renal artery.

left renal artery may require ligation and division of the left adrenal and gonadal veins to provide adequate mobilization of the left renal vein (Fig. 28.3).

– *The right renal artery courses posterior to the vena cava:*

- It can be exposed proximally through the base of the small bowel mesentery. Ligation and division of 2 or more pairs of lumbar veins may be required to adequately retract the vena cava to the right of midline. Further visualization is facilitated by cephalad retraction of the left renal vein.
- Exposure of the distal right renal artery is accomplished via medial mobilization of the ascending colon and duodenum. The renal vein lies anterior to the artery and is retracted cephalad to expose the artery (Fig. 28.4).

– Bilateral renal artery exposure is facilitated by complete cephalad mobilization of the right colon and small bowel along the right lateral peritoneal reflection.

– Bypass from the aorta to the right, left, or bilateral renal arteries with saphenous vein requires vein of appropriate length and typically >4 mm in diameter:
  - *End-to-side anastomosis*: The end of saphenous vein to side of renal artery anastomosis is completed first.

• Proximal and distal control of the renal artery is obtained with Silastic vessel loops. Tightening the loops allows control for creation of the anastomosis:

– The renal artery intima is easily injured therefore many surgeons prefer judiciously applied small vascular clamps on the renal artery to achieve control.

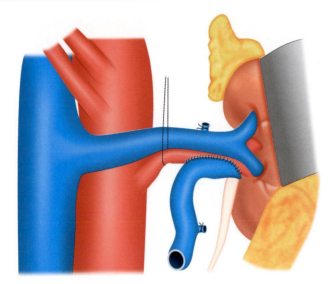

Fig. 28.5: Arteriotomy.

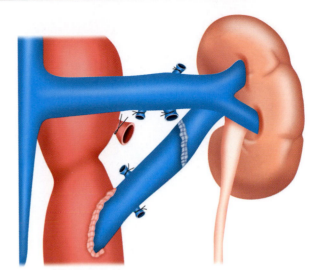

Fig. 28.6: The renal artery and vein graft are cut to appropriate length and spatulated.

- An arteriotomy is created with a #11 blade and extended with Potts' scissors to a length —two to three times the diameter of the vein graft. The anastomosis is sewn with 6-0 polypropylene suture (Fig. 28.5).
- Inflow to the kidney is re-established and the graft is occluded with a bulldog or Heifetz clamp.
- The aorta is clamped below the renal arteries and above the inferior mesenteric artery. On the left, the vein graft is positioned posterior to the left renal vein, whereas on the right, the vein graft is typically tunneled posterior to the vena cava.
- *An aortotomy is created and the anastomosis completed with 6-0 polypropylene suture*:
  - *End-to-end anastomosis*: The proximal aortic anastomosis is performed first to limit renal ischemia time.
- The aorta is clamped below the renal arteries and the saphenous vein graft sewn to the aorta as described above. The vein graft is controlled with a bulldog or Heifetz clamp, and the aortic clamp is removed.
- The native renal artery is ligated proximally with 2-0 braided permanent suture and transected.
- The renal artery and vein graft are cut to appropriate length and spatulated. Right and left renal artery bypasses are tunneled as described above. An end-to-end anastomosis is created with 6-0 polypropylene suture (Fig. 28.6):
  - *Extra-anatomic bypass from the common hepatic artery to the right renal artery may be utilized for bypass to the right renal artery*:

- The approach may be via a midline or subcostal incision.
- *A Kocher maneuver is performed to expose the inferior vena cava and right renal pedicle*:
  - The common hepatic artery is controlled within the hepatoduodenal ligament using vessel loops.
- The gastroduodenal artery is ligated and divided near its origin from the hepatic artery:
  - The right renal artery and vein are controlled with vessel loops.
  - Beginning at the amputated stump of the gastroduodenal artery, a saphenous vein graft is sewn to the hepatic artery in an end-to-side fashion using 6-0 polypropylene suture. The distal end is controlled with a bulldog clamp.
  - The right renal artery is ligated and divided near its origin from the aorta.
  - The proximal end of the renal artery is spatulated and sewn in an end-to-end fashion to the saphenous vein graft (Fig. 28.7).
- *Left retroperitoneal approach*:
  - Peritoneum retracted anterior and to the right, while the plane between left colon and left kidney is developed.
  - Dissection continues superiorly to expose left renal vein, which is mobilized to expose the aorta. Distal dissection extends to the origin of the inferior mesenteric artery:
    - The right renal artery may be accessed via a left retroperitoneal approach, though additional

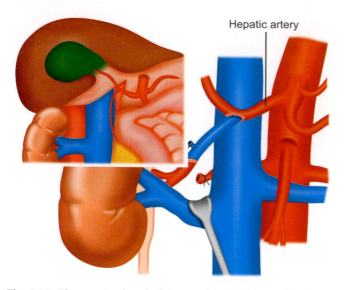

Hepatic artery

Fig. 28.7: The proximal end of the renal artery is spatulated and sewn in an end-to-end fashion to the saphenous vein graft.

anterior, cephalad and right-sided dissection may be required.

– If concurrent aortic replacement in required, proximal control of the aorta is achieved below the involved renal artery or arteries unless there is a juxtarenal component to the aneurysm that would require suprarenal clamp to perform the proximal aortic anastomosis. Distal control may be obtained between the level of the renal arteries and the inferior mesenteric artery:

▪ If a suprarenal clamp is required, saphenous vein grafts should be sewn to the aortic tube graft prior to aortic cross-clamping to minimize renal ischemia times.

– When aortic replacement is not required, the proximal anastomosis between the saphenous vein graft and aorta is created on the infrarenal aorta. Clamps can be applied proximally below the renal arteries and distally above the level of the inferior mesenteric artery. An aortotomy two to three times the diameter of the vein graft is created. The vein graft is spatulated and the anastomosis is created with 5-0 monofilament polypropylene suture. After the proximal anastomosis is completed, the graft(s) is/are flushed of debris and controlled with a small bulldog or Heifetz vascular clamp.

– The right renal artery is further dissected and controlled distally with a curved Cooley clamp. The

proximal artery is ligated with 2-0 permanent braided suture and divided near its origin on the aorta. Prosthetic grafts to the right renal artery are typically tunneled in a retrocaval position to avoid contact with the duodenum. However, vein grafts can generally be placed anterior to the vena cava without major adverse effects.

– The anastomosis is created with 6-0 monofilament polypropylene suture. Prior to completion of the anastomosis, the clamp on the proximal vein graft is temporarily released to flush any debris from the lumen. The clamps are removed and the anastomosis inspected for hemostasis.

– The left renal artery anastomosis is completed in similar fashion. Alternatively, an anastomosis from end of vein to side of renal artery can be created using vessel loops to obtain proximal and distal control of the renal arteries.

2.3 Closure

• *Midline transperitoneal approach*:
  – The posterior peritoneum is closed using 3-0 braided absorbable suture in a running fashion.
  – The abdominal fascia is closed in the midline using #1 slow-absorbing monofilament suture.
  – Skin is closed with staples.
• *Left retroperitoneal approach*:
  – The abdominal fascia is closed using #1 slow-absorbing monofilament suture.
  – Skin is closed with staples.

3 POSTOPERATIVE

3.1 Complications

• *Common complications*:
  – *Cardiovascular*: arrhythmia (5–9%), myocardial infarction (3%), stroke (1–2%)
  – *Pneumonia*: 7.5%
  – *Postoperative renal insufficiency requiring permanent dialysis*: 4–9%
• *Rare complications*:
  – Vein graft aneurysm
  – Graft-enteric fistula
• *Operative mortality*:
  – 3.3–8% in series from high volume centers[1,2,6]
  – 10% in large administrative database.[7]

3.2 Outcomes

- *Hypertension*: cured (8–12%), improved (73–85%), worsened (15–21%)
- *Renal function*:
  - Improved (42–76%), unchanged (41–47%), worsened (10–24%)
  - Dialysis eventually required in 15–38% of long-term survivors
  - *5-year dialysis free survival*: 50%[8]
- *Graft patency*:
  - *At 4–5 years*: primary patency 80–88%, secondary patency 87–90%
- *5-year overall survival*: 52–69%
  - Most deaths due to cardiovascular disease
  - 5-year survival 94% for fibromuscular disease or Takayasu's arteritis.

3.3 Follow-up

- Renal artery duplex prior to hospital discharge
- Office follow-up for wound check in 2–3 weeks
- Repeat office visit with surveillance renal artery duplex every 3 months for 1 year, yearly thereafter.

3.4 E-mail an Expert

- *E-mail address*: monetag@ohsu.edu

SUGGESTED READING

Benjamin ME, Dean RH. Techniques in renal artery reconstruction: Part I. Ann Vasc Surg. 1993;10:306-14.

Benjamin ME, Dean RH. Techniques in renal artery reconstruction: Part II. Ann Vasc Surg. 1993;10:409-14.

Calligaro KD, Dougherty MJ. Renal Artery Revascularization. In: Ascher E (Ed). Haimovici's Vascular Surgery, 6th edition. Chichester, West Sussex: Wiley-Blackwell; 2012.

Ham SW, Kumar SR, Wang BR, et al. Late outcomes of endovascular and open revascularization for nonatherosclerotic renal artery disease. Arch Surg. 2010;145(9):832-9.

Levy MM, Kiang W, Johnson JM, et al. Saphenous vein graft aneurysm with graft enteric fistula after renal artery bypass. J Vasc Surg. 2008;48:738-40.

Reilly JM, Rubin BG, Thompson RW, et al. Revascularization of the solitary kidney: A challenging problem in a high risk population. Surgery. 1996;120:732-7.

Saifi J, Shah DM, Chang BB, et al. Left retroperitoneal exposure for distal mesenteric artery repair. J Cardiovasc Surg. 1990; 31:629-33.

Wind GG, Valentine RJ. Anatomic Exposures in Vascular Surgery, 3rd edition. Philadelphia: Lippincott, Williams and Wilkins; 2013.

Zarins CK, Gewertz BL. Atlas of Vascular Surgery, 2nd edition. Philadelphia: Elsevier; 2005.

REFERENCES

1. Cambria RP, Brewster DC, L'Italien GJ, et al. Renal artery reconstruction for the preservation of renal function. J Vasc Surg. 1996;24:371-82.
2. Cherr GS, Hansen KJ, Craven TE, et al. Surgical management of atherosclerotic renovascular disease. J Vasc Surg. 2002;35:236-45.
3. Balzer KM, Pfeiffer T, Rossbach S, et al. Prospective randomized trial of operative vs interventional treatment for renal artery ostial occlusive disease (RAOOD). J Vasc Surg. 2009;49
4. ASTRAL investigators. Revascularization versus medical therapy for renal-artery stenosis. N Engl J Med. 2009;361: 1953-62.
5. Cooper CJ, Murphy TP, Cultip DE, et al. Stenting and medical therapy for atherosclerotic renal artery disease. N Engl J Med 2014; 370:13-22.
6. Darling RC, Shah DM, Chang BB, et al. Retroperitoneal approach for bilateral renal and visceral artery revascularization. Am J Surg. 1994;168:148-51.
7. Modrall JG, Rosero EB, Smith ST, et al. Operative mortality for renal artery bypass in the United States: Results from the National Inpatient Sample. J Vasc Surg. 2008;48:317-22.
8. Marone LK, Clouse WD, Dorer DJ, et al. Preservation of renal function with surgical revascularization in patients with atherosclerotic renovascular disease. J Vasc Surg. 2004;39:322-9.

QUIZ

Question 1. What percentage of patients will be cured of hypertension (i.e. normal blood pressure with no antihypertensive medications) as a result of renal artery bypass?

a. <15%
b. 33%
c. 50%
d. >85%

Question 2. In the usual anatomic configuration, the renal artery is typically found .... to the left renal vein.

a. Cephalad
b. Caudad
c. Superficial
d. Deep

Question 3. Based on single institution studies, what is the expected 5-year dialysis-free survival following renal artery bypass?

a. 25%
b. 40%
c. 50%
d. 80%

Question 4. Surveillance following renal artery bypass is best achieved using:

a. Renal artery duplex-ultrasonography
b. Contrast CT angiography
c. Magnetic resonance angiography
d. Clinical monitoring of blood pressure and renal function

chapter 29

Aortorenal Endarterectomy

Tod M Hanover, Mark P Androes, John Eidt

1 PREOPERATIVE

1.1 Indications/Contraindications

- The frequency of open renal revascularization has decreased in concert with the rise of endovascular alternatives.

General indications for renal revascularization (open or endovascular):

- Uncontrollable hypertension and significant unilateral or bilateral renal artery stenosis
- Ischemic nephropathy and significant bilateral renal artery stenosis or unilateral stenosis with a solitary kidney
- Flash pulmonary edema and/or refractory heart failure associated with renovascular hypertension
- Loss of functional renal mass associated with significant renal artery stenosis

Indications for open surgical renal revascularization:

- Anatomy not suitable for endovascular therapy (e.g. multiple small renal arteries, early primary branching of the main renal artery or plaque extending into the mid or distal renal artery)
- Failed endovascular procedure
- Aortic surgery adjacent to the renal arteries (e.g. aneurysm repair or aortoiliac occlusive disease) with indication for renal revascularization

Indications for endarterectomy:

- Renal artery plaque localized to the origins of the renal arteries
- Multiple small renal arteries

Contraindication to renal revascularization:

- Asymptomatic renal artery stenosis (prophylactic renal revascularization)
- Medically-controlled hypertension
- End-stage renal disease as suggested by severe renal atrophy (<6–7 cm length) and/or elevated renal resistive index (>0.8)

Contraindication to endarterectomy:

- Renal plaque extending into the mid or distal renal artery
- Patient unable to tolerate aortic occlusion
- Aneurysm involving renal arteries (relative)

1.2 Evidence

- Atherosclerotic renovascular disease may be associated with severe hypertension and decreased renal function.
- Atherosclerotic renovascular disease is predictive of cardiovascular morbidity and mortality.
- There are limited data to guide therapy. In particular, there are no level one studies (large, prospective, randomized) that directly compare treatments of atherosclerotic renovascular disease.
- Uncontrolled data suggest that select patients with significant renal artery stenosis may benefit from surgical revascularization: uncontrolled hypertension, flash pulmonary edema, and rapid decline in renal function.[1]

1.3 Materials Needed

- Self-retaining abdominal retractor (e.g. Omnitrac or Bookwalter)
- Intraoperative Duplex Ultrasound (15/7.5 MHz linear array probe), sterile sheath with coupling gel
- *Prosthetic grafts*: Dacron, polytetrafluoroethylene
- Standard vascular surgical set
- Preoperative vein mapping if vein patch or venous conduit anticipated

1.4 Preoperative Risk Assessment

It is critical to identify significant patient-specific risks prior to surgical revascularization

- *Cardiac*: Due to the consequences of long-standing hypertension, most patients should be evaluated for underlying cardiac disease. Echocardiography is recommended to evaluate signs of left ventricular hypertrophy and global pump function. Patients with symptomatic cardiac disease should undergo comprehensive cardiac assessment according to current recommendations for aortic surgery.

- *Renal*: Every effort should be made to normalize or improve renal function prior to surgery. In particular, nephrotoxic drugs including iodinated contrast should be avoided in the preoperative period
- Perioperative medications including statins, β-blockers, anticoagulants, and antiplatelet agents should be appropriately managed.
- Significant volume contraction is common secondary to chronic diuretic therapy and preoperative hydration should be considered.
- *Anatomic risks*: Due to the complexity of renal revascularization, preoperative imaging should be of high quality and provide views of the aorta and all visceral arteries. In addition, the quality of potential donor vessels (atherosclerotic plaque, calcification, and thrombus) should be evaluated.

1.5 Preoperative Checklist

- In addition to the identity of the patient, the side of planned renal reconstruction must be consistent with preoperative notes and imaging, and confirmed by verbal consent of the patient.
- Confirm availability of cross-matched blood and cell saver (if needed).
- Review with anesthesia team plans regarding the anticipated level of aortic clamping, administration of vasopressors, and renal protective medications.

1.6 Decision-Making Algorithm

- *See* Flowchart 29.1.

1.7 Pearls and Pitfalls

Pearls:
- The renal artery should be sufficiently mobilized to allow eversion of the renal artery into the aorta.
- Avoid excessive traction on the plaque to prevent fracture prior to completion of the endarterectomy.
- A compliant balloon catheter may be inserted into the renal artery and retracted toward the aorta to facilitate visualization of the endpoint of the endarterectomy.
- Intraoperative duplex may be used to confirm technical success.

Pitfalls:
- Avoid endarterectomy in aorta or renal artery that is frankly aneurysmal.
- Endarterectomy is discouraged in the setting of heavy calcification in the renal artery or aorta since the remaining adventitia may be very thin and structurally unsound. Conversion to a renal artery bypass may be indicated in this setting.
- Avoid blind avulsion endarterectomy. Every effort should be made to visualize the distal endpoint of the plaque.
- Isolated transrenal endarterectomy is discouraged.

1.8 Surgical Anatomy

- The kidneys and renal arteries are located in the retroperitoneum along with the overlying pancreas and duodenum (Fig. 29.1A).
- The renal arteries are deep to the renal veins (Fig. 29.1B).

1.9 Positioning

- Supine position is most commonly used for aortorenal intervention (Fig. 29.2A).
- Left flank approach allows single cavity abdominal exposure which is useful when performing transaortic endarterectomy for combined renal and mesenteric disease (Fig. 29.2B).

1.10 Anesthesia

- Preoperative hydration
- General anesthesia
- Radial arterial line
- Pulmonary artery catheter and/or transesophageal echo as applicable
- Establish diuresis prior to aortic clamping with Mannitol 12.5–25 g IV and repeat as needed to maintain diuresis
- Anticoagulation with heparin 100 u/kg prior to clamping aorta and monitored to maintain therapeutic aPTT (250–290s)

2 PERIOPERATIVE

2.1 Incision

- Midline incision allows extensive dissection of aorta for combined aorta and renal procedures (Fig. 29.2A).
- Left flank incision for retroperitoneal or transabdominal exposure may be an advantage in obese patients, those with multiple previous abdominal surgeries, and allows aortic clamping at any level (Fig. 29.2B).

Flowchart 29.1: Algorithm for the treatment of symptomatic atherosclerotic renovascular disease.

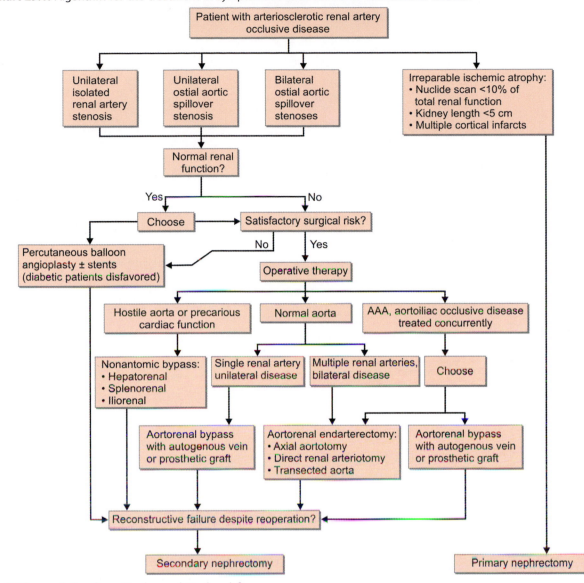

Source: With permission from Stanley and Upchurch.[2]

2.2 Steps

Step 1: Transverse colon is reflected cephalad and the small bowel retracted to the patient's right (Fig. 29.3A).

Step 2: The duodenum is mobilized by incising the peritoneum overlying the aorta and dividing the ligament of Treitz. The underlying aorta and left renal vein are exposed by dividing the periaortic fat and lymphatic tissue. Large lymphatics should be ligated. Ligation of the lumbar, gonadal, and adrenal veins allow for mobilization of the left renal vein for enhanced exposure of the left renal artery. The upper limit of dissection with this approach

is defined by the origin of the superior mesenteric artery (Fig. 29.3B).

Step 3: The left renal vein is mobilized by dividing the left adrenal vein superiorly, the left gonadal vein inferiorly, and the lumbar vein posteriorly. Additional small venous tributaries should be carefully dissected and divided to avoid avulsion with retraction (Fig. 29.3C). The aorta and left renal artery are mobilized sufficiently to facilitate eversion of the renal artery.

Step 4: Access to the proximal portion of the right renal artery is gained by mobilization of the inferior vena cava (Fig. 29.3D). This is accomplished by dividing the lumbar

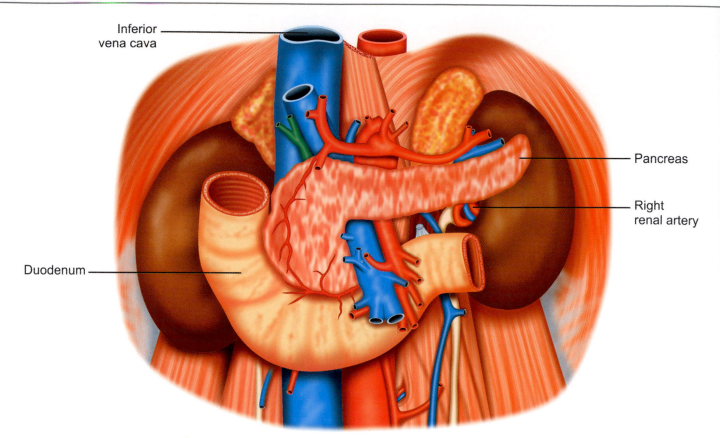

Fig. 29.1A: (A) Overlying retroperitoneal viscera. Duodenum, pancreas, and IVC are superficial to the right renal artery.

branches of the IVC and retraction of the IVC to the right taking care to avoid excessive traction on the junction between the left renal vein and the IVC.

More extensive exposure of the mid and distal right renal artery is obtained by incising the white line of Toldt of the cecum and ascending colon (Brasch-Cattell maneuver) and retracting the right colon and small bowel toward the chest (Fig. 29.3E). The duodenum is mobilized (Kocher maneuver) allowing cephalad retraction of the right colon, small bowel, duodenum, and pancreas. Avoid excessive retraction on the origin of the SMA to prevent avulsion or intimal dissection (Fig. 29.3F).

Step 5: After systemic heparinization, (80–100 u/kg), the aorta is cross-clamped proximal and distal to the intended endarterectomy. A curvilinear aortotomy is made with an 11 blade and Potts scissors (Fig. 29.3G). Traction sutures in the cut edge of the aorta may be used to facilitate visualization of the renal orifices. If the plaque is confined to the origin of the renal arteries, an endarterectomy plane is developed at the junction of the plaque and the normal aortic wall. More commonly, a discrete boundary between the renal plaque and more diffuse aortic disease cannot be defined, and it is necessary to initiate the endarterectomy by circumferentially inscribing the origin of the renal artery with a 15 blade (Fig. 29.3H). Occasionally, the severity of the aortic plaque will necessitate cylindrical endarterectomy of the entire visceral aortic segment including the renal arteries. Aortic endarterectomy continuing into the renal artery is then performed. Care must be taken to ensure that the integrity of the residual aortic wall is maintained. The eversion of the renal artery is accomplished as the first assistant gently grasps the renal artery distal to the plaque and everts it into the aorta. The distal endpoint of the plaque can be identified by using a combination of gentle traction on the plaque combined with eversion of the mobilized renal artery (Fig. 29.3I).

Transaortic renal endarterectomy may be performed through either a longitudinal aortotomy (Figs. 29.3J and K) or transverse aortotomy that extends into the origins of the renal arteries (Fig. 29.3L). The transverse aortotomy has the theoretical advantage of allowing visualization of the distal endpoint of the renal plaque. However, due to the time required for patch closure of the transverse

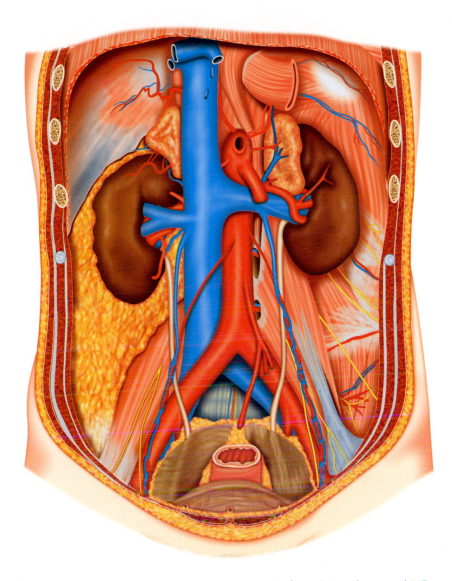

Fig. 29.1B: (B) Exposed IVC and aortic anatomy. From the anterior approach, the right renal vein and IVC are mobilized to approach the right renal artery, and the left renal vein is mobilized with division of branches as needed to approach the left renal artery and origin of the right renal artery.

aortotomy, the longitudinal technique is preferred. The longitudinal arteriotomy also permits endarterectomy of multiple accessory renal arteries.

Combined aortic and renal disease. Aortic occlusive or aneurysmal disease combined with renal disease can be approached through a transverse infrarenal aortotomy. If additional exposure is needed for visualization of the renal orifices, a longitudinal aortotomy may be extended proximal to the renal arteries. As depicted previously, the left renal vein and IVC are mobilized to allow access to the renal arteries. After wide mobilization of the renal arteries, eversion endarterectomy of the origins of

the renal arteries is performed. The aortic graft is then beveled for an end-to-end anastomosis. The renal arteries should be back bled and clamped prior to aortic flushing to minimize the risk of embolization of atherosclerotic debris (Figs. 29.3M to O). The aortic clamp is then replaced in an infrarenal position, taking care to avoid clamping the polypropylene suture that can weaken or fracture the suture.

Combined mesenteric and renal disease (Figs. 29.3L and M). Transaortic mesenteric and renal endarterectomy is usually performed through a flank approach. Left medial visceral rotation (Mattox maneuver) is performed by dividing the lateral peritoneal attachments of the left colon and spleen (Fig. 29.3P). The left colon, spleen, and tail of the pancreas are rotated medially allowing access to the entire abdominal aorta. The left kidney is usually not mobilized (Fig. 29.3Q). The left crus of the diaphragm may be incised to allow supraceliac aortic exposure and control. The celiac, SMA and left renal arteries are sufficiently mobilized to allow eversion into the aorta during endarterectomy. Exposure is usually limited to the origin of the right renal artery. All visceral arteries are controlled with vessel loops to prevent back bleeding and assure excellent visibility. Dense perivisceral neural and lymphatic tissue is common when exposing the origins of the celiac and SMA. Care should be taken to avoid avulsion of small phrenic branches arising at the base of the celiac artery.

Combined mesenteric and renal disease (Figs. 29.3N to P). Prior to clamping, diuresis is established with mannitol and systemic anticoagulation with heparin. Proximal and distal control is confirmed. Lumbar arteries can be controlled with hemoclips or ties prior to aortotomy. A curvilinear incision is made in the aorta starting approximately 1–2 cm proximal to the celiac artery and extending to just between the renal arteries in the midline. It is important to leave sufficient distance between the aortotomy

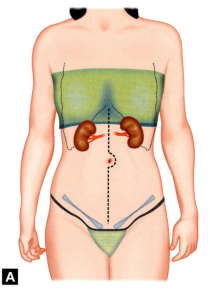
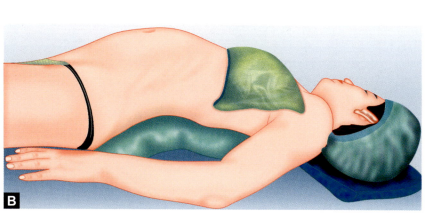

Figs. 29.2A and B: (A) Supine position. (B) Left flank position.

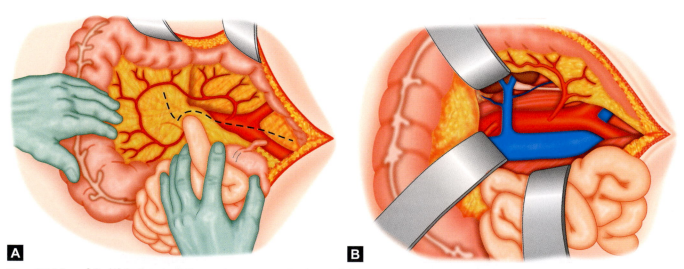

Figs. 29.3A and B: (A) Incise posterior peritoneum at the base of the mesentery. (B) IVC and aortic exposure.

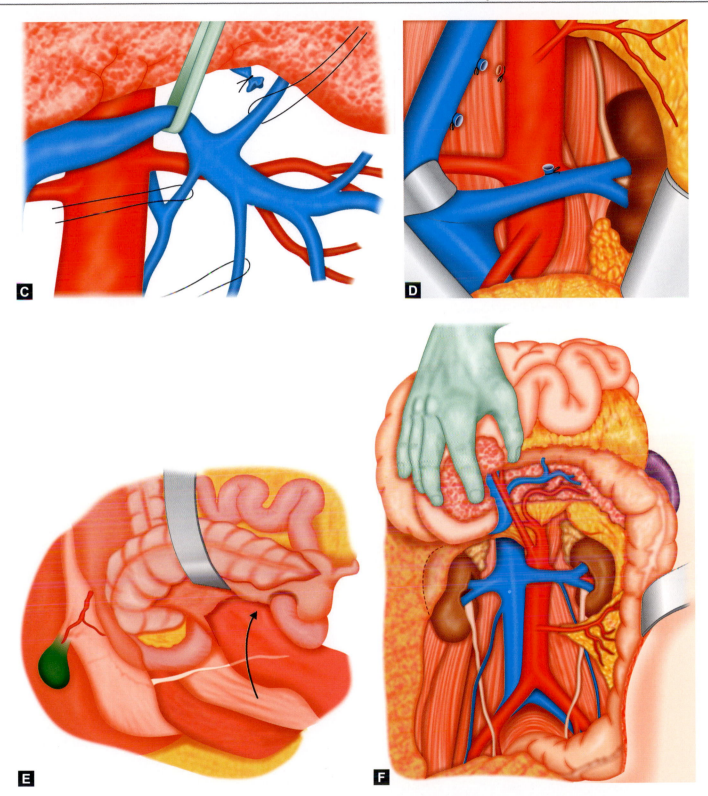

Figs. 29.3C to F: (C) Branches of left renal vein are divided for mobilization of the vein and exposure of the left renal artery. (D) Mobilize the inferior vena cava (IVC) for exposure of the proximal right renal artery. (E) Right visceral rotation. Reflect the right colon medially and perform Kocher's maneuver to allow exposure of entire right renal artery and kidney. (F) Extensive exposure obtained for bilateral renal artery reconstruction by mobilization of the cecum and ascending colon.

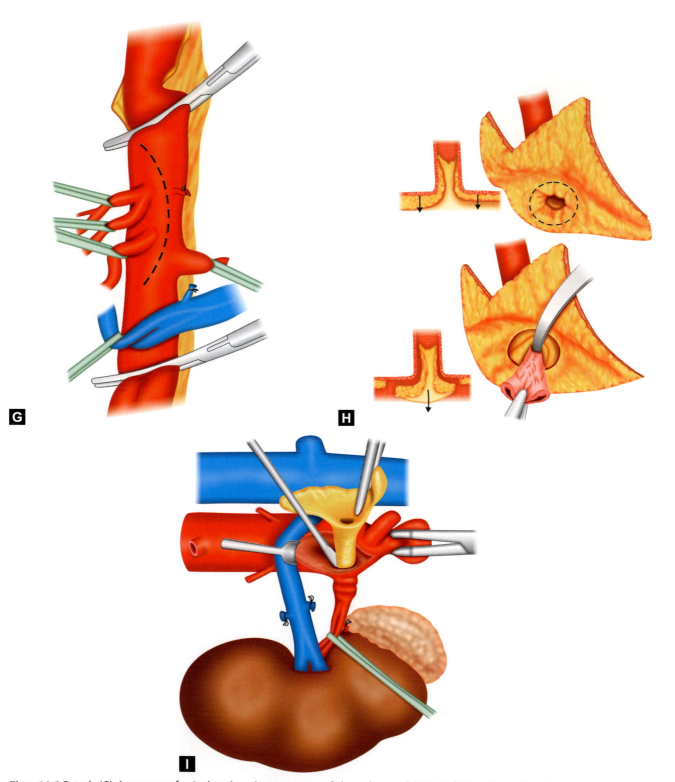

Figs. 29.3G to I: (G) Aortotomy for isolated endarterectomy of the celiac and SMA. Additional renal endarterectomy accomplished with extention of aortotomy inferiorly. (H) Sharply inscribe plaque circumferentially to initiate endarterectomy plane. (I) Distal endpoint visualized with gentle traction on the plaque and eversion of the renal artery into the aorta. Transaortic endarterectomy may be accomplished through longitudinal aortotomy.

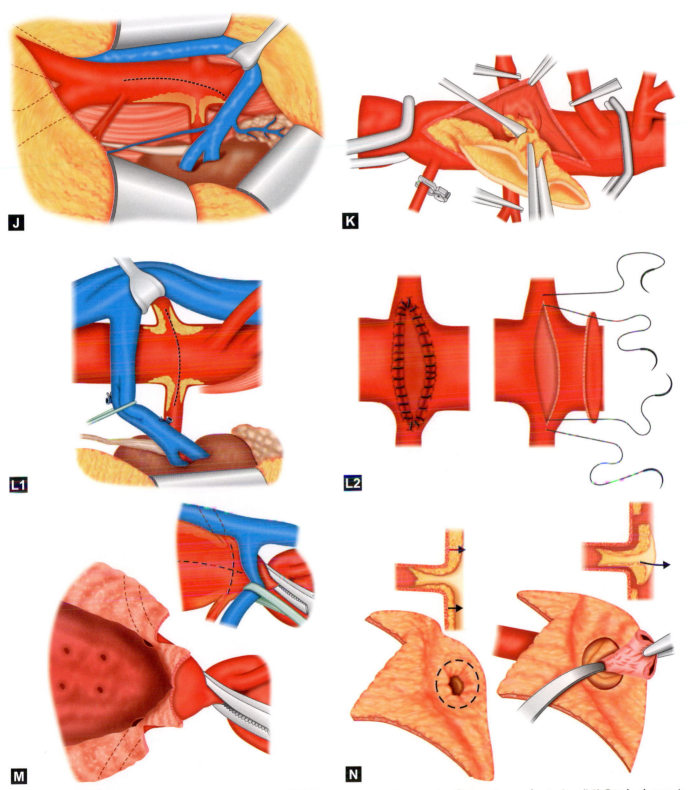

Figs. 29.3J to N: (J and K), or transverse aortotomy. (L1) Transverse aortotomy extending onto renal arteries. (L2) Patch closure is recommended to avoid narrowing renal arteries. (M and N) Infrarenal transverse aortotomy for infrarenal aortic occlusive disease may be combined with a longitudinal incision proximal to the renal orifice.

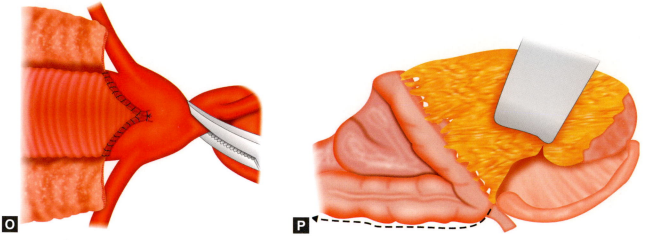

Figs. 29.3O and P: (O) Aortic graft is then beveled for end to end anastomosis. Renal arteries are back bled and occluded prior to flushing the aorta. (P) Combined mesenteric and renal endarterectomy approached through a left flank incision by dividing the lateral peritoneal attachments and reflecting the left colon, spleen, and tail of the pancreas medially.

and the orifices of the visceral arteries to accommodate the suture line without encroachment on the lumen of the visceral arteries (Fig. 29.3R). Bolus infusion of cold normal saline or Ringer's lactate into the renal arteries may be performed. An endarterectomy plane is developed and eversion of the plaque from the visceral and renal vessels is performed (Fig. 29.3S). Precision is more important than speed. After back-bleeding and flushing, the aortotomy is closed with running 5-0 Prolene (Fig. 29.3T).

2.3 Closure

- Intraoperative duplex evaluation performed with a 15.0/7.0 MHz probe:
  - Minor defect <60% diameter-reducing stenosis <200 cm/sec, peak systolic velocity (PSV)
  - Major defect >60% diameter-reducing stenosis >200 cm/sec, PSV and turbulent waveform
  - Occlusion no Doppler signal
- Major defects are found in 10% of cases and required revision
- Fascial closure performed in a standard fashion[2]

3 POSTOPERATIVE

3.1 Complications

- Most common complications:
  - Myocardial infarction
  - Renal failure
  - Graft thrombosis

  - Stroke
  - Arrhythmia
  - Pneumonia
- Least common complications:
  - Death

3.2 Outcomes

- Perioperative mortality 3% to 8%
- Increased perioperative mortality with combined aortic and renal revascularization
- Perioperative complications 7% to 30%
- Postoperative renal function
  - Improved 26% to 58%
  - Worsened 3% to 27%
  - Dialysis 4%
- Hypertension
  - Up to 85% improved or cured[1,3]

3.3 Follow-Up

- Duplex scanning is performed if deterioration in the control of hypertension or renal function occur
- Scan in early morning after overnight fast.
- Unsatisfactory visualization of the renal arteries occurs in 10% to 24% of reported series and most commonly is secondary to obesity, ileus, or postsurgical scarring.
- Positive results include increased PSV >200 cm/s and renal to aortic ratio >3.5; decreased diastolic flow may represent distal disease or flap, or increased renovascular resistance.

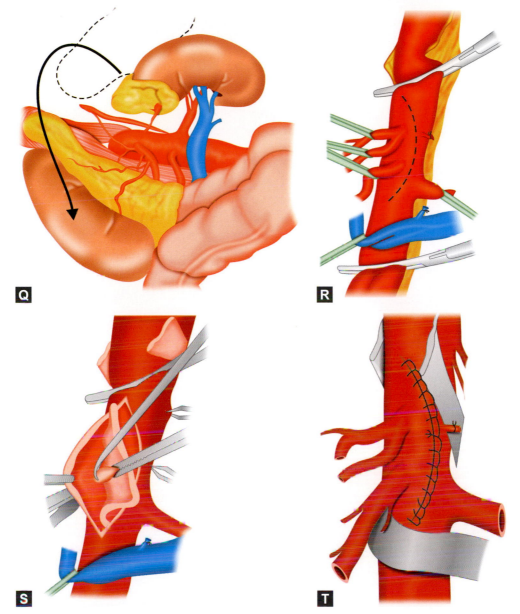

Figs. 29.3Q to T: (Q) Left kidney is not mobilized. Crus of diaphragm incised for supraceliac control. (R) Aortotomy begins cephalad to celiac and extends to renal arteries. Leave sufficient distance between aortotomy and visceral orifice to avoid visceral luminal encroachment with closure. (S) Endarterectomy with eversion of the plaque from the visceral and renal arteries. (T) Aortotomy closure with 5-0 prolene.

- Poor visualization, abnormal duplex, or worsening HTN or renal function warrants arteriogram or CTA.[4]

3.4 E-mail an Expert

- *E-mail address*: jeidt@ghs.org

3.5 Web Resources/References

- www.uptodate.com

REFERENCES

1. Edwards MS, Corriere MA. Contemporary management of atherosclerotic renovascular disease. J Vasc Surg. 2009;50: 1197-210.
2. Stanley JC, Upchurch GR. Renovascular occlusive disease: treatment. Decis Making Vasc Surg. 2001;247.
3. Hansen KJ, Deitch JS. Transaortic mesenteric endarterectomy. Surg Clin North Am. 1997;77(2): 397-407.

4. Cherr GS, Hansen KJ, Craven TE, et al. Surgical management of atherosclerotic renovascular disease. J Vasc Surg. 2002;35:236-45.

5. Eidt JF, Fry RE, Clagett GP, et al. Postoperative follow-up of renal artery reconstruction with duplex ultrasound. J Vasc Surg. 1988;8:667-73.

6. Benjamin ME, Dean RH. Techniques in renal artery reconstruction part 1. Ann Vasc Surg. 1996;10(3):306-14.

7. ACC/AHA 2005 Practice guidelines for the management of patients with peripheral vascular disease. Circulation. 2006; 113:e463-654.

QUIZ

Question 1. While performing an aortogram with runoff for claudication, the right renal artery is found to have a 70% stenosis at the origin. The patient has hypertension well controlled on one medication. What is the appropriate course of action?

a. Refer to a cardiologist for renal artery stent placement
b. Refer to a vascular surgeon for renal artery reconstruction
c. Either A or B is appropriate
d. Continue best medical care

Question 2. A 60-year-old male is scheduled for an aortobifemoral bypass for aortoiliac occlusive disease. He also has bilateral 60% renal artery stenosis. His creatinine is normal and he is not hypertensive. What is the best option?

a. Obtain intraoperative renal ultrasound and if >80% stenosis repair renal arteries

b. Perform bilateral renal artery endarterectomy at the time of ABF
c. Do not repair the renal arteries
d. Refer to cardiologist to stent the renal arteries preoperatively

Question 3. Bilateral renal artery endarterectomy is performed. Intraoperative duplex reveals left renal artery PSV 120 cm/s and right renal artery PSV 300 cm/s at the endarterectomy endpoint. Appropriate care includes:

a. Right renal arteriotomy, tack down the endpoint and perform angioplasty closure of the right renal artery
b. Aortotomy and repeat eversion endarterectomy of renal artery
c. Renal artery is patent and no further intervention or evaluation is warranted
d. Repeat renal duplex in 1 month, and if significant stenosis remains, renal stent at that time

ANSWERS: 1. d   2. c   3. a

Splenic Aneurysm Repair

Rachel C Danczyk, Greg Moneta

1 PREOPERATIVE

1.1 Indications

Nearly all splenic artery aneurysms warrant repair because of their potential for rupture, however, indications generally are based on diameter and symptoms:[1-3]

- Enlarging or >2 cm asymptomatic aneurysms
- Any ruptured or symptomatic aneurysm (e.g. epigastric pain, left upper quadrant pain, and back pain)
- Pregnant women or women of childbearing age
- Planned liver transplantation
- Pseudoaneurysm of any size
- Presence of portal hypertension

1.2 Evidence

Repair is aimed at preventing or treating rupture:

- Incidence of rupture is unknown.
- Mortality associated with rupture is ≥25%.
- Pregnancy is associated with 20% to 50% of ruptures and maternal/fetal mortality rates are >80% when associated with splenic aneurysm rupture.

1.3 Materials Needed

- Materials needed vary based upon the therapeutic approach chosen.
- Options include open aneurysm repair, endovascular embolization, or stent-graft repair depending on the size and location(s) of the aneurysm(s).
- Special materials to be considered are:
  - Endoscopic vascular stapler
  - Endoscopic harmonic scalpel (Ethicon)/LigaSure (Covidien)
  - *N*-butyl-2-cyanoacrylate (for glue embolization, alone or with coils)

- Balloon-expandable covered stent graft or self-expanding covered stent graft, 5–6 Fr guiding catheter system

1.4 Preoperative Risk Assessment

The overall risk of elective aneurysm repair should be <0.5% to proceed electively:

- *Low-intermediate risk*:
  - Age <50
  - Women of childbearing age
  - Asymptomatic, stable aneurysm
- *High risk*:
  - Extensive comorbidities (CHF, recent MI, pulmonary hypertension)
  - Ruptured aneurysms
  - Pregnant women
  - Portal hypertension

1.5 Preoperative Checklist

Special considerations to add to the Surgical Safety Checklist:

- *Sign in*:
  - Anticipate blood loss, especially if ruptured or aneurysm enlarging
  - Perinatology/OB-GYN may potentially need to participate in management if patient is pregnant
- *Time out*:
  - Discuss critical events including exposure of aneurysm, gaining proximal and distal control
  - Imaging available for review
- *Sign out*:
  - Postanesthesia laboratories including hematocrit and screening for coagulopathy
  - Coordinate resuscitation with anesthesia and critical care teams.

1.6 Surgical and Interventional Approaches

- If ruptured and hemodynamically unstable, usually proceed with emergent open surgical repair (ligation ± splenectomy)
- If ruptured and hemodynamically stable, can consider embolization, stent-graft repair, or open surgical repair (ligation ± splenectomy)
- If not ruptured, can consider multiple therapeutic approaches
  - Proximal/mid-arterial
    - Open exclusion
- Proximal/distal ligation
- Aneurysmectomy (if within the pancreas)
  - Laparoscopic exclusion
  - Embolization
  - Stent graft
  - Distal/hilar
    - Embolization (single aneurysm and distal flow preserved)
    - Open exclusion + splenectomy
    - Laparoscopic exclusion + splenectomy

1.7 Pearls and Pitfalls

Pearls:
- Proximal and mid-arterial ligation does not usually require distal revascularization or splenectomy due to the presence of collateral flow to the spleen from the short gastric arteries.
- If there are multiple distal aneurysms at or within the hilum, splenectomy is generally the preferred approach.
- Distal pancreatectomy may be required at the time of splenectomy.
- Embolization or stent grafts are a good option in those patients who cannot tolerate an open operation. Catheter-based techniques are associated with lower morbidity and mortality than open surgical techniques.[3]
- Laparoscopic splenectomy can also be considered for those patients with distal aneurysms who desire a less-invasive approach.

Pitfalls:
- Patients with aneurysmal disease due to Ehlers–Danlos syndrome should be treated with careful ligation to avoid rupture associated with a normal-appearing artery.
- Stent grafts should be placed only if arterial tortuosity is not prohibitive to prevent migration of the graft or recanalization of the aneurysm.
- If distal pancreatectomy is performed, a surgical drain should be considered to control enzymatic secretions from the pancreatic parenchyma.

- Postembolization syndrome (pain, fever, nausea, pancreatitis, and pleural effusion) should be expected in 20–30% of patients undergoing embolization. This usually resolves without sequelae.

1.8 Surgical Anatomy

- *See* Figure 30.1.

1.9 Positioning

- Supine for open splenic aneurysm repair or for endovascular repair
- Forty-five-degree right semidecubitus position for laparoscopic splenic aneurysm repair (Fig. 30.2)

1.10 Anesthesia

- Anticipate blood loss
- Provide adequate pressure point padding to avoid nerve injury

2 PERIOPERATIVE

2.1 Open Surgical Repair of Splenic Artery Aneurysm

This section covers open surgical exclusion of splenic artery aneurysms.[1]

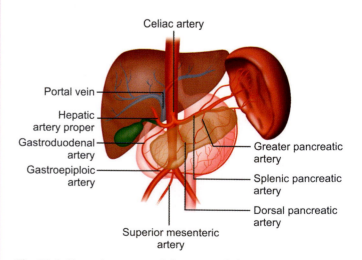

Fig. 30.1: Normal anatomy of the upper abdomen illustrating the splenic artery and its branches.

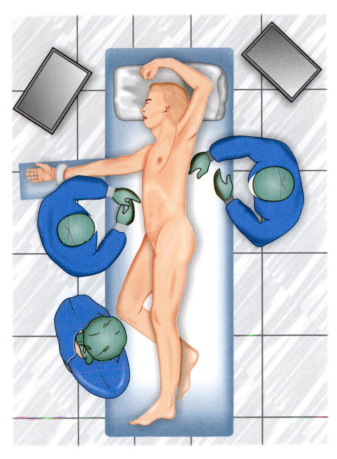

Fig. 30.2: Patient positioned in 45° right semidecubitus position for laparoscopic exclusion/splenectomy.

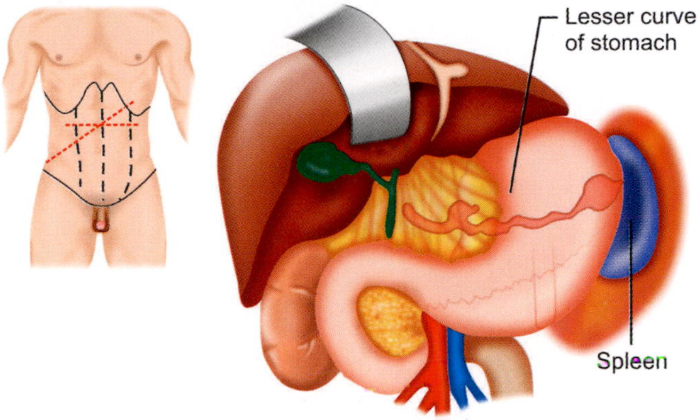

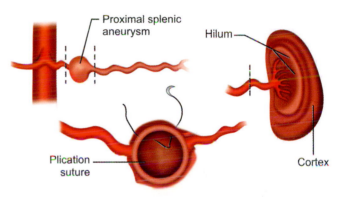

Fig. 30.3: Surgical approaches for open repair of splenic artery aneurysms can include vertical midline, chevron, or left subcostal incisions. The specific exposure chosen depends on the location of the aneurysm.

Fig. 30.4: Surgical exclusion of splenic artery aneurysms vary based upon location.

Incision and Exposure

- Central or mid-splenic aneurysms can be approached either via vertical midline or chevron incisions. Distal splenic artery aneurysms are best approached via a left subcostal incision (Fig. 30.3).
- Once within the peritoneum, access to the proximal splenic artery is gained by opening the lesser sac. Access to the midsplenic artery can be approached by elevating the pancreas cephalad or caudad depending on the relationship between the pancreas and the aneurysm. Aneurysms in the distal artery or hilum can be exposed by mobilizing the spleen (Fig. 30.3).

Exclusion

- Proximal aneurysms can be ligated without arterial reconstruction. Once exposed, bulldog clamps can be applied proximally and distally. An endoscopic vascular load stapler device can be used to transect the artery proximal and distal to the aneurysm. Alternatively, the ligation can be performed using suture ligatures (Fig. 30.4).
- Midsplenic aneurysms, which are embedded in the pancreas, can be treated by ligating the artery from within the aneurysm following vascular control proximal and distal to the aneurysm (Fig. 30.4).
- Distal splenic aneurysms, especially those within the splenic hilum, often are best treated by splenectomy. With the spleen mobilized to gain exposure, the endoscopic vascular load stapler device can then be used to transect the distal splenic artery and the spleen can be removed (Fig. 30.4).

Closure

- A standard, layered closure of the abdomen can be performed using either permanent or absorbable suture material.

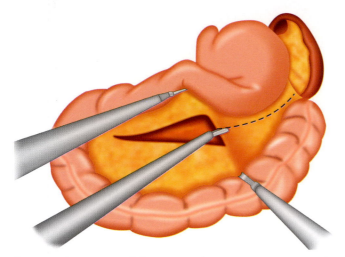

Fig. 30.5: Transection of the gastrocolic omentum to access the lesser sac.

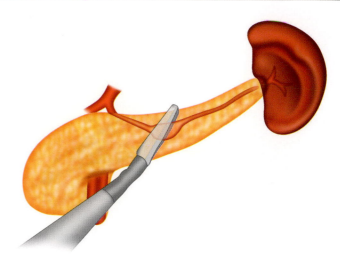

Fig. 30.6: Laparoscopic Doppler ultrasonography (US) can be used to identify the aneurysm and its tributaries. Confirmation of exclusion can also be performed after ligation of the aneurysm.

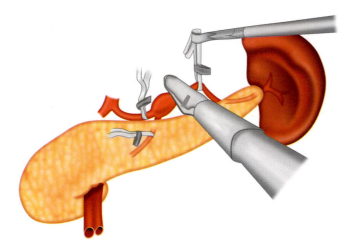

Fig. 30.7: Exclusion of a splenic aneurysm using an endoscopic vascular load stapler device Umbilical tape or vessel loops can be used to aid in ligation.

2.2 Laparoscopic Repair of Splenic Artery Aneurysms

This section covers laparoscopic surgical exclusion of splenic artery aneurysms.[4,5]

Incision

- Four trocars are placed with the patient positioned as shown in Figure 30.2. Two 12-mm trocars, one 10-mm trocar, and a 5-mm trocar (for assistance) are chosen.

- A 10-mm, 30-degree laparoscope is used for visualization.

Exposure of the Splenic Aneurysm

- The lesser sac is entered to gain exposure of the splenic artery (Fig. 30.5).
- Proximal or mid-splenic aneurysms can be ligated without arterial reconstruction. Once exposed, vessel loops or umbilical tape can be applied proximally and distally. Alternatively, vascular bulldogs can be applied. An endoscopic vascular load stapler device can be used to transect the artery proximal and distal to the aneurysm (Figs. 30.6 and 30.7).
- Distal splenic aneurysms, especially those within the splenic hilum, can be treated by aneurysmectomy and splenectomy. With the spleen mobilized laterally, the endoscopic vascular load stapler device can be used to transect the distal splenic artery and the spleen can be removed using a specimen retrieval bag (Fig. 30.8).

Closure

- The fascial defects associated with 12-mm trocar sites should be closed using 0-Vicryl suture. These sites can be closed using a Carter Thomason inlet closure device (Fig. 30.9) or anteriorly using standard closure techniques.
- Skin incisions may be closed with absorbable suture with or without skin glue.

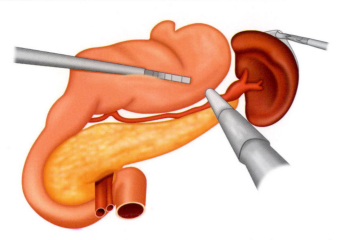

Fig. 30.8: Laparoscopic aneurysmectomy and splenectomy is indicated for distal or hilar aneurysm disease. An endoscopic vascular load stapler device is shown here.

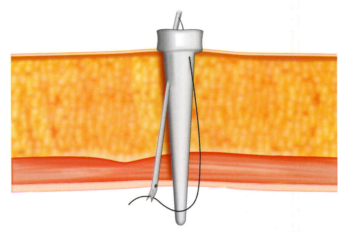

Fig. 30.9: The Carter Thomason-CloseSure System (Cooper Surgical, Inc.).

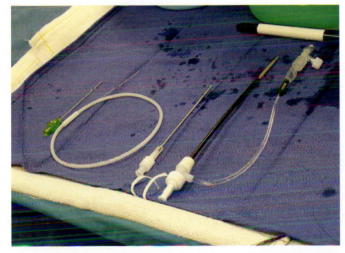

Fig. 30.10: Micropuncture access kit with 20-gauge access needle, 18-G floppy-tipped wire, dilator, and 5 Fr sheath with side port.

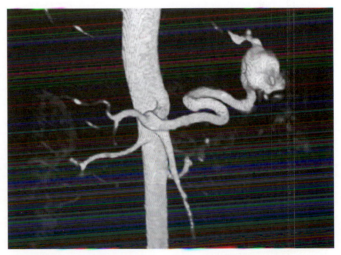

Fig. 30.11: Saccular aneurysm of the splenic artery (arrow).

2.3 Endovascular Repair of Splenic Artery Aneurysms

This section covers endovascular embolization and stent-graft placement for treatment of splenic artery aneurysms.

Access

- Right percutaneous femoral artery access with micropuncture kit (Fig. 30.10)
- Placement of an 8 Fr sheath to allow for angiography
- Selective angiogram of the splenic artery is performed (Fig. 30.11)

Exclusion

- Using a guidewire and 5 Fr catheter, the efferent artery is accessed and the guide wire exchanged for a stiff wire.
- Transcatheter embolization method-embolization coils are placed distal and proximal to the neck of the aneurysm ("sandwich" technique)[3] (Fig. 30.12).
- *Stent-Graft Method*: A balloon expandable stent graft is loaded onto the wire, advanced and inflated, bridging the aneurysmal neck. Self-expanding stent grafts can also be chosen if the artery is tortuous at the location of the aneurysm (Fig. 30.13).[6]

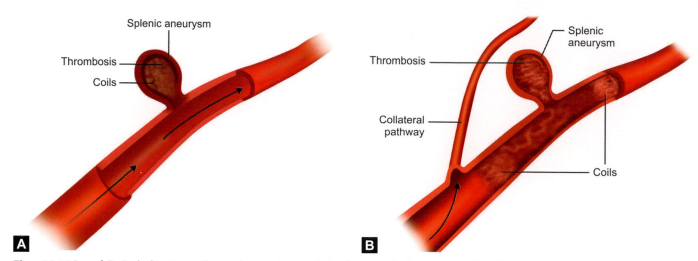

Figs. 30.12A and B: Embolization coils can be used to exclude the pseudo-/aneurysm either by placing coils within the sac (A) or by placing coils distal and proximal to the aneurysm sac, causing thrombosis of the aneurysm (B).

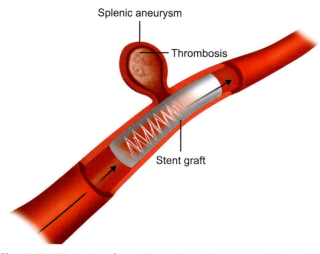

Fig. 30.13: A stent graft can be employed to successfully exclude blood flow from the pseudo-/aneurysm sac while maintaining flow through the splenic artery.

- Completion angiography is performed to demonstrate exclusion of the aneurysm.
- *N*-butyl-2-cyanoacrylate can also be used as an adjunct to coiling aneurysms or can be substituted for coils.

Closure

- Open access
  - Closure of superficial femoral artery with interrupted 5–0 or 6–0 Prolene sutures
  - Incision closed in three layers–two layers of absorbable suture, subcuticular skin suture, and skin glue

- Percutaneous access
  - Closure with percutaneous closure device of choice
  - Manual pressure

3 POSTOPERATIVE

3.1 Complications

In addition to the common postprocedure complications (wound infection, DVT, PE, etc.), these are specific complications associated with splenic aneurysm repair:[1,3]

Most common complications:
- Postembolization syndrome
- Splenic infarction
- Recanalization after endovascular intervention
- Pancreatitis

Least common complications:
- Pancreatic fistula
- Splenic/subphrenic abscesses
- Postsplenectomy sepsis

3.2 Outcomes

- Risk of rupture significantly decreased
- Shorter length-of-stay with endovascular or laparoscopic approaches

3.3 Follow-Up

- Postsplenectomy vaccinations (*Streptococcus* pneumoniae, *Hemophilus* influenzae, *Neisseria meningitidis*) prior to discharge for those patients who have undergone splenectomy. There is no reported data to support vaccinations for those patients who undergo catheter-based treatment and experience splenic infarction; however, the risk of vaccination is low and can be considered on a case-by-case basis.[3]

- Clinic visit 2–3 weeks after procedure for inspection of incision(s).
- Postembolization/stent-graft CT angiogram at 3,6,12, 24 months; if no change at 24 months, can extend imaging to every 2–3 years thereafter.[7]
- No follow-up imaging required for open/laparoscopic repair.

3.4 E-mail an Expert

- *E-mail address*: monetag@ohsu.edu

REFERENCES

1. Stanley JC, Upchurch GR, Henke PK. Treatment of splanchnic and renal artery aneurysms. In: Zelenock, et al. (Eds). Mastery of Vascular and Endovascular Surgery. Philadelphia: Lippincott Williams & Wilkins; 2006. pp. 177-8.
2. Rockman C, Maldonado T. Splanchnic artery aneurysms. In: Cronenwett J, Johnston W (Eds). Rutherford's Vascular Surgery, 7th edition. Philadelphia, PA: Saunders; 2010. pp. 2140-55.
3. Madoff DC, Denys A, Wallace MJ, et al. Splenic arterial interventions: anatomy, indications, technical considerations, and potential complications. Radiographics. 2005; 25:S191-211.
4. Arca MJ, Gagner M, Heniford T, et al. Splenic artery aneurysms: methods of laparoscopic repair. J Vasc Surg. 1999; 30:184-8.
5. Poulin EC. Laparoscopic surgery of the spleen. In: Soper NJ, Swanstrom LL, Eubanks WS (Eds). Mastery of Endoscopic and Laparoscopic Surgery. Philadelphia: Lippincott Williams & Wilkins; 2009. pp. 395-409.
6. Rossi M, Rebonato A, Greco L, et al. Endovascular exclusion of visceral artery aneurysms with stent-grafts: technique and long-term follow-up. Cardiovasc Intervent Radiol. 2008;31(1):36-42. Epub 2007 Oct 6.
7. Lakin, RO, Bena JF, Sarac TP, et al. The contemporary management of splenic artery aneurysms. J Vasc Surg. 2011; 53:958-65.

CHAPTER 31

Endovascular Treatment of Renal Artery Aneurysm

John Eidt, Bruce Gray

Most renal artery aneurysms (RAA) are discovered during the workup for hypertension or as an incidental finding with abdominal imaging. The natural history of RAA is poorly defined. Most renal aneurysms are small, asymptomatic and do not warrant treatment other than observation. While many remain asymptomatic, some renal aneurysms are associated with pain, hematuria, hypertension, and rupture. Rupture may result in marked hematuria, arteriovenous fistula formation, or retroperitoneal hemorrhage. RAA are most commonly atherosclerotic, post-traumatic, or mycotic. Others may be associated with fibromuscular dysplasia, Ehler–Danlos syndrome, vasculitis, or neurofibromatosis. Endovascular treatment has become the primary approach for most RAA because most have a saccular morphology. Fusiform aneurysms at the bifurcation and main RAA aneurysms that are not amenable to stent graft exclusion might be more ideally treated with open surgical techniques. The goals of therapy are to prevent rupture and preserve renal function.

1 PREOPERATIVE

1.1 Indications/Contraindications

- *Indications*:
  - Asymptomatic aneurysm > 1.5–2.0 cm in diameter; without delay in women of childbearing age
  - Symptomatic aneurysm of any size
  - Pseudoaneurysm of any size
- *Contraindications*:
  - Occluded (thrombosed) aneurysm
  - Aneurysm that with endovascular treatment would sacrifice significant renal parenchyma

1.2 Evidence and Classification System

- Recent data (since 2008) consists of retrospective observational studies and case reports of ~200 patients treated with coil embolization, balloon assisted coil embolization, stent assisted coil embolization, glue embolization, and stent graft exclusion. There are no prospective comparative trials comparing endovascular strategies to open surgical repair nor between each of these strategies. The reported technical success rates are +95% with a combination of these strategies.
- Classification system[1-5]
  - Type 1 RAAs are saccular aneurysms arising from the main renal artery or a large segmental branch and are particularly amenable to stent graft treatment.
  - Type 2 RAAs are fusiform aneurysms frequently involving branch points of the renal artery and therefore usually requiring open repair due to the risk of losing renal parenchyma.
  - Type 3 RAAs are distal aneurysms that can be treated with coil embolization without danger of sacrifice of significant parenchyma.

1.3 Materials Needed

- Fluoroscopic imaging capable of high quality contrast studies with iodinated contrast
- Intravascular ultrasound or optimal coherence tomography catheter (0.014" compatible)
- Preshaped sheath (5 or 6 Fr), catheters, and wires (0.035" and 0.014") appropriate for renal anatomy (Figs. 31.1)
- Complete array of bare and covered stents (balloon-expandable and self-expandable)
- Coils (0.035", 0.021", and 0.018"), detachable
- *N*-Butyl cyanoacrylate, ethylene vinyl copolymer glue (Onyx, ev3 Inc., Plymouth, MN), or gelfoam

1.4 Preoperative Assessment of the Risk of Adverse Aneurysm-related Event

- *Low risk*:
  - Calcified RAA

– Aneurysm in main renal artery (Rundback type I)
– Normal glomerular filtration rate (GFR) (>60 cm/s)
• *Intermediate risk*:
– Symptomatic RAA, but hemodynamically stable
– Aneurysm in small segmental or intralobar artery (Rundback type III)
– Mild-moderate reduction in GFR (30–60 cm/s)
• *High risk*:
– RAA in patient with connective tissue disease (Ehlers–Danlos syndrome) or unstable symptomatic RAA
– Aneurysm in proximal artery bifurcation (Rundback type II)
– Severe reduction in GFR (<30 cm/s) or solitary functioning kidney

1.5 Preoperative Checklist

Sign in:
– Patient has confirmed identity, site, procedure, and consent
– Identify significant allergies (iodinated contrast) and premedicate if present
– Serum creatinine measured and patient appropriately hydrated
– Pulse oximetry on patient
Time out:
– Confirm team members and reconfirm patient, site, and procedure
– Describe preoperative assessment and intended endovascular strategy
– Delineate procedural concerns and possible tactical alternatives to care

Sign out:
• Confirm (physician) the endovascular treatment performed
• Review key concerns for recovery and management of the patient (pain, hydration, antibiotics)

1.6 Decision-Making Algorithm

• *See* Flowchart 31.1.

1.7 Pearls and Pitfalls

Pearls:

• Intravascular ultrasound provides accurate detail to facilitate the sizing of aneurysms for stent grafts, stents, and coils.
• Take multiple arteriographic images prior to treatment to assess inflow and outflow, renal artery branches, and size of the aneurysm neck.
• Anatomic candidates for a stent graft:
– Be able to create seal proximal and distal to RAA
– No significant exclusion of branch renal arteries
– Must be deliverable
• Narrow-necked saccular aneurysms are amenable to coil embolization without a stent or balloon assistance by first using a framing coil followed by coils that fill in the spaces (i.e. hydrocoils).

Pitfalls:

• Wide-necked aneurysms that are coiled should be done with stent or balloon assistance that minimizes the risk of coil misplacement and protrusion into the arterial lumen.
• Avoid coil embolization of pseudoaneurysms since coil expansion can lead to rupture.

1.8 Surgical Anatomy

• *See* Figure 31.2.

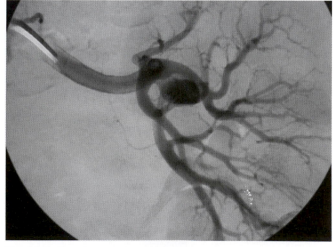

Fig. 31.1: Renal artery aneurysm.

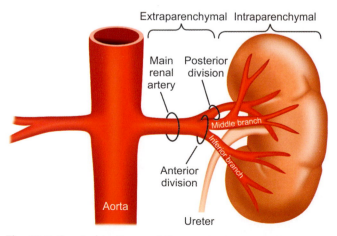

Fig. 31.2: Surgical anatomy of the renal artery aneurysm.

Flowchart 31.1: Decision-making algorithm.

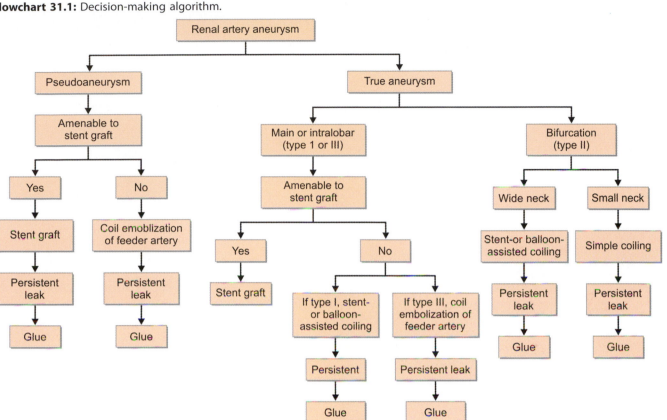

1.9 Angiographic and Ultrasound Imaging and Classification

- *See* Figures 31.3 to 31.7.

1.10 Anesthesia

- Conscious sedation with local anesthesia at the access site.
- Antibiotic within 30 minutes of the start of the procedure.
- Heparin bolus (50–80 units/Kg) after sheath insertion; rebolus if procedure >60 minutes
- Hydration before and after the procedure to minimize contrast nephropathy.

2 PERIOPERATIVE

2.1 Stent Graft Exclusion of a Main Renal Artery Aneurysm

- *See* Figures 31.8A to F.

2.2 Coil Embolization of a 3-cm Bifurcation Aneurysm of the Right Renal Artery

- *See* Figures 31.9A to C.

2.3 Stent-Assisted Coil Embolization of a Bifurcation Aneurysm in a Patient with Fibromuscular Dysplasia

- *See* Figures 31.10A to E.

2.4 Stent Graft of a Branch Renal Artery Aneurysm with Distal Coil Embolization and Sacrifice of the Branch

- *See* Figures 31.11A to C.

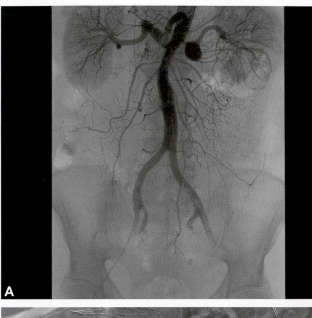

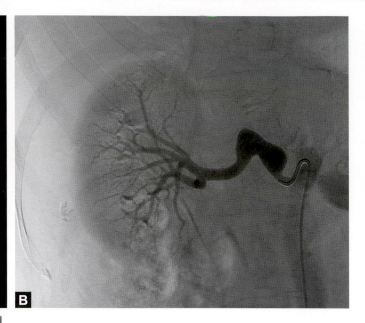

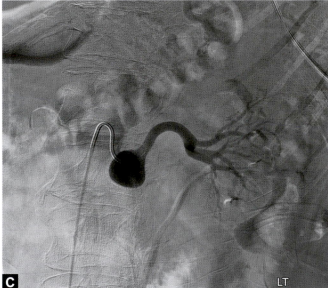

Figs. 31.3A to C: Arteriogram showing bilateral main renal artery aneurysm from aortogram (A), selective right renal artery (B), selective left renal artery (C).

2.5 Stent Graft Exclusion of Main and Intralobar Aneurysm with Ultrasound and CT Follow-Up

- *See* Figures 31.12A to L.

2.6 Balloon-Assisted Coil Embolization of a Bifurcation RAA

- *See* Figures 31.13A to E.

3 POSTOPERATIVE

3.1 Complications

Most common complications:
- Access site bleeding, infection, occlusion
- Renal infarction
- Persistent flow and growth of aneurysm
- Stent graft thrombosis
- Inability to catheterize the feeding vessel
- Contrast nephropathy

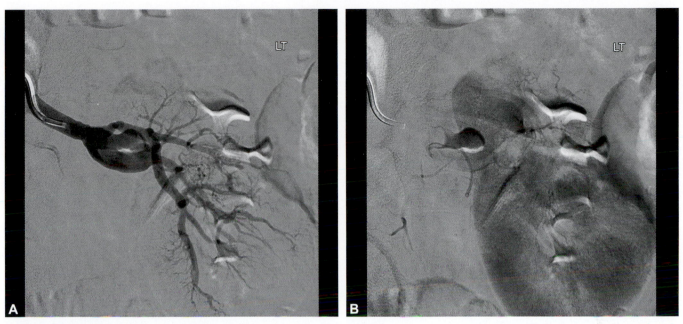

Figs. 31.4A and B: Selective arteriogram of bifurcation aneurysm of left renal artery showing dilation of inferior renal artery. (A) Early and (B) delayed emptying of aneurysm.

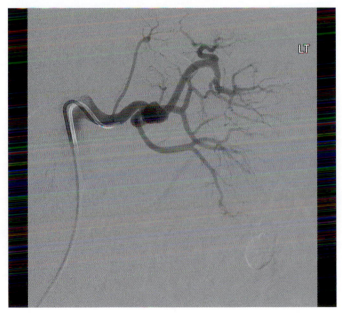

Fig. 31.5: Arteriogram of left renal artery showing a fusiform bifurcation aneurysm with involvement of both the anterior and posterior division (treated with open surgery).

Least common complications:
- Loss of kidney
- Renal artery dissection or perforation
- Misplacement of coils or stent (geographic miss) in the target artery
- Embolization of wrong artery

3.2 Outcomes

Expected outcomes:
- Thrombosis and regression of aneurysm sac
- Maintenance of baseline renal function
- Rarely develop "new" true aneurysms in the renal parenchyma

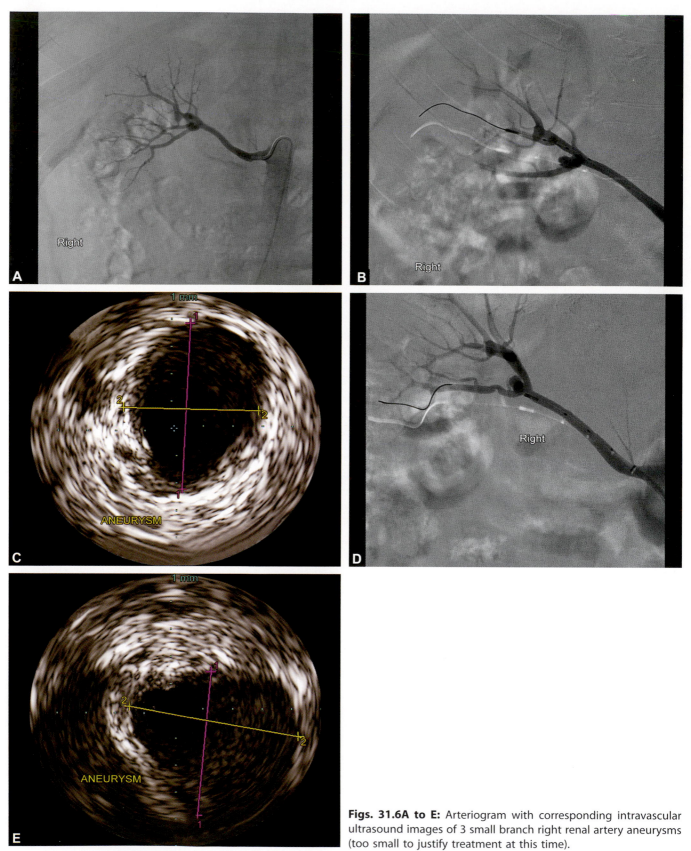

Figs. 31.6A to E: Arteriogram with corresponding intravascular ultrasound images of 3 small branch right renal artery aneurysms (too small to justify treatment at this time).

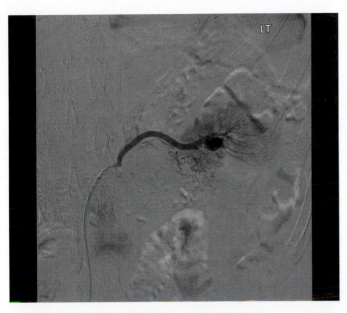

Fig. 31.7: Arteriogram of intralobar aneurysm of an accessory left renal artery.

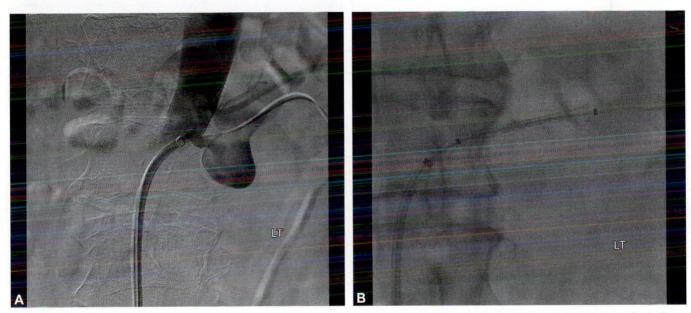

Figs. 31.8A and B: (A) Selective left renal arteriogram of a main renal artery aneurysm before treatment. (B) Delivery of a balloon expandable [ICAST stent (6 mm), Atrium Medical Corporation, NH] through a 6 Fr Destination sheath (Terumo, Japan) over n 0.035" Versacore wire (Abbott Vascular, CA).

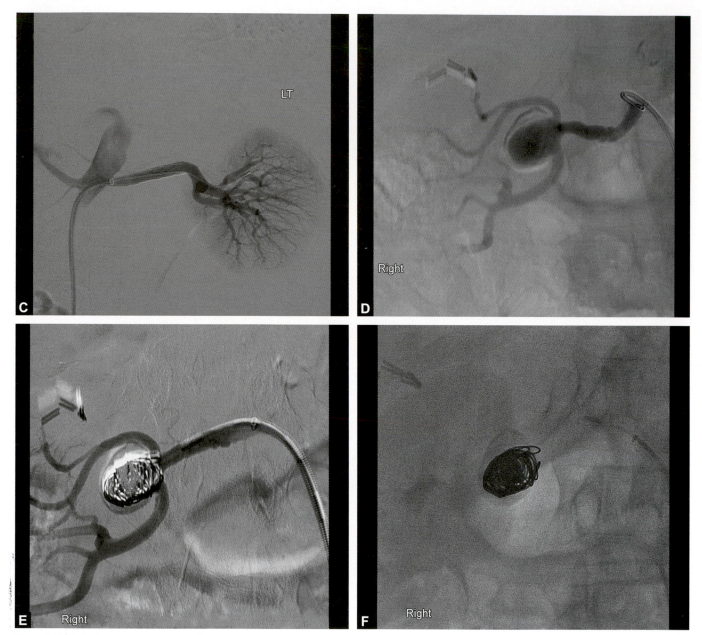

Figs. 31.8C to F: (C) Arteriogram of aneurysm exclusion. (D) Example of using a caging coil initially (16 mm x 40 cm, Penumbra, California, USA) in a 15 mm aneurysm placed through an Expert stent (Abbott Vascular, CA) with a Progreat catheter (2.8 Fr, Terumo). (E) Packing coil into the caging coil (12 mm x 30 mm). (F) Nice tight packing with complete exclusion of the aneurysm.

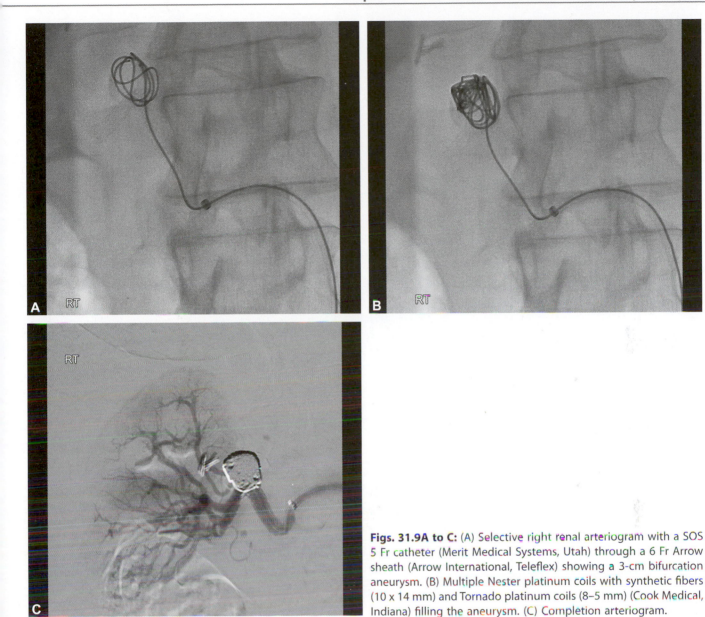

Figs. 31.9A to C: (A) Selective right renal arteriogram with a SOS 5 Fr catheter (Merit Medical Systems, Utah) through a 6 Fr Arrow sheath (Arrow International, Teleflex) showing a 3-cm bifurcation aneurysm. (B) Multiple Nester platinum coils with synthetic fibers (10 x 14 mm) and Tornado platinum coils (8–5 mm) (Cook Medical, Indiana) filling the aneurysm. (C) Completion arteriogram.

3.3 Follow-Up

- Dual antiplatelet regimen for patients with stent graft, otherwise standard of care
- Medical reevaluation for antihypertension therapy
- Imaging after endovascular treatment is quite variable
  - Ultrasound can be used to follow kidney size and main renal artery patency (RAP), but not RAA size and exclusion.
  - Arteriography is the most accurate test to confirm RAP and RAA exclusion, but not size.
  - Computed tomography angiography (CTA) can demonstrate, RAP, RAA size, and exclusion:
    - Once full exclusion is confirmed on the CTA then yearly clinical evaluation with renal ultrasound may be sufficient.
    - Persistent aneurysm with no regression or enlargement then arteriography and possible reintervention
  - MRA has a limited role in follow-up of the treated RAA since metallic material (coil, stent graft, nitinol, stainless steel) creates artifact. But, may be useful to screen or follow other aneurysms. Serial radiation exposure with CTA can be avoided by use of MR for those patients requiring frequent follow-up cross-sectional imaging studies.

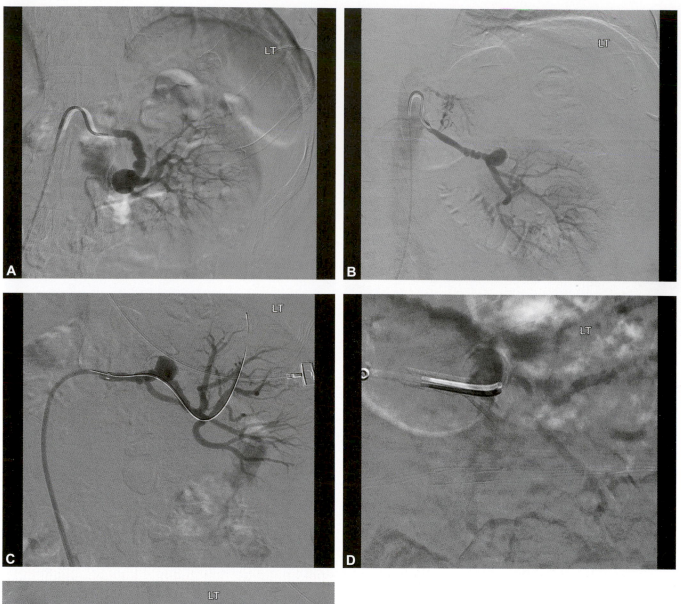

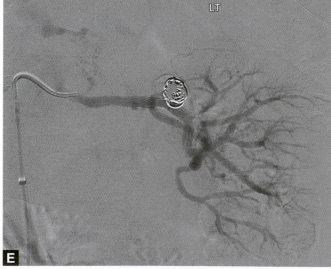

Figs. 31.10A to E: (A) Selective arteriogram of left renal artery aneurysm in a patient with medial fibromuscular dysplasia in the AP plane. (B) Arteriogram with caudal and right anterior oblique (RAO) angulation. (C) Arteriogram with cranial and RAO angulation and wire traversal (0.014^2 Grand Slam, Abbott Vascular) into the appropriate distal branch. (D) Berenstein shaped catheter (Merit Medical) into aneurysm through balloon expandable stent (Valeo, Bard Medical, 5 mm) to deliver coils into aneurysm. (E) Completion arteriogram after Nester and Tornado coils.

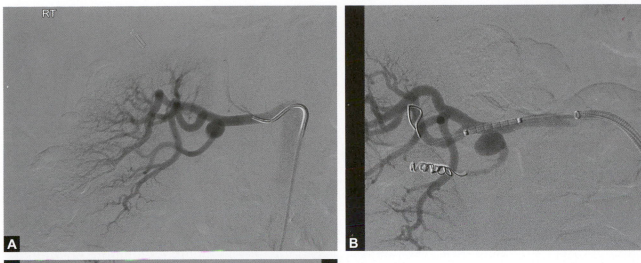

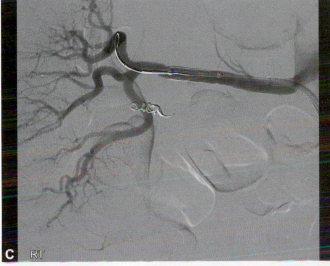

Figs. 31.11A to C: (A) Selective arteriogram of branch aneurysm of the inferior branch of right renal artery. (B) Nester coil (5 mm, Cook Medical) in distal branch with pre-deployed balloon expandable ICAST stent (Atrium Medical, 5 x 16 mm) over branch. (C) Completion arteriogram with exclusion of the RAA and lack of flow in distal branch. (RAA: Renal artery aneurysm).

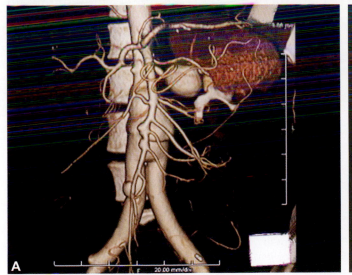

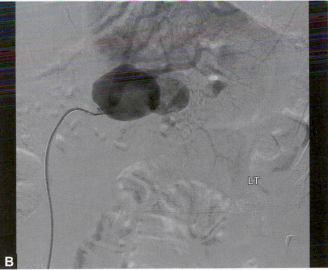

Figs. 31.12A and B: (A) Computed tomography reconstruction of a patient with a solitary left kidney (S/P right nephrectomy after failed aneurysm bypass) with renal artery aneurysms (RAAs). Notice previous aortobifemoral bypass. (B) Selective arteriogram of main left RAA seen on CT to be 5 cm in diameter.

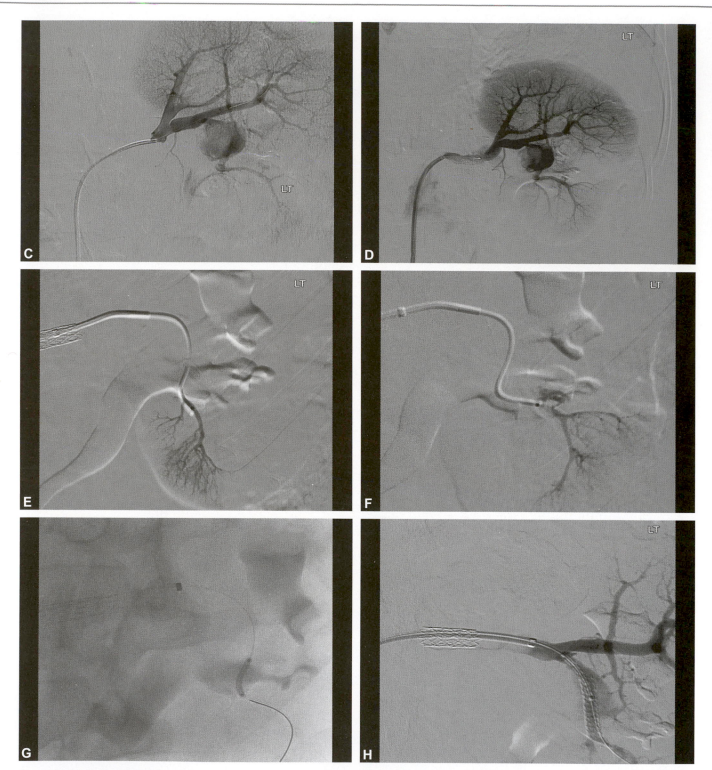

Figs. 31.12C to H: (C) Catheter placed beyond the main left RAA to document integrity of distal main renal artery and to demonstrate the intralobar aneurysm in the inferior portion of the left kidney. (D) Placement of 5 x 16 mm ICAST stent graft through a 6 Fr Ansel sheath (Cook Medical) to exclude the main RAA. (E) Progreat 2.8 Fr (Terumo) into small branch distal to the intralobar aneurysm that was 3.5 cm in diameter. Note this catheter is telescoped through the angled 5 Fr catheter in the main RA. (F) Same Progreat catheter into a larger outflow branch. (G) Delivery of 3 x 19 mm Graftmaster stent graft (Jomed, Abbott Vascular) over a 0.014" BMW coronary wire. (H) Delivery of a 3.5 x 19 mm Graftmaster more proximal to the first stent graft with angiographic guidance to avoid protrusion into middle renal artery branch.

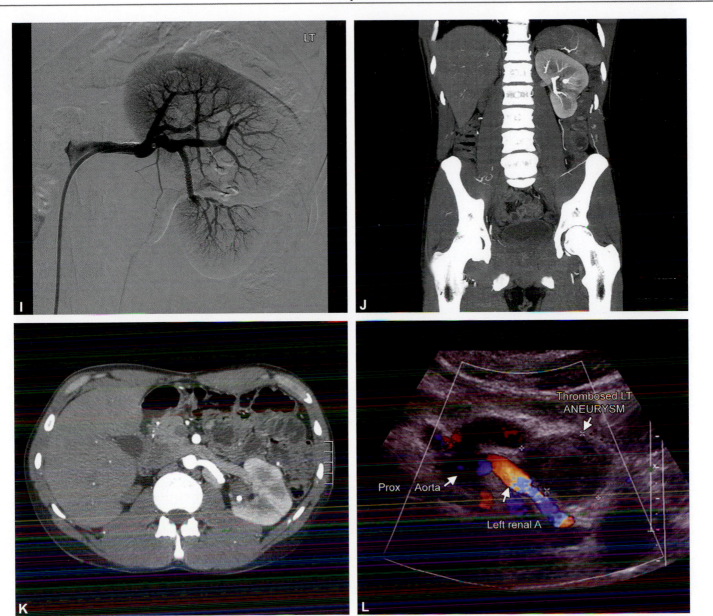

Figs. 31.12I to L: (I) Completion arteriogram. (J), (K) Computed tomography images demonstrating regression of both aneurysms. (L) Ultrasound image showing exclusion of main RA aneurysm.

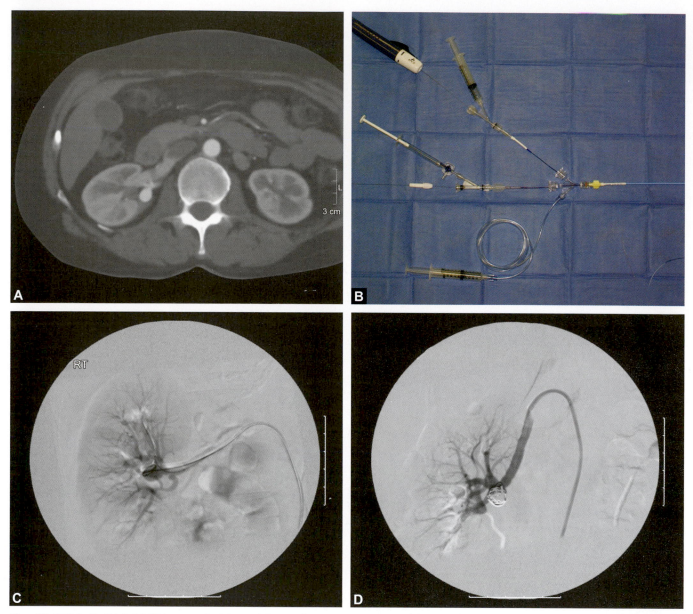

Figs. 31.13A to D: (A) Axial CT image of a 1.5 cm right renal artery aneurysms (RAA) at the bifurcation. (B) Equipment used including an 8 Fr renal double curve guide (Cordis, NJ), Hyperglide conformable (compliant) balloon (eV3, Minneapolis), and Guglielmi detachable coils (Target Therapeutics, California). (C) Selective arteriogram of branch aneurysm of the right renal artery with balloon in place and access catheter into the RAA. (D) Completion arteriogram with exclusion of the RAA.

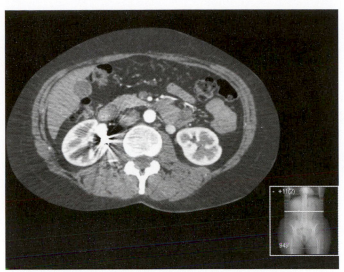

Figs. 31.13E: (E) Axial CT image demonstrating the metal artifact after coiling of the right RAA.

3.4 E-mail an Expert

- *E-mail address*: bhgray@ghs.org

3.5 Web Resources/References

- http://emedicine.medscape.com/article/463015-overview
- http://radiographics.highwire.org/content/26/6/1687.full.pdf
- http://vaware.org/visceral-arteries/renal-artery-aneurtsm.html
- http://www.sirweb.org/patients/renal-artery-aneurysms
- http://www.youtube.com/watch?v=4u15hN4czaU

REFERENCES

1. Zhang Z, Yang M, Song L, et al. Endovascular treatment of renal artery aneurysms and renal arteriovenous fistulas. J Vasc Surg. 2013;57:765-70.
2. Manninen HI, Berg M, Vanninen RL. Stent-assisted coil embolization of wide-necked renal artery bifurcation aneurysms. J Vasc Interv Radiol. 2008;19:487-92.
3. Hislop SJ, Patel SA, Abt PL, et al. Therapy of renal artery aneurysms in New York State: outcomes of patients undergoing open and endovascular repair. Ann Vasc Surg. 2009; 23:194-200.
4. Sedat J, Chau Y, Baque J. Endovascular treatment of renal aneurysms: a series of 18 cases. Eur J Rad. 2012; 81:3973-8.
5. Rundback JH, Rizvi A, Rozenblit GN, et al. Percutaneous stent-graft management of renal artery aneurysms. J Vasc Interv Radiol. 2000;9:1189-93.

QUIZ

Question 1. The diagnosis of renal artery aneurysm is best made with:
a. Digital subtraction arteriography
b. Plain radiograph of the abdomen
c. Duplex ultrasound
d. Computed tomography angiography

Question 2. The best treatment for a pseudoaneurysm of the distal main renal artery is:
a. Coil embolization
b. Stent graft
c. Glue embolization
d. Stent-assisted embolization

Question 3. The most accurate way to determine renal aneurysm exclusion on follow-up study after endovascular treatment is:
a. Digital subtraction arteriography
b. Plain radiograph of the abdomen
c. Duplex ultrasound
d. Computed tomography angiography

ANSWERS: 1. d   2. b   3. a

SECTION
5

Peripheral Vascular

Diagnostic Angiography

Justin Hurie

1 PREOPERATIVE

1.1 Indications

Indications
- Arterial evaluation
- Endovascular intervention

Relative Contraindications
- Type 4 Ehlers–Danlos syndrome
- Anaphylaxis to contrast media

1.2 Evidence

- As the only imaging modality that allows intervention, angiography is often viewed at the gold standard for arterial evaluation. There is controversy regarding the best initial work up for patients that have evidence of peripheral arterial disease as illustrated in the following references.[1,2]

1.3 Materials Needed

- *See* Figures 32.1A to D.

1.4 Preoperative Planning and Risk Assessment

Planning:
- Assess patient for a history of a contrast allergy and risk of renal dysfunction.

Risk assessment:
- Contrast induced nephropathy occurs in 1–2% of patients with normal renal function. Preoperative hydration with normal saline appears to be the most effective method to prevent contrast-induced nephropathy. Sodium bicarbonate and *N*-acetylcysteine may also provide benefit.
- *Low risk*:
  - Young, healthy patients with normal renal function

- *Intermediate risk:*
  - Advanced age, congestive heart failure, dehydration, hyperosmolar states
  - Diabetes may be a marker for underlying renal dysfunction
- *High risk:*
  - Pre-existing renal dysfunction

1.5 Preoperative Checklist

Sign in:
- Location of imaging, pregnancy status, allergies, renal function
- Position of patient and level of anesthesia

Time out:
- Confirmation of procedure
- Antibiotics and DVT prophylaxis (if indicated)

Sign out:
- Postoperative location, pulse examination
- Need for anticoagulation or antiplatelet agent

1.6 Pearls and Pitfalls

Pearls:
- Ultrasound guided access may decrease the risk of an external iliac or superficial femoral artery puncture.
- Always mark preprocedural pedal Doppler signals in order to avoid postoperative uncertainty.
- Follow As Low As Reasonably Achievable (ALARA) guidelines in order to minimize the risk of radiation injury.
- Carbon dioxide may serve as an alternative contrast medium for patients with a contrast allergy or renal dysfunction undergoing abdominal or lower extremity intervention.

Pitfalls:
- French size of a sheath refers to the inner diameter, while the French size of a catheter refers to the outer diameter.
- Increasing distance from source and minimizing the duration of exposure are the most effective way to decrease radiation dose.

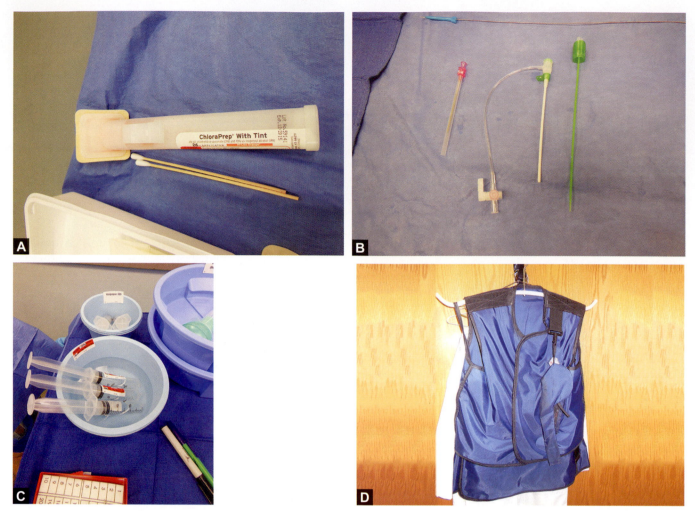

Figs. 32.1A to D: (A) Chlorhexadine gluconate and alcohol for skin preparation. (B) Setup for arterial access including needle, sheath, and starter wire. (C) Back table setup including heparin and contrast. (D) Follow your institutional guidelines for radiation safety. Proper lead protective gear includes a lead apron and glasses.

- Hold metformin for 48 hours after contrast administration in order to minimize the risk of lactic acidosis.
- Absolute care must be taken to ensure that no air is introduced with injection of carbon dioxide.

1.7 Surgical Anatomy

- *See* Figures 32.2A and B.

1.8 Positioning

- The patient is placed supine. Optimal imaging of the hypogastric artery is accomplished with rotation of the image intensifier to 20–30° to the contralateral anterior oblique. Imaging of the profunda femoral artery is best accomplished with rotation of the image intensifier to 20–30° to the ipsilateral anterior oblique.

1.9 Anesthesia

- Place Foley catheter in order to allow adequate urinary drainage while patient is supine and immobile.
- Place an arterial line if frequent blood samples are need or hemodynamic instability is expected.
- Plan on using light sedation if breath-holding is required.
- Despite steroid prophylaxis, patients may still have an adverse reaction to contrast administration.

2 PERIOPERATIVE

2.1 Access

- *See* Figures 32.3A to C.

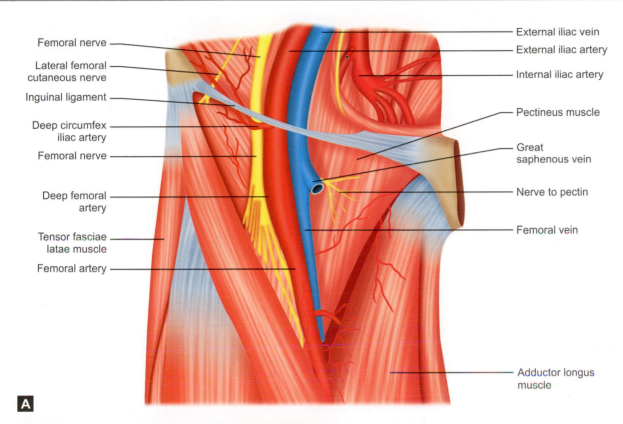

Femoral nerve

Lateral femoral cutaneous nerve

Inguinal ligament

Deep circumfex iliac artery

Femoral nerve

Deep femoral artery

Tensor fasciae latae muscle

Femoral artery

External iliac vein

External iliac artery

Internal iliac artery

Pectineus muscle

Great saphenous vein

Nerve to pectin

Femoral vein

Adductor longus muscle

A

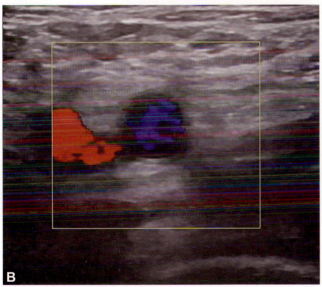

B

Figs. 32.2A and B: (A) Illustrates the relative location of the femoral artery between the femoral nerve and the femoral vein. The inguinal ligament is located between a line drawn between the anterior superior iliac spine and the pubic tubercle. (B) Ultrasound image of the femoral artery and vein that allows arterial puncture under direct visualization.

2.2 Catheter Selection

- *See* Figures 32.4A to C and Table 32.1.

2.3 Closure

- *See* Figures 32.5.

3 POSTOPERATIVE

3.1 Complications

Most common complications:

- Hematoma
- Pseudoaneurysm

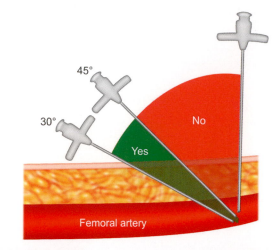

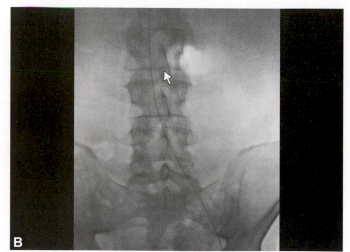

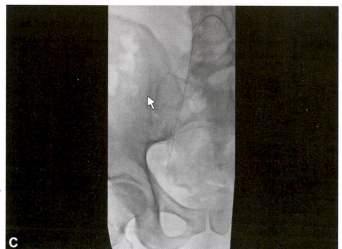

Figs. 32.3A to C: (A) Puncture the femoral artery at an angle between 30° and 45°. (B) Initial wire placement after sheath insertion. (C) Selection of the contralateral iliac artery using a wire and cobra catheter.

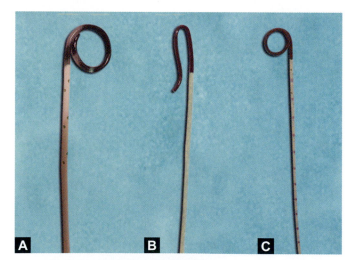

Figs. 32.4A to C: Flush catheters (A) have multiple side holes that allow better opacification with a power injector compared to an end-hole catheters (B). (C) Marker catheters allow direct measurement of length, but increase cost.

Table 32.1: A guide to usual vessel diameter and a suggested rate of injection for various vascular beds.

Location	Vessel diameter (mm)	Rate (mL/s)	Total volume (mL)
Aorta	Up to 20	20	40
Iliac	6–10	10	10
Femoral	5–8	4	8
Popliteal	3–5	Hand	6
Tibial	2–4	Hand	6

- Nephrotoxicity

Least common complications:

- Peripheral embolization
- Dissection
- Anaphylaxis
- Radiation injury

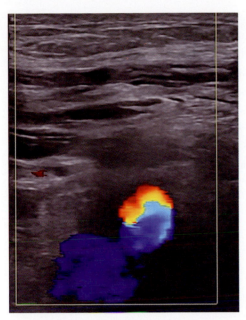

Fig. 32.5: Hemostasis is obtained with manual compression related to the sheath size. A general rule of thumb is 3 minutes per French (i.e. 6 Fr needs compression of at least 18 minutes). Inadequate compression may result in pseudoaneurysm formation. Pseudoaneurysms may contain to-and-fro flow as seen in the following image.

3.2 Follow-Up

- Check postprocedure Doppler signals and evaluate the lower extremities for evidence of distal embolization.
- Monitor the patient for the development of an adverse reaction.
- Have the patient lie flat depending on the method of closure.

3.3 E-mail an Expert

- *E-mail address*: jhurie@wakehealth.edu

3.4 Web Resources/References

Web resources:

- http://www.acr.org/Quality-Safety/Standards-Guidelines
- http://www.e-radiography.net/
- http://www.sirweb.org/clinical/cpg/PADExecSumm.pdf
- http://www.scai.org/SecondsCount/Test/SecondsCountGuidetoRadiationSafety.aspx

REFERENCES

1. Collins R, Burch J, Cranny G, et al. Duplex ultrasonography, magnetic resonance angiography, and computed tomography angiography for diagnosis and assessment of symptomatic, lower limb peripheral arterial disease: systematic review. BMJ. 2007;334:1257.
2. Ouwendijk R, de Vries M, Stijnen T, et al. Multicenter randomized controlled trial of the costs and effects of noninvasive diagnostic imaging in patients with peripheral arterial disease: the DIPAD trial. Am J Roentgenol. 2008; 190:1349-57.
3. Maki DG, Ringer M, Alvarado CJ. Prospective randomized trial of providone-iodine, alcohol, and chlorhexidine for prevention of infection associated with central venous and arterial catheters. Lancet. 1991;338:339-43.
4. Briguori C, Airoldi F, D'Andrea D, et al. Renal Insufficiency following contrast media administration trial (REMEDIAL): a randomized comparison of 3 preventive strategies. Circulation. 2007;115:1211-17.
5. Morcos S, Thomsen HS, Webb JAW. Prevention of generalised reactions to contrast media: a consensus report and guidelines. Eur Radiol. 2001;11:1720-8.
6. Kadir S. Diagnostic Angiography, 1st edition. Philadelphia: W.B. Saunders; 1986.
7. Rana NR, McLafferty RB. Arteriography. In: Cronenwett JL, Johnston KW (Eds). Rutherfords's Vascular Surgery, 7th edition. Philadelphia: Saunders; 2010.

QUIZ

Question 1. How long should you hold metformin after angiography?
a. 24 hours
b. 48 hours
c. 72 hours
d. Metformin is a contraindication to contrast administration

Question 2. What is the expected rate of renal dysfunction after contrast administration in the general population?
a. 1–2%
b. 3–5%
c. 6–10%
d. 11–15%

Question 3. What is the most effect method to decrease the risk of contrast-induced nephropathy?

a. 150 meq NaBicarb in 1 L of D5W infusion 1 mL/kg/h × 18 hours
b. Mucomyst 600 mg PO BID × 4 doses
c. Vitamin C 3 g PO prior to the procedure and 2 g PO after procedure
d. 0.9% NaCl infusion 1 mL/kg/h × 18 hours

Question 4. In most patients, what is the best to image the profunda femoral artery?

a. Anterior posterior
b. 20° contralateral anterior oblique
c. 20° ipsilateral anterior oblique
d. Lateral

Question 5. What angle of entry should be used for the access needle?

a. <30%
b. 40%
c. 50%
d. >50%

Femoral Embolectomy

Michael Brewer, Karen Woo

1 PREOPERATIVE

1.1 Indications

- Aortic saddle embolus
- Acute iliofemoral thrombosis or embolism
- Acute femoropopliteal thrombosis or embolism
- Acute lower extremity bypass graft thrombosis
- Contraindications
  - Chronic occlusion iliofemoral arteries
  - Chronic occlusion femoropopliteal arteries
  - Aneurysmal degeneration of the iliac, femoral, or popliteal arteries

1.2 Evidence

- Accepted standard of care for acute limb ischemia (nonaneurysmal) with emergent or urgent revascularization is based on the clinical stage of acute limb ischemia.
- Patients categorized as Rutherford class IIA can be treated with catheter-directed thrombolysis or thromboembolectomy.
- Patients categorized as Rutherford class IIB require emergent thromboembolectomy.
- Large randomized trials (STILE, TOPAS) showed no significant difference in outcomes between surgical thromboembolectomy and thrombolysis for acute limb ischemia.[1-3]

1.3 Materials Needed

- Standard peripheral vascular surgery instrument tray
- *Standard balloon embolectomy catheters*: #3-Fogarty to #7-Fogarty, 60–100 cm in length
- Silicone vessel loops
- 5-0 and 6-0 polypropylene suture

1.4 Preoperative Planning and Risk Assessment

Planning:
- Arterial duplex
- Conventional angiogram
- CT angiogram

Risk assessment:
- *Low risk*:
  - Short ischemia time (<6 hours)
  - Audible pedal arterial Doppler signals
  - Motor and sensation intact
- *Intermediate risk*:
  - Intermediate ischemia time (6–24 hours)
  - Audible pedal venous Doppler signals only, arterial signals inaudible
  - Diminished/absent sensation but motor intact
- *High risk*:
  - Prolonged ischemia time (>24 hours)
  - No audible pedal arterial or venous Doppler signals
  - Diminished/absent sensation and motor

1.5 Preoperative Checklist

Sign in:
- Confirm patient, procedure, site, laterality, and imaging
- Surgical consent and site marking complete
- Allergies reviewed
- Blood products available
- Confirm intraoperative angiography readily available

Time out:
- Confirm patient, procedure site, and side
- Ensure antibiotics given
- Ensure availability of heparin
- Address any concerns from all team members
- Display imaging

Sign out:

- Confirm procedure actually performed
- Document procedural outcomes
- Store intraoperative imaging
- Review specimen labeling

1.6 Pearls and Pitfalls

Pearls:

- Prep and drape for potential axillofemoral artery bypass in the setting of iliofemoral thromboembolus.
- Prep and drape both groins and lower extremities in the setting of femoropopliteal thromboembolus.
- Always assess the greater saphenous veins with Duplex ultrasonography in preparation for bypass should the thromboembolectomy be unsuccessful.
- Gently inflate the Fogarty balloon while withdrawing the catheter back so as to prevent arterial intimal injury or rupture.
- Inflate the balloon with heparinized saline, not air.
- Continue to make passes with the Fogarty catheter until you have a negative pass (no thrombus); then make one more.
- If aortic thrombus is seen on imaging, bilateral femoral thromboembolectomy is necessary.
- If a leg fasciotomy is considered, it should be performed.
- Completion angiography should be performed to confirm absence of residual thrombus or underlying disease.
- The patient should remain on anticoagulation after thromboembolectomy, with duration and dose dependent on etiology of the thromboembolus. Surgical drain placement may be required.

Pitfall:

- Do not be overly aggressive with balloon inflation.

1.7 Surgical Anatomy

- *See* Figure 33.1.

1.8 Positioning

- *See* Figures 33.2A and B.

1.9 Anesthesia

- Adequate intravenous access with two large bore catheters or a central venous catheter should be established
- Arterial catheter blood pressure monitoring
- General endotracheal anesthesia unless patient has major cardiopulmonary risk factors
- Spinal or regional nerve block if risk of general anesthesia is too great

2 PERIOPERATIVE

2.1 Incision

Either a longitudinal or oblique incision over the common femoral artery can be used based on surgeon preference (*See* Figs. 33.3A and B).

2.2 Steps

See Figures 33.4A to D.

- Pedal Doppler signals should be auscultated at completion to delineate procedural success.
- Consider angiography if a strong doppler signal or pulse is not obtained following embolectomy.
- Separate popliteal and tibial artery thromboembolectomy may be required for tibial trifurcation thromboembolus.

2.3 Closure

- The wound is closed in at least four layers. The deep investing fascia and the subcutaneous layers are closed with 2-0 running absorbable braided suture. The deep dermal layer is closed with 3-0 running absorbable braided suture. The skin is closed using 4-0 running subcuticular absorbable monofilament suture or staples.

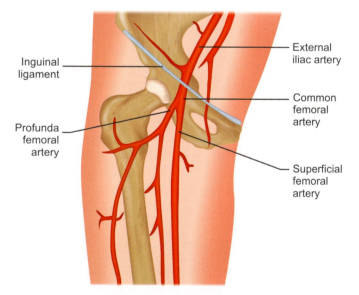

Fig. 33.1: The external iliac artery becomes the common femoral artery at the level of the inguinal ligament. The common femoral artery divides into the profunda femoral artery and the superficial femoral artery.

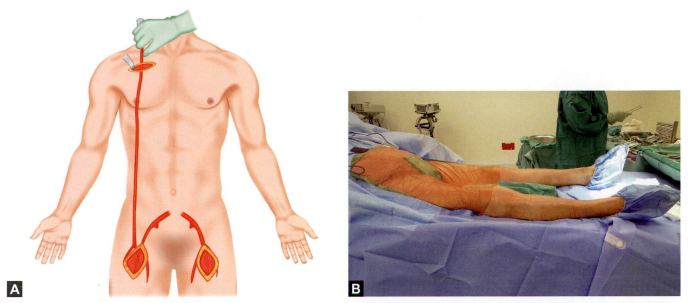

Figs. 33.2A and B: (A) Position patient supine with right arm at 90° for iliofemoral thromboembolism. Both lower extremities should be circumferentially prepped and draped (umbilicus to the toes). (B) Position patient supine with arms alongside the torso for patients with isolated femoropopliteal thromboembolism. Both lower extremities should be circumferentially prepped and draped (umbilicus to the toes).

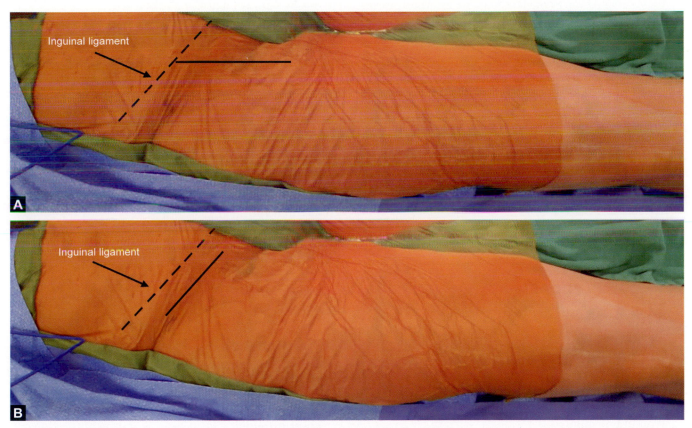

Figs. 33.3A and B: (A) 6–8 cm longitudinal incision over the course of the femoral artery with the proximal aspect starting at the level of the inguinal ligament. (B) 6–8 cm oblique incision, centered over the femoral artery, parallel to and 1–2 fingerbreadths below the inguinal ligament.

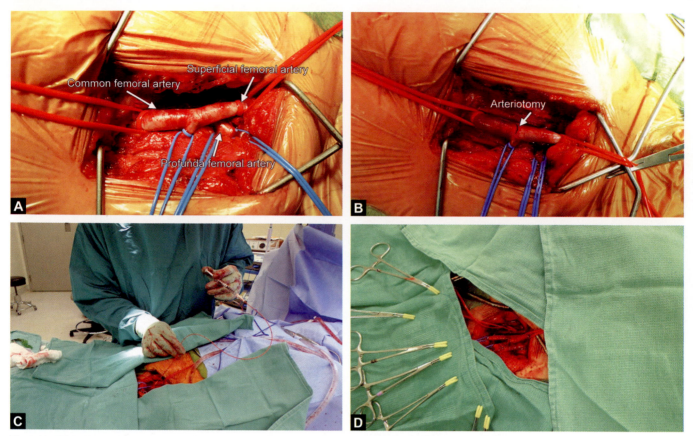

Figs. 33.4A to D: (A) The common femoral artery, superficial femoral artery, and profunda femoral artery are dissected out from the level of the inguinal ligament. Care is taken to perform a circumferential dissection and identify all branches. The profunda femoral artery should be dissected out to its first bifurcation. Proximal and distal control of all arteries and branches is obtained using double looped vessel loops. (B) A transverse arteriotomy is made with a #11 scalpel just proximal to the bifurcation of the common femoral artery. (C) A large diameter (5–7 Fr) balloon embolectomy catheter is passed proximally to remove any thrombus from the distal aorta and iliac arteries to establish inflow. Care should be taken whenever using the embolectomy catheter to only inflate the balloon while pulling back on the catheter to avoid rupturing the vessel. The balloon should only be inflated to a volume such that there is minimal resistance when pulling the catheter. If any increase in resistance is felt, the volume in the balloon should be decreased. Smaller (3–4 Fr) balloon embolectomy catheters are passed distally to remove thrombus from the superficial femoral, popliteal, and profunda femoral arteries to establish outflow. (D) The arteriotomy is closed with interrupted 5-0 or 6-0 polypropylene sutures. All vessel loops are removed.

3 POSTOPERATIVE

3.1 Complications

Most common complications:
- Bleeding or hematoma – risk increased by need for postoperative anticoagulation
- Recurrent thrombosis
- Reperfusion injury
- Compartment syndrome
- Wound infection

Least common complications:
- Seroma
- Lymphocele
- Arterial perforation or rupture
- Long-term aneurysm or arteriovenous fistula formation

3.2 Outcomes

Expected outcomes:
- Successful removal of thrombus or embolus with re-establishment of inline arterial blood flow to the lower extremity
- Resolution of any preoperative pain or discoloration
- Restoration of neurologic function

3.3 Follow-Up

- The patient is monitored in the intensive care unit to evaluate for recurrent ischemia, myocardial depression, or development of compartment syndrome in patients who did not undergo fasciotomy.
- Therapeutic heparin is resumed within 12 to 24 hours of operation if there is no evidence of bleeding.
- Heparin is transitioned to warfarin prior to discharge.
- Warfarin is continued for at least 3 months. The total duration of warfarin therapy is determined by the etiology of the thrombus/embolus.
- Surgical follow-up visit in 2 weeks to inspect surgical site.

3.4 E-mail an Expert

- *E-mail address*: karen.woo@med.usc.edu

REFERENCES

1. Rutherford RB. Clinical staging of acute limb ischemia as the basis for choice of revascularization method: when and how to intervene. Semin Vasc Surg. 2009;22:5-9.
2. The STILE Investigators: Results of a prospective randomized trial evaluating surgery versus thrombolysis for ischemia of the lower extremity. The STILE trial. Ann Surg. 1994;220:251-66.
3. Ouriel K, Veith FJ, Sasahara AA. A comparison of recombinant urokinase with vascular surgery as initial treatment for acute arterial occlusion of the legs. Thrombolysis or Peripheral Arterial Surgery (TOPAS) Investigators. N Engl J Med. 1998;338:1105-11.

QUIZ

Question 1. Emergent femoral embolectomy is indicated in a patient with which Rutherford classification of acute limb ischemia?
a. Rutherford I
b. Rutherford IIA
c. Rutherford IIB
d. Rutherford III

Question 2. The least common complication of femoral thromboembolectomy is:
a. Bleeding/hematoma formation
b. Wound infection
c. Recurrent thrombosis
d. Arterial rupture

Question 3. Which of the following should NOT be performed during a femoral thromboembolectomy?
a. Obtain proximal and distal control of the vessels using vessel loops
b. Inflate the balloon of the embolectomy catheter prior to pulling the catheter
c. Make a transverse arteriotomy in the common femoral artery
d. Close the incision in multiple layers

ANSWERS:

1. c   2. d   3. b

Iliac Artery Angioplasty and Stenting

Christopher Smolock

1.1 PREOPERATIVE

1.1 Indications and Contraindications

- Indications for iliac angioplasty and stenting are anatomic lesions in symptomatic patients with a suitable lesion who fail optimal medical therapy, including smoking cessation, weight loss, a monitored exercise regimen, β-blockers, antiplatelet agents, and statins:
  - *Anatomic guidelines*:
    - Trans Atlantic Inter Society Consensus (TASC) II Criteria A and B lesions as well as many TASC C lesion
    - *See* Figure 34.1
  - *Symptomatic arterial occlusive disease*:
    - Lifestyle-liming claudication
      - Calf, thigh, or buttock pain reproducible by walking and relieved by rest
    - *Critical limb ischemia (CLI)*:
      - Spectrum of pathology due to impaired blood flow that cannot meet metabolic demands of tissue. Ranges from rest pain to tissue loss (Rutherford category 4–6)
  - *See* Table 34.1
  - Residual dissection, ulcerated plaques, acute occlusion secondary to thromboembolism, >30% stenosis, or a persistent pressure gradient 5–10 mm Hg post-dilation
  - Adjunctive stenting during EVAR (endovascular abdominal aorta aneurysm repair)
- Relative contraindications
  - TASC D Lesions
  - Technical considerations precluding endovascular intervention
    - Juxtarenal aortic occlusion and disease
    - >1 mm circumferential calcification
    - Renal insufficiency (GFR <30 mL/min per 1.73 m^2)

1.2 Evidence

- Recommendations for iliac angioplasty and stenting from the TASC II guidelines on the management of patients with peripheral arterial disease (PAD) are graded according to the level of evidence.[1]
- *See* Table 34.2
- No prospective randomized trials exist comparing aortoiliac stenting versus open surgery for lower extremity revascularization.

1.3 Materials Needed

- *See* Figures 34.2 to 34.9.
- *There are several FDA approved stents for use in iliac arteries. Some examples are the following*:
- Product name (company)
  - E-Luminexx (Bard)
  - Wallstent (Boston Scientific)
  - Zilver 518 and 635 (Cook)
  - SMART (Cordis)
  - Express LD Iliac (Boston Scientific)
  - Palmaz-premounted and unmounted (Cordis)
  - Viabahn (W.L. Gore)
  - Visi-Pro (EV3)

1.4 Preoperative Planning and Risk Assessment

- Preoperative planning and risk assessment is the single most important step in endovascular surgery.
- *History and physical examination*:
  - Claudication/rest pain/tissue loss
  - Quality-of-life impairments
  - Pulse examination
  - Inspection for lower extremity ulcers

Type A lesions
- Unilateral or bilateral stenoses of CIA
- Unilateral or bilateral single short (≤ 3 cm) stenosis of EIA

Type B lesions
- Short (≤ 3 cm) stenosis of infraronal aorta
- Unilateral CIA occlusion
- Single or multiple stenosis totaling 3-10 cm involving the EIA not extending into the CFA
- Unilateral EIA occlusion not involving the origins of internal iliac or CFA

Type C lesions
- Bilateral CIA occlusions
- Bilateral EIA stenosis 3-10 cm long not extending into the CFA
- Unilateral EIA stenosis extending into the CFA
- Unilateral EIA occlusion that involves the origins of internal iliac and/or CFA
- Heavily calcified unilateral ELA occlusions with or without involvement of origins of internal iliac and/or CFA

Type D lesions
- Intra-renal aorta iliac occlusion
- Diffuse disease involving the aorta and both iliac arteries requiring treatment
- Diffuse multiple stenoses involving the unilateral CIA, EIA, and CFA
- Unilateral occlusions of both CIA and EIA
- Bilateral occlusions of EIA
- iliac stenoses in patients with AAA requiring treatment and not amenable to endograft placement or other lesions requiring open aortic or iliac surgery

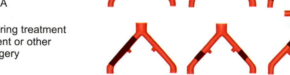

Fig. 34.1: TASC II criteria based on the TASC for the management of peripheral arterial disease.

Table 34.1: Rutherford's classification of peripheral arterial disease (PAD). The higher category or grade with more severe clinical manifestations suggests more severe arterial disease.

Fontaine		Rutherford			
Stage	Clinical	Grade	Category	Clinical	
I	Asymptomatic	0	0	Asymptomatic	
IIa	Mild claudication	I	1	Mild claudication	
IIb	Moderate-severe claudication	I	2	Moderate claudication	
		I	3	Severe claudication	
III	Ischemic rest pain	II	4	Ischemic rest pain	
IV	Ulceration or gangrene	III	5	Minor tissue loss	
		III	6	Major tissue loss	

Table 34.2: Level of evidence and treatment recommendations for aortoiliac disease.

Grade	Criteria	Recommendation
A	At least 1 randomized controlled trial (RCT)	
B	Well-conducted clinical studies without good quality RCT	Endovascular therapy is preferred to open surgery when both options yield equivalent short- and long-term symptomatic improvement
C	Expert committee reports or opinions and/or clinical experience	Endovascular therapy is preferred for TASC A and B lesions. Open surgery is preferred for TASC C lesions in patients without severe comorbid medical illnesses. Open surgery is preferred for TASC D lesions.

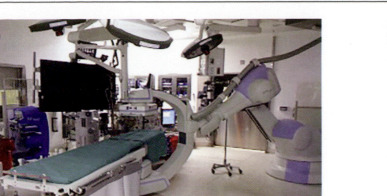

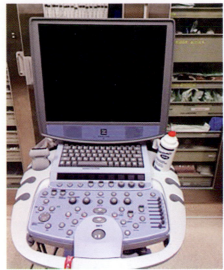

Fig. 34.2: Hybrid interventional suite at the Cleveland Clinic with the capability to perform endovascular and open surgery. The imaging equipment and C-arm are built into the room to optimize the use of the technology.

Fig. 34.3: Vascular duplex with a pulse wave probe (left) for visualization of the femoral artery during puncture.

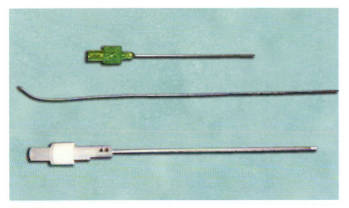

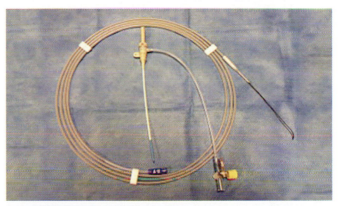

Fig. 34.4: A micropuncture needle (top) is used to gain access into the femoral artery. A micropuncture wire (middle) is cannulated into the artery. The needle is removed and then the artery is dilated with the 4-Fr micropuncture sheath (bottom).

Fig. 34.5: The 4-Fr micropuncture sheath is removed over a hydrophilic wire and exchanged for a 10-cm 5-Fr sheath.

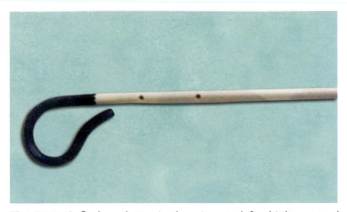

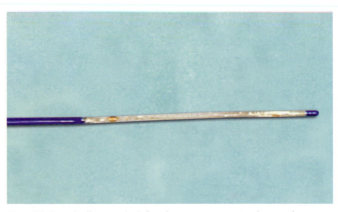

Fig. 34.6: A flush catheter is then inserted for high-powered contrast injection and aortogram.

Fig. 34.7: A balloon used for iliac artery angioplasty. There are radiopaque metallic clips at the ends of the balloon to facilitate fluoroscopic visualization.

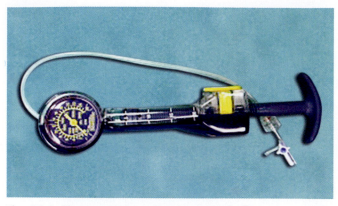

Fig. 34.8: The insufflator is used to tack balloon expandable stents to the wall of the aorta. The balloon inflation pressures vary by manufacturer.

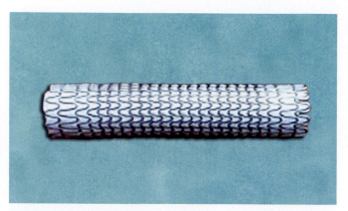

Fig. 34.9: Iliac stent (Viabahn, GORE). The Viabahn stent is a self-expanding stent-graft made of nitinol with PTFE graft material. It is approved for use in the iliac artery and the superficial femoral artery. (PTFE: Polytetrafluoroethylene).

- *Preoperative testing*:
  - Ankle-brachial index (ABI)
  - Arterial duplex
  - CTA
  - MRA

1.5 Preoperative Checklist

- *Sign in*:
  - Before induction of anesthesia, the patient confirms their name, the procedure being performed, and the affected extremity.
- *Time out*:
  - All team members present and accounted for. The surgeon repeats the indicated procedure and any special equipment, such as fluoroscopy and duplex, and confirmation of antibiotic prophylaxis.
- *Sign out*:
  - The nurse verbalizes the procedure performed, verifies the instrument count is correct, and the surgeon reviews the plan for the patient, including antiplatelet and anticoagulation regimen.

1.6 Decision-Making Algorithm

- *See* Flowchart 34.1.

1.7 Pearls and Pitfalls

Pearls:
- Factors that negatively affect the outcome of aortoiliac angioplasty include the long lesions with heavy thrombus

burden, circumferential calcium, as well as patients that continue to smoke and patients with renal failure.
- The hypogastric artery can be crossed with an uncovered bare metal stent during iliac stenting with minimal consequence. One hypogastric artery may be sacrificed by a covered stent and the incidence of buttock claudication or necrosis is minimal due to collaterals from the contralateral hypogastric and the ipsilateral profunda, inferior mesenteric, and middle sacral arteries.
- The stent diameter is estimated from the normal arterial segment next to the diseased segment or on the contralateral iliac. Slight oversizing of the stent by 5–10% is recommended.

Pitfalls:
- Mild pain during dilation indicates adventitia stretching, but severe pain along with hypotension may indicate arterial rupture.
- The common iliac artery is generally treated through an ipsilateral retrograde approach. An acute aortic bifurcation or lesions near the CFA may require access from the contralateral femoral artery or antegrade access from the brachial artery.
- Predilation with balloon angioplasty prior to stenting is recommended for tight iliac lesions to prevent dislodgment of the balloon expandable stent.

1.8 Surgical Anatomy

- *See* Figures 34.10A to C.

1.9 Positioning

See Figure 34.11
- Anesthesia
- Monitored anesthesia care is preferred using fentanyl and versed for pain control and sedation. The patient

Flowchart 34.1: Decision-making algorithm for treatment of aortoiliac disease.

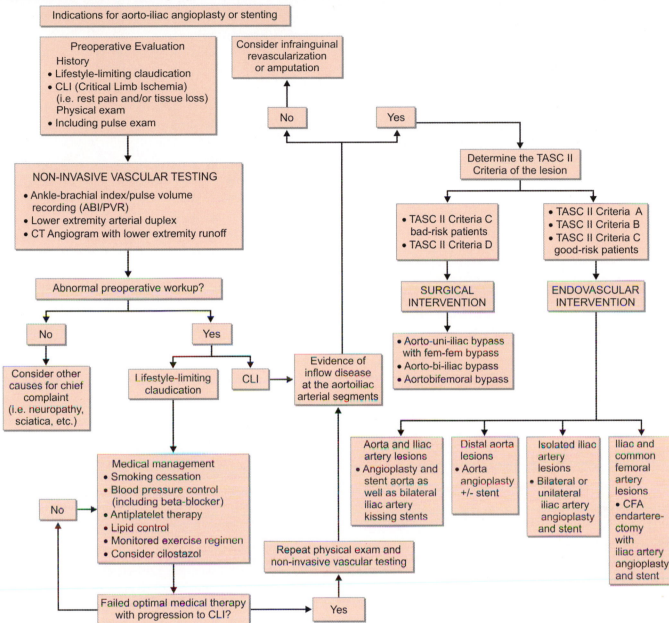

should be alert and responsive to breath-hold during abdominal and pelvic angiograms, which reduces the motion artifact.

- Local anesthesia with lidocaine at the groin puncture site as well as near the adventitia reduces pain.

- General anesthesia is used in selected patients or if iliac angioplasty and stenting is combined with another procedure, such as common femoral endarterectomy or femoral–popliteal bypass.

2 PERIOPERATIVE

2.1 Incision

- *See* Figures 34.12A and B.

2.2 Steps

- *See* Figures 34.13 to 34.15.

Typically, iliac angioplasty utilizes a 75-cm shaft, 5–10 mm diameter, 2–4 cm length balloon angioplasty

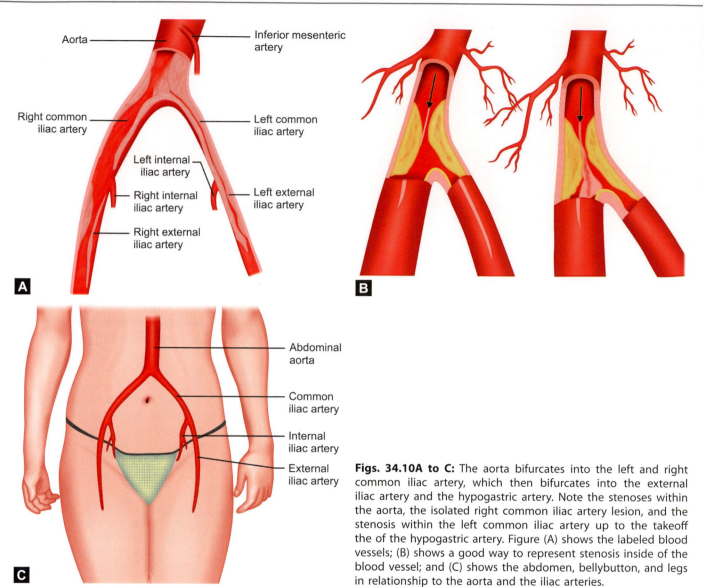

Figs. 34.10A to C: The aorta bifurcates into the left and right common iliac artery, which then bifurcates into the external iliac artery and the hypogastric artery. Note the stenoses within the aorta, the isolated right common iliac artery lesion, and the stenosis within the left common iliac artery up to the takeoff the of the hypogastric artery. Figure (A) shows the labeled blood vessels; (B) shows a good way to represent stenosis inside of the blood vessel; and (C) shows the abdomen, bellybutton, and legs in relationship to the aorta and the iliac arteries.

catheter that tracks over a 0.035-in. guidewire through a 5–7 Fr sheath.

Completion angiogram (*See* 📹 34.3).

An angiogram at the end of the case may demonstrate new pathology, including arterial rupture or dissection, stent dislodgment or malposition, or inadequate treatment.

2.3 Closure

- Groin pressure for 3–5 minutes for every French size dilated up to 8 Fr. If 9 Fr or greater is used, a cutdown and direct arterial closure is preferred. If pressure is held, the patient must lay flat for 6 hours to allow the clot to form and stabilize.

- Alternatively, a percutaneous closure device can be used. This reduces the amount of time that pressure has to be held, allows the patient earlier mobility, but has a 1.5% incidence of infection.

3 POSTOPERATIVE

3.1 Complications

- *Most common complications*:
  - Contrast-induced nephropathy in patients with renal insufficiency (serum Cr >1.5) is the third most common cause of acute renal failure in hospitalized patients.

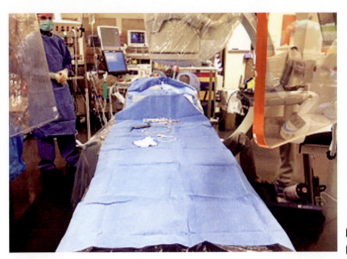

Fig. 34.11: Patient in the interventional suite with bilateral groins prepped and draped for an endovascular intervention.

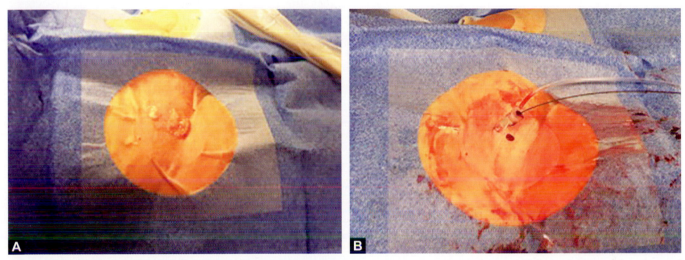

Figs. 34.12A and B: The 5-Fr sheath with access into the common femoral artery overlying the medial third of the common femoral artery distal to the takeoff of the inferior epigastric artery. IV heparin is administered to approximately double the patient's baseline activated clotting time (ACT) to reduce clot on the sheath and wires.

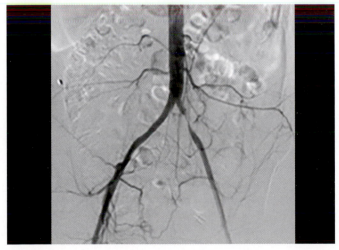

Fig. 34.13: A flush catheter in the infrarenal aorta showing the aorta, aortoiliac bifurcation, in an anterior-posterior projection.

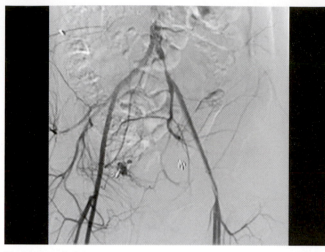

Fig. 34.14: Pelvic angiogram at 24° right anterior oblique to get a better projection of the right hypogastric origin from the common iliac artery. Note the focal stenosis proximal to the hypogastric artery and distal to the aortoiliac bifurcation providing a landing zone for the stent.

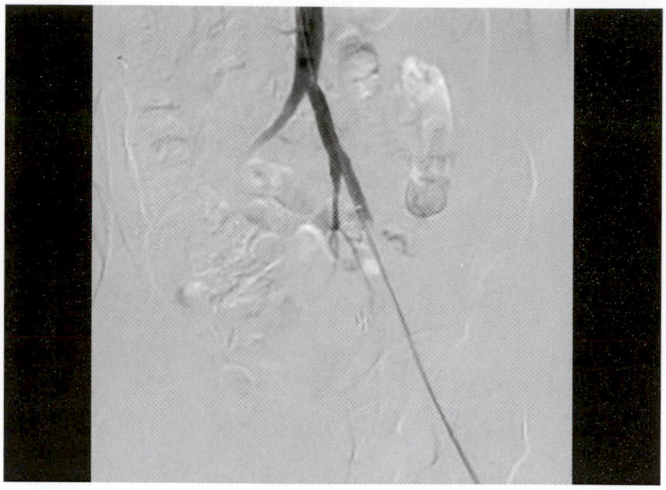

Fig. 34.15: Deployment of an 8 mm diameter, 37-mm-long express stent. The stenosis is no longer present and the hypogastric artery is still patent. There is no evidence of pseudoaneurysm, dissection, or arterial rupture.

- Local wound complications at the groin puncture site occur in 1–3% of cases. The most feared complication is retroperitoneal hematoma, which occurs in "high" sticks in the external iliac artery.
  - Other common complications include pseudoaneurysm, dissection, vessel spasm, and thrombus formation
- *Least common complications*:
  - Periprocedural cardiovascular or cerebrovascular incidents
  - Stent infection
  - Arteriovenous fistula
  - Symptomatic distal embolization
  - Arterial rupture
  - Stent misplacement, migration, or embolization

3.2 Outcomes

- According to the FDA, technical success is defined as <30% residual stenosis or >5 mm Hg systolic pressure gradient.
- A postoperative increase in the ABI of 0.1 or an improvement in at least 1 level on Rutherford's category as well as a physical examination with improvement in the postintervention pulse examination is considered a clinical success.
- Patients with intermittent claudication have a 10-year shorter life expectancy than the general population.

- Angioplasty performed primarily for claudicants has a 96% technical success rate, 86% 1-year patency, and 71% 5-year patency:
  - Patients with CLI have worse outcomes than claudicants.
  - Primary or selective stenting of the iliac arteries has better outcomes than angioplasty alone.
- Intimal hyperplasia, vessel recoil, and progression of atherosclerosis lead to restenosis and occlusion of iliac arteries. Smokers are at a higher risk for re-intervention compared to nonsmokers.
  - According to Murphy et al., technical success and overall limb salvage rate of iliac stenting is 98% with 89% 1-year primary patency, 75% 5-year primary patency, 7% major complications, and 0.5% 30-day mortality.[2]

3.3 Follow-Up

- Recommendations for follow-up include a duplex and ABI/PVRs at 1 month, 3 months, 6 months, and 1-year postintervention as well as yearly thereafter.
- Patients with worsening symptoms/decreasing quality of life due to progression of disease or restenosis on imaging with a diameter reduction >50%, a doubling of peak systolic velocity, or an ABI drop >0.1 mandate repeat CT or angiogram for further evaluation and intervention.

3.4 Video Clips 📹

- 📹 **34.1:** Initial aortogram with the flush catheter positioned in the infrarenal aorta showing lumbar arteries from the aorta, the aortoiliac bifurcation, and a stenosis in the left common iliac artery.
- 📹 **34.2:** Pelvic angiogram showing a stenosis within the left common iliac artery, with patency of bilateral hypogastric and common femoral arteries as well as the proximal bilateral superficial femoral and profunda arteries.
- 📹 **34.3:** Completion angiogram after deployment of a 8 × 37 mm express stent showing improved flow in the left common iliac artery.

3.5 E-mail an Expert

- *Email addresses*: smolocc@ccf.org; milerr@ccf.org; rangell@ccf.org

SUGGESTED READINGS

Bosch JL, Hunink MG. Meta-analysis of the results of percutaneous transluminal angioplasty and stent placement for aortoiliac occlusive disease. Radiology. 1997;204:87-96.

Galaria II, Davies MG. Percutaneous transluminal revascularization for iliac occlusive disease: long-term outcomes in TransAtlantic Inter-Society Consensus A and B lesions. Ann Vasc Surg. 2005;19:352-60.

Hirsch AT, Haskal ZJ, Hertzer NR, et al. ACC/AHA 2005 practice guidelines for the management of patients with peripheral arterial disease (lower extremity, renal, mesenteric, and abdominal aortic): a collaborative report from the American Association for Vascular Surgery/Society for Vascular Surgery, Society for Cardiovascular Angiography and Interventions, Society for Vascular Medicine and Biology, Society of Interventional Radiology, and the ACC/AHA Task Force on Practice Guidelines (Writing Committee to Develop Guidelines for the Management of Patients With Peripheral Arterial Disease): endorsed by the American Association of Cardiovascular and Pulmonary Rehabilitation; National Heart, Lung, and Blood Institute; Society for Vascular Nursing; TransAtlantic Inter-Society Consensus; and Vascular Disease Foundation. Circulation. 2006; 113 (11): e463-e654.

Klein WM, van der Graaf Y, Seegers J, et al. Long-term cardiovascular morbidity, mortality, and reintervention after endovascular treatment in patients with iliac artery disease: the Dutch iliac stent trial study. Radiology. 2004;232:491-8.

Leville CD, Kashyap VS, Clair DG, et al. Endovascular management of iliac artery occlusions: extending treatment to TransAtlantic Inter-Society Consensus class C and D patients. J Vasc Surg. 2006;43:32-39.

Rzucidlo EM, Powerll RJ, Zwolak RM, et al. Early results of stent-grafting to treat diffuse aortoiliac occlusive disease. J Vasc Surg. 2003;37:1175-80.

Tetteroo E, van der Graaf Y, Bosch JL, et al. Randomised comparison of primary stent placement versus primary angioplasty followed by selective stent placement in patients with iliac-artery occlusive disease: Dutch Iliac Stent Trial Study Group. Lancet. 1998;351(9110):1153-9.

REFERENCES

1. Norgren L, Hiatt WR, Dormandy JA, et al. Inter-society consensus for the management of peripheral arterial disease (TASC II), J Vasc Surg. 2007;45(Suppl S):S5eS67.
2. Murphy TP, Ariaratnam NS, Carney WI Jr, et al. Aortoiliac insufficiency: long-term experience with stent placement for treatment. Radiology. 2004;231(1):243-9.

QUIZ

A 72-year-old woman presents to you in clinic with 100-feet claudication that is preventing her from going food shopping. She must rest for 5 minutes for the pain to subside before she can continue walking. She smokes 1 pack per day for 50 years. She had an MI 3 years ago, leading to a CABG x1. She had a heart catheterization 6 months ago and a bare metal stent was deployed. Her past medical history also includes diverticulitis. She states that she stubbed her little toe on her right foot 2 weeks ago on the curb and she had a small cut on her foot, which has healed.

Question 1: What is your next step with the appropriate reason?

a. Biopsy the healed cut on her foot to exclude any atypical disease.

b. Perform a CT scan with lower extremity runoff because her history is compelling for PAD and you want to map her arterial tree to determine which TASC criteria she falls in and whether she should be treated open or endovascular.

c. Take her to the catheter laboratory for a diagnostic angiogram with possible intervention because her symptoms are mild, so she likely falls under TASC A or B, so she warrants an endovascular intervention for her PAD.

d. Take a physical examination, including pulse examination, and perform noninvasive tests such as ABI/

PVR because her history is compelling for PAD and you need to further characterize it.

Question 2: The patient returns to clinic. She quit smoking and has been exercising with minimal improvement. Her physical examination is unchanged. You perform a CT angiogram of the abdominal aorta with bilateral lower extremity runoff and note an 80% stenosis that extends from the aortoiliac bifurcation on the right to the takeoff of the right hypogastric artery with extensive calcification that involves 50% of the circumference of the common iliac artery. Her baseline creatinine is 1.4. What TASC grade does this patient have and should she be treated with open surgery or an endovascular intervention?

a. TASC A; open
b. TASC A; endovascular
c. TASC B; open
d. TASC B; endovascular

Question 3: You take the patient to the interventional suite and place bilateral kissing iliac stents. On your completion angiogram you see a dissection that was not present during your initial pelvic angiogram. The dissection tracks from the distal right common iliac artery and involves the hypogastric artery. What do you do next?

a. Convert to open surgery by having the anesthesiologist intubate the patient for general anesthesia and perform a retroperitoneal incision to directly repair the dissection.
b. Insert a stent.
c. Embolize the hypogastric artery.
d. No further acute intervention is necessary. Closely follow the patient as an outpatient.

Question 4: Immediately after the case, the patient has palpable right lower extremity dorsalis pedis and posterior tibial pulses. Her ABI improves to 0.9 on the right lower extremity. She has immediate improvement and is able to go shopping without experiencing pain and her wound heals within days. Under which scenario would you take the patient back to the catheter laboratory for a diagnostic angiogram with a possible intervention.

a. During the 1-year follow-up, the patient has started to smoke again and is no longer in a supervised exercise program. The patient denies symptoms, but requests an angiogram since that's the gold-standard test.
b. She shows up in the local ER with purulent, foul-smelling discharge from her right groin, with fever, chills, and night sweats.
c. The patient follows up in 3 years due to pain in her right leg that wakes her up from sleep and she must dangle her feet from the side of the bed for the pain to go away.
d. All of the above.

Femoropopliteal Angioplasty and Stenting

Steven Satterly, Niten Singh

1 PREOPERATIVE

1.1 Indications

- Failure of Exercise Program and/or Failure of Medical Management
- Atherosclerotic Stenosis of femoropopliteal artery, causing lifestyle limiting claudication
- Traversable occlusion of femoropopliteal artery
- Rest pain, tissue Loss, Gangrene with high-risk patient for open bypass
- *Contraindications*:
  - Poor anatomical candidate
  - Impassable lesion
  - Endovascular treatment failure
  - Acute limb ischemia/Trauma
  - Noncompliant patient

1.2 Evidence

- *TASC A and B lesions*: Single stenosis < 10 cm of length, single occlusion < 5 cm of length; multiple lesions (stenoses or occlusions) < 5 cm, single stenosis or occlusion < 15 cm not involving infrageniculate arteries, single or multiple lesions in the absence of continuous tibial vessels to improve inflow for distal bypass, calcified occlusion < 5 cm length; single popliteal stenosis—*Endovascular therapy is treatment of choice [C]*
- *TASC C lesions*: Multiple stenoses or occlusions totaling > 15 cm, recurrent stenoses or occlusions following two endovascular interventions—*Open surgery for good risk patients[C]*
- *TASC D lesions*: Chronic total occlusions of common femoral artery or superficial femoral artery (SFA) > 20 cm and involving popliteal artery, chronic total occlusion of popliteal artery, and proximal trifurcation vessels—*Open surgery [C]*[1–3]

1.3 Materials Needed

- Angiography suite with digital subtraction angiography
- 5-Fr micropuncture kit (Fig. 35.1)
  - 5-Fr corrugated needle
  - Starting guidewire
  - Dilator
  - Flush catheter
- 5-Fr sheath (Fig. 35.2)
- 0.035 Floppy tip wire (J-wire, Bentson wire); 180 cm (Fig. 35.3)
- Flush catheter, exchange catheter, selective catheter (Figs. 35.4A and B)
- Hydrophilic glidewire, stiff hydrophilic glidewire (180 cm and 260 cm) (Fig. 35.5)
- Longer sheath (55 cm, 70 cm, etc.) (Fig. 35.6)
- Self-expanding nitinol stent (5–7 mm in lengths that are 40–100 cm) (Fig. 35.7)
- 4–7 mm balloon angioplasty catheter in various lengths (Fig. 35.8)
  - Inflation device (Fig. 35.9)

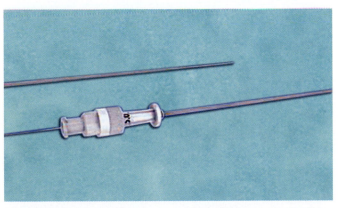

Fig. 35.1: Micropuncture access set (depicted here is the Set from Cook Medical, Bloomington, IN.

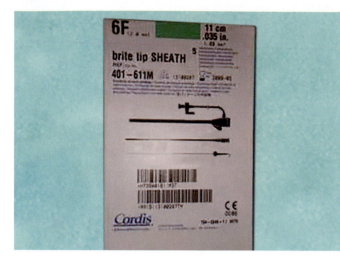

Fig. 35.2: 6 Fr access sheath.

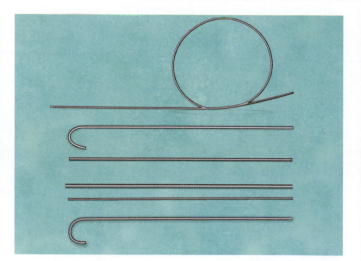

Fig. 35.3: Starter wire (depicted here Bentson wire, Cook Medical, Bloomington, IN).

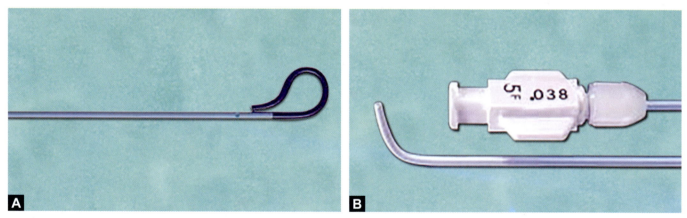

Figs. 35.4A and B: (A) Flush angiographic catheter for aortograms and useful to crossover to Contralateral iliac artery. (B) Selective or end-hole catheter utilized for lower extremity angiographic imaging.

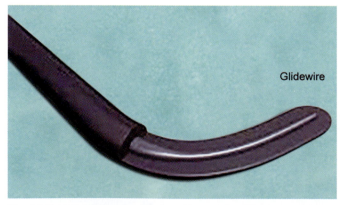

Glidewire

Fig. 35.5: Hydophilic wire (depicted here is the Glidewire, Terumo, Somerset, NJ).

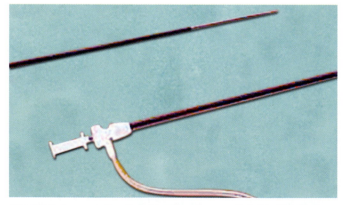

Fig. 35.6: Longer sheath for performing contralateral procedure. Generally 55 cm or 70 cm will be adequate for femoropopliteal procedures.

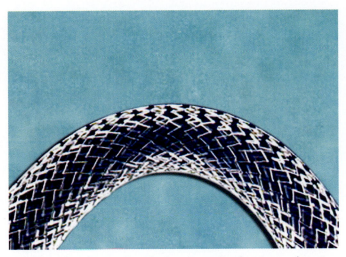

Fig. 35.7: Nitinol stent. Sizes for femoropopliteal region are between 5 mm and 7 mm in diameter.

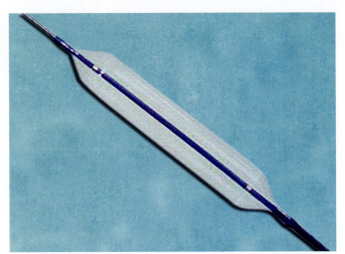

Fig. 35.8: Angioplasty catheter—balloons for this region can range anywhere from 3 mm for predilation to 7 mm for treatment.

– Heparinized saline
– Contrast (Fig. 35.10)
– Protective gear (e.g. lead apron and lead glasses) (Figs. 35.11 and 35.12)

1.4 Preoperative Risk Assessment

Planning:
• Coronary risk assessment, particularly in those with claudication symptoms
• In patients with critical limb ischemia, optimal medical management of cardiac factors along with expeditious repair
• Preoperative noninvasive studies [ABI, tissue perfusion (TcPO$_2$)]
• Arteriogram clearly identifying distal target (above or below knee popliteal artery) as well identifying any disease in the inflow femoral artery (*See* Figs. 35.5A and B)
• *Low risk*:
  – Most patients would not be considered low risk as they all have associated coronary disease.
• *Intermediate risk*:
  – Patients with stable coronary and pulmonary comorbid conditions
• *High risk*:
  – Unstable cardiac disease
  – Unstable pulmonary disease
  – Lower extremity contractures preventing exposure

1.5 Preoperative Checklist

Sign in:
• Correctly identify patient and mark correct extremity
• Review patient's medical history and medications
• Review relevant laboratories (creatinine, hematocrit, prothrombin time, partial thromboplastin time, and platelets count)

Time out:
• Name and identification of patient
• Anticipated procedure
• Ensure preprocedure antibiotics have been administered.
• Ensure equipment that will be required is present.
• Review laboratories and allergies.

Sign out:
• Debrief on procedure
• Identify improvements that can be made

1.6 Decision-Making Algorithm

• *See* Flowcharts 35.1 and 35.2.

1.7 Pearls and Pitfalls

Pearls:
• Remember to utilize your noninvasive information to help prepare for the case and save contrast (i.e. you do not need to perform aortography if a duplex or CT has given you the information and no treatment is required).
• Dilute your contrast to half-strength or less to achieve suitable images and contrast load.

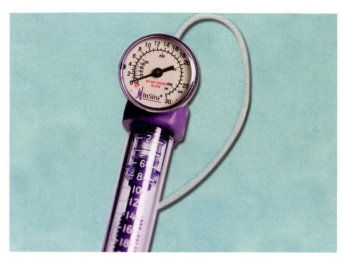

Fig. 35.9: Endoflator device allows for controlled expansion of the balloon and close monitoring of the ATM to avoid burst.

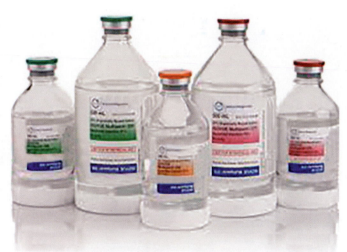

Fig. 35.10: Contrast agent which should be diluted to limit the amount of exposure.

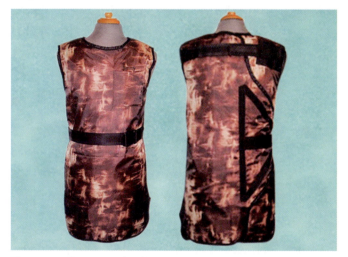

Fig. 35.11: Protective lead apron.

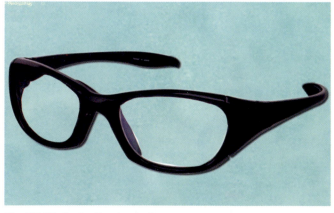

Fig. 35.12: Protective lead glasses.

Flowchart 35.1: Overall treatment strategy for peripheral arterial disease.

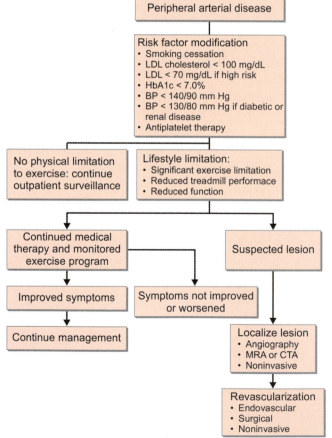

(BP: Blood pressure; HbA1c: Hemoglobin A1c: LDL: Low density lipoprotein; MRA: Magnetic resonance angiography; CTA: Computed tomographic angiography). *Source*: Hiatt.[2]

Flowchart 35.2: Intraoperative decision-making algorithm.

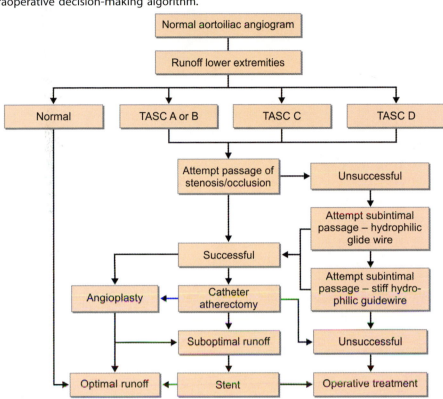

- Longer sheaths from a contralateral approach allows for a stable platform to perform the procedure.
- Crossing the lesion with wire is the key and once achieved the lesion should be treatable.
- For sequential lesions, angioplasty proximal lesions first.
- Predilate heavily calcified lesions with small balloon first to assess behavior of plaque.
- Angioplasty creates a controlled dissection of a lesion and does not always require stenting.
- Single, small lesions will respond more favorably to stenting.
- Entering a subintimal plane is beneficial in crossing chronic total occlusions.
- Remember a nitinol stent will expand when warmed to its nominal size given the constraint imposed by the lesion.
- Extravasation of contrast in a chronic total occlusion (CTO) does not mandate open repair as the area will likely not be perfused once the wire is removed.

Pitfalls:

- An access arteriogram is an easy way to ensure correct access. A high access can lead to a retroperitoneal hematoma and a low access can lead to a pseudoaneurysm. Removing the microaccess and applying pressure if this is noted prior to upsizing the sheath and anticoagulation can prevent these complications.
- Losing wire access can lead to procedural failure especially with tough CTOs.

- Unnecessary arteriographic runs can lead to contrast-induced nephropathy.
- Inability to re-enter the true lumen is the limiting factor of a subintimal dissection.
- Not reading the instructions for use can result in suboptimal results (i.e. stent deployment technique).

1.8 Surgical Anatomy

- *See* Figure 35.13.

1.9 Positioning

- *See* Figure 35.14.

1.10 Anesthesia

- Mallampati score
- Oxygen source
- Intravenous sedation and pain medications
- Intubation kit

2. PERIOPERATIVE

2.1 Assess Access Site

- *See* Figures 35.15.

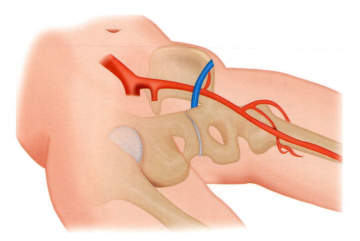

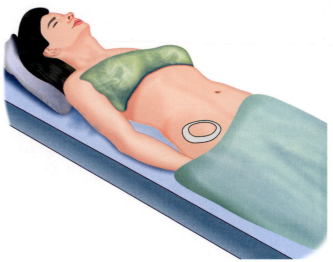

Fig. 35.13: Surgical anatomy. Femoral access—palpate the lateral corner of the pubis. Then palpate the anterior superior iliac spine. The relevant surgical anatomy on physical examination helps triangulate the position of the common femoral pulse.

Fig. 35.14: Positioning. The patient is placed in the supine position. The patient's hair in the inguinal region is clipped and prepped with chlorhexidine or preferred aseptic solution. A groin towel is placed and circumferential sterile towels around ipsilateral leg. The leg is then draped, keeping the access site available.

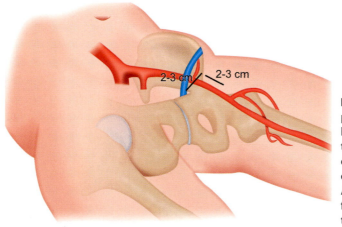

Fig. 35.15: Assess access site. Palpate corner of pubic symphysis, palpate anterior superior iliac spine and draw or imagine a dotted line connecting these two structures. One third distance lateral to the pubic bone and 2–3 cm inferior to this line will locate the common femoral artery pulse and your desired access point. Use of fluoroscopy can be used as an adjunct to locate proper access. A metal object can be positioned on the skin and adjusted with fluoroscopy to overlie the apex of the femoral head. At this location, the common femoral artery is typically appreciated.

2.2 Procedure

• *See* Figures 35.16 to 35.19.

2.3 Closure

The size of sheath utilized and the amount of atherosclerotic disease within the artery will dictate closure. An appropriate percutaneous closure device, interval sheath withdrawal, and arterial compression should be used. Postoperative clinical evaluation for color/pulse and Doppler examinations should be annotated in the chart on bilateral limbs.

3 POSTOPERATIVE

3.1 Complications

Complications:
• Discomfort
• Hematoma/bleeding
• Vessel rupture or dissection
• Pseudoaneurysm
• Distal embolization
• Stent thrombosis
• Stent kinking
• Contrast allergy

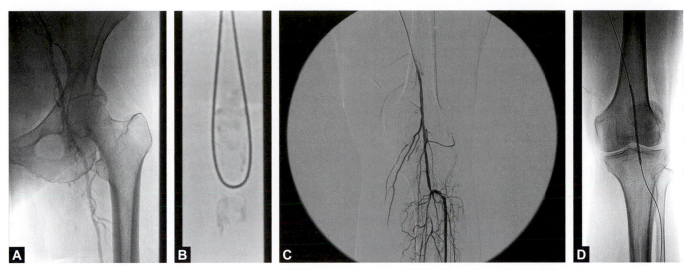

Figs. 35.16A to D: The contralateral iliac artery is selected and the wire is advanced to the contralateral common femoral artery. Next, the Flush catheter is exchanged for a selective or end-hole catheter and the contralateral lower extremity runoff is performed. 25–75 U/kG systemic heparin is given for femoropopliteal lesions. The superficial femoral artery is occluded (A). Using subintimal passage of the wire the lesion is crossed (B) and the catheter is able to re-enter the true lumen distally as confirmed in the arteriogram (C). The lesion distally is predilated with a 4 mm balloon (D).

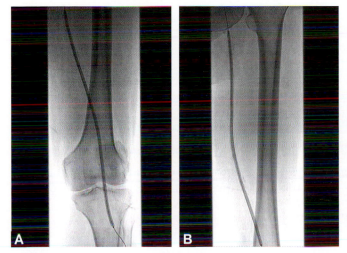

Figs. 35.17A and B: The entire occluded SFA is dilated with a long 6-mm balloon distally (A) and proximally (B).

Fig. 35.18: Completion arteriogram reveals a good angiographic result and no flow limiting dissection therefore a stent was not placed.

- Contrast-induced renal failure
- Reperfusion pain
- Compartment syndrome

3.2 Outcomes

- Improved distal perfusion
- Decreased claudication
- Improved wound healing
- Improved ABI

3.3 Follow-Up

- Ankle brachial index postoperatively and in short interval (i.e. approximately 4 weeks)
- Duplex imaging of area of treatment at short interval and annually
- Exercise program/counseling
- Primary care provider for medical optimization
- Risk factor modification

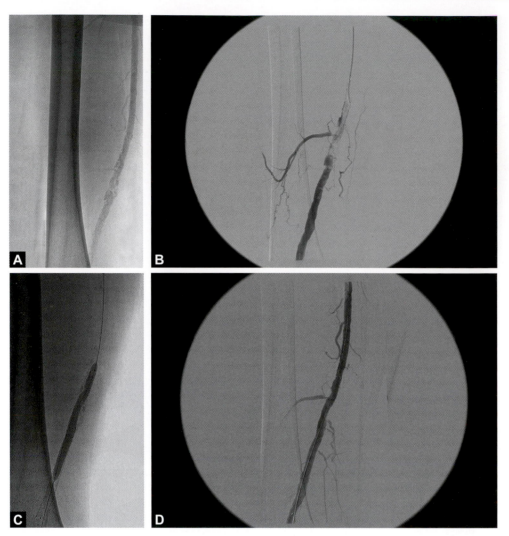

Figs. 35.19A to D: Angioplasty and stenting of a lesion. Using the similar technique described above the lesion is visualized (A). With more proximal positioning of the catheter the lesion appears very high-grade and calcified (B). 6-mm self-expanding nitinol stents were placed and postdilated with a 6-mm balloon (C). Completion arteriogram reveals good angiographic success (D).

REFERENCES

1. Norgren L, Hiatt WR, Dormandy JA. Inter-society consensus for the management of peripheral arterial disease (TASC II). J Vasc Surg. 2007;45:S5-S67.

2. Hiatt WR. Medical treatment of peripheral arterial disease and claudication. N Engl J Med. 2001;344:1608-21.

3. Schneider PA. Endovascular Skills: Guidewire and Catheter Skills for Endovascular Surgery, 3rd edition. Informa Healthcare; 2008.

QUIZ

Question 1. Which of the following statements is true regarding indication for femoropopliteal angioplasty and stenting?

a. The indications are markedly different than the indication for open revascularization.

b. A noncompliant patient is likely a better candidate for endovascular procedures

c. A trial of risk factor modification and exercise is not necessary in patients that are candidates for an endovascular procedure.

d. Failure of medical management and an exercise program is an indication for endovascular intervention in a patient with lifestyle limiting claudication.

Question 2. Which of following is true regarding femoral access?

a. Obtaining access is often best obtained simply by palpating a pulse and placing a needle in the vessel.
b. Ultrasound guidance not helpful in obtaining access and adds to the procedural time.
c. A local arteriogram can prevent postoperative complications.
d. The skin fold in the groin area is the landmark for femoral access.

Question 3. Which of the following is true regarding femoropopliteal angioplasty and stenting?

a. All lesions of the SFA require stenting.
b. The limiting step in subintimal dissection is entry into the subintimal plane.
c. If a stent is to be utilized a self- expanding nitinol stent is preferred in this region.
d. A chronic occlusion cannot be treated with angioplasty and stenting.

Open Repair of Femoral Artery Aneurysm

CHAPTER 36

Robert Molnar, Maria Molnar

1 PREOPERATIVE

1.1 Indications

- *Symptomatic*: pain; venous obstruction; acute thrombosis with claudication, embolization, rest pain or gangrene; rupture (rare yet life-threatening)
- Asymptomatic: size > 2.5 cm
- Failed compression therapy or ultrasound-guided thrombin injection of a pseudoaneurysm
- *Contraindications*: Asymptomatic small aneurysm in high-risk surgical patient. These should be followed for future enlargement or symptoms.

1.2 Evidence

- Due to limited published data on the natural history of femoral aneurysms as well as the rare occurrence of isolated true aneurysms, most surgeons have a adopted a strategy for repairing aneurysms > 2.5 cm in size in low-risk patients.

1.3 Materials Needed

- In general, standard vascular surgical instruments for open surgical procedures are sufficient.
- Graft materials of appropriate size [Dacron or polytetrafluoroethylene (PTFE)].
- In cases where there is proximal extension above the level of the inguinal ligament, balloon occlusion either from the contralateral femoral approach or using intraluminal balloons with a three-way stopcock can be utilized to allow for proximal control rather than performing a retroperitoneal approach in high-risk patients. Any standard angioplasty balloon with adequate radiologic imaging can be employed for the contralateral approach to obtain proximal inflow control.

1.4 Preoperative Planning and Risk Assessment

Planning:
- Imaging with ultrasound, CT, or MRI to evaluate the true extent of the aneurysmal dilatation and to rule out associated aneurysms involving the Aorta, iliacs, contralateral femoral or popliteal arteries that might take priority for operative repair.[1,2] Figure 36.1A—duplex images of a large left common femoral aneurysm.
- Vascular imaging by conventional angiography, computed tomography angiography (CTA) or magnetic resonance angiography (MRA) to assess for occlusive disease processes and establish adequate arterial inflow and outflow vessels especially after distal embolization. Figure 36.1B—angiogram 5-cm true right femoral aneursym.
- Type and Cross for 2 units of PRBCs to be available in the event of significant blood loss or preoperative anemia.
- Perioperative antibiotics
- Baseline arterial doppler

Risk assessment:
- Careful assessment and optimization of medical comorbidities to include cardiac and respiratory risk factors, bleeding diatheses or hypercoagulable states.
- For pseudoaneurysms related to cardiac interventions with the use of drug-eluting stents, Plavix should not be held and consultation with cardiology should be obtained regarding optimal antiplatelet management.
- For aneurysms that appear to be inflamed or are suggestive of an infection, use appropriate antibiotics and obtain cultures during the repair. For suspected infected aneurysms, vein map prior to surgery and use autogenous vein for the repair. Consider cryopreserved vein or artery if autogenous conduit is not adequate or available.

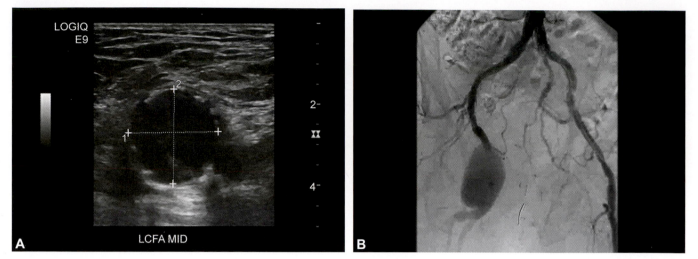

Figs. 36.1A and B: (A) Duplex image of a large true femoral aneurysm; (B) Angiogram of a true 5 cm right femoral aneurysm. *Source*: Michigan Vascular Center.

1.5 Preoperative Checklist

- Follow the WHO (World Health Organization) preoperative checklist including patient identification, right site surgery, appropriate consent, needed equipment and supplies, preoperative antibiotics and anticipated concerns.

1.6 Pearls and Pitfalls

Pearls:

- Prep and drape wide for extension of incisions or to allow for retroperitoneal exposure for adequate proximal control.
- For large aneurysms, it is not necessary to resect the aneurysm sac, as this can lead to nerve or venous injury. The walls of the aneurysm sac can be closed over the graft as an added layer of graft protection.
- For large pseudoaneurysms due to a percutaneous catheter injury associated with significant hematoma and difficult dissection, avoiding injury to surrounding structures can be accomplished by entering the large pseudoaneurysm directly and applying digital control above and below the catheter induced hole while suture repair is accomplished.
- For iatrogenic, catheter-induced pseudoaneurysms, be sure to suture through full thickness arterial wall and not through the weak pseudoaneurysm wall. Sutures not through all layers of the arterial wall can pull through at a later time, thus leading to recurrent pseudoaneurysm formation or uncontrolled bleeding.
- For iatrogenic, catheter-induced pseudoaneurysms, inspect the artery circumferentially to avoid missing a posterior wall catheterization injury.

Pitfalls:

- Avoid postoperative lymphatic leaks by meticulously ligating lymph nodes or lymphatic channels. Consider a lateral approach to the dissection, sweeping the more lymphatic containing subcutaneous tissue medially to avoid transecting lymphatic channels.
- Avoid postoperative wound healing complications by resecting any nonviable subcutaneous tissue or compromised skin edges prior to closing.

1.7 Surgical Anatomy

The common femoral artery courses from below the inguinal ligament approximately half way between the pubic symphysis and the anterior superior iliac spine. It branches at variable distances below the inguinal ligament (usually about 4 cm) into the superficial femoral artery and the profunda artery.

1.8 Positioning

The patient should be positioned supine with an indwelling Foley catheter, with the arms either out to the side on arm boards or tucked depending on surgeon and anesthesia preference. Prepping and draping should be from the costal margin superiorly, lateral to the iliac crest, medially to the pubic symphysis and distally to the knee.

1.9 Anesthesia

General or spinal anesthesia is preferred. However, sedation and a local anesthesia with an appropriate field block can be utilized for patients with excessive anesthesia risks.

2 PERIOPERATIVE

2.1 Incision

- The common femoral artery can be approached either through a longitudinal incision following the course of the artery or via an oblique incision coursing from lateral to medial. In an obese patient with a large pannus, it is often helpful to retract the abdominal wall toward the opposite upper abdominal quadrant with tape prior to prepping and draping. The oblique incision can be carried laterally and deepened along the inguinal ligament, freeing the inguinal ligament laterally to allow exposure of the proximal common femoral artery and distal external iliac artery under the inguinal ligament. Alternatively, if more proximal exposure of the common femoral artery is needed with the longitudinal incision, the inguinal ligament can be incised and repaired at closure. Figure 36.2A—preoperative marking for open repair of a 6 centimeter false femoral artery aneurysm, Figure 36.2B—proposed incision to allow lateral extension along the inguinal ligament for higher proximal control during operative exposure.

2.2 Steps

- The proximal artery above the aneurysm is dissected free and a vessel loop is placed around the normal caliber artery above the aneurysm (Fig. 36.3A).
- Dissection is then directed below the aneurysm where the superficial femoral and profunda arteries are dissected free for distal control (Fig. 36.3B). Side branches can be controlled either with vessel loops or clips which are to be removed following the repair.
- Once adequate proximal and distal control is obtained, the patient is administered heparin or another anticoagulation regimen per surgeon preference.
- The proximal and distal vessels are clamped with vascular clamps or occluded by use of the vessel loops and the aneurysm sac is opened longitudinally (Fig. 36.3C):
  - In a type I aneurysm (involving only the common femoral artery), the proximal and distal neck of the aneurysm are prepared and a prosthetic graft of reference vessel size is placed as an interposition graft using standard vascular techniques (Figs. 36.2 C and D). The walls of the aneurysm can be folded over the graft and secured with either running or interrupted sutures as is employed for aortic aneurysm grafting.
  - In a type II aneurysm (involving both the common femoral artery and the profunda artery), the interposition graft can be anastomosed distally to the profunda artery with the superficial femoral artery being reimplanted to the side of the interposition graft, or a second graft used end-to-side from the initial graft to the superficial femoral artery. Any configuration of grafts can be employed depending on anatomical findings and surgeon preference (Figs. 36.2E to H).
  - In an iatrogenic pseudoaneurysm (Fig. 36.2I), the arterial wall defect will often be seen at the base of the aneurysm cavity and can be repaired with simple suture closure. Direct suture repair of the arterial

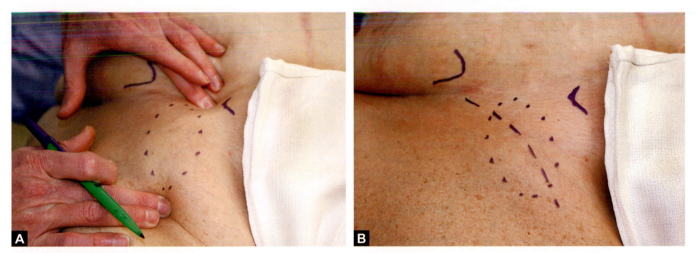

Figs. 36.2A and B: Incisions marked.

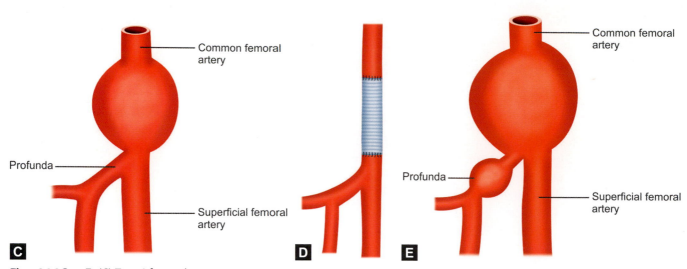

Figs. 36.2C to E: (C) Type I femoral artery aneurysm. (D) Type I repair. (E) Type II femoral artery aneurysm involving profunda artery.

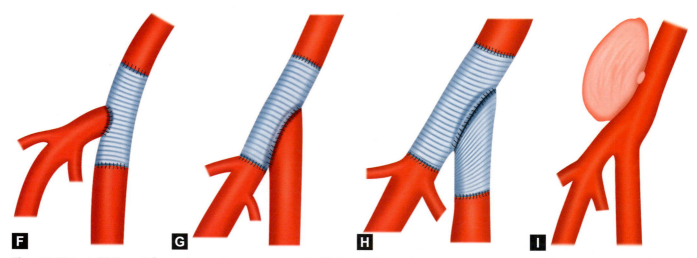

Figs. 36.2F to I: (F) Type II femoral artery aneurysm repair. (G) Type II femoral artery aneurysm repair. (H) Type II common femoral artery aneurysm repair. (I) Iatrogenic pseudoaneurysm from arterial injury.

defect can be employed being sure to incorporate full-thickness sutures to the arterial wall (Fig. 36.3D and E). Many surgeons will resect either all of the pseudoaneurysm cavity or portions of the cavity depending on the technical difficulty (Fig. 36.3F).

- In an infected field or suspected infection, autogenous vein should be utilized with or without a sartorius muscle flap covering the repair. The sartorius muscle can be detached from its insertion to the anterior iliac spine, freed along its lateral border and rotated over with tacking sutures to the inguinal ligament to provide a vascularized muscle flap coverage to the repair.[6]

- Following the repair, the wound should be inspected for any lymphatic leaks and these appropriately suture ligated. Any necrotic or nonviable/poorly perfused tissue should be resected including compromised skin. The wound should be closed in multiple layers and the skin closed by surgeon preference with attention to avoiding undue tension on the skin edges (Fig. 36.3G).

- If a drain is to be used, it should be brought through a separate skin incision laterally and secured by suture.

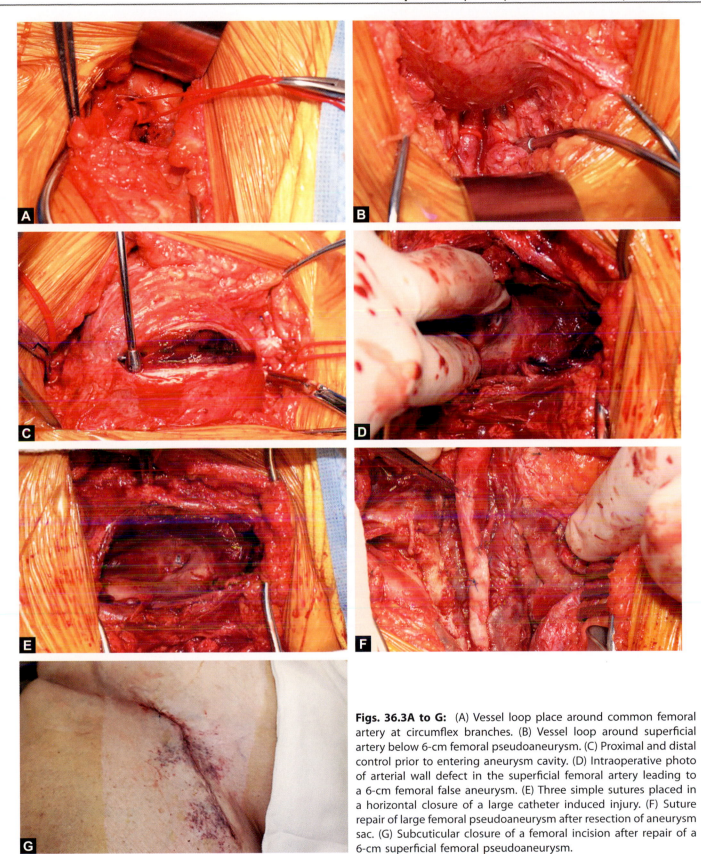

Figs. 36.3A to G: (A) Vessel loop place around common femoral artery at circumflex branches. (B) Vessel loop around superficial artery below 6-cm femoral pseudoaneurysm. (C) Proximal and distal control prior to entering aneurysm cavity. (D) Intraoperative photo of arterial wall defect in the superficial femoral artery leading to a 6-cm femoral false aneurysm. (E) Three simple sutures placed in a horizontal closure of a large catheter induced injury. (F) Suture repair of large femoral pseudoaneurysm after resection of aneurysm sac. (G) Subcuticular closure of a femoral incision after repair of a 6-cm superficial femoral pseudoaneurysm.

3 POSTOPERATIVE

3.1 Complications

Most common complications:
- Cardiac: Appropriate preoperative evaluation and management of cardiac risk factors including perioperative blood pressure control is necessary
- Lymphatic leak and lymphocele
- Skin necrosis or wound break down
- Infection
- Bleeding

Least common complications:
- Graft thrombosis
- Embolization
- Nerve injury
- Venous thrombosis

3.2 Outcomes

- Generally excellent
- Perioperative mortality ranges from 0% to 4% heavily influenced by comorbidities[4,5]
- 5-year patency for interposition grafts and saphenous vein grafts of 80%[5]

3.3 Follow-Up

- Postoperative evaluation of distal circulation and wound healing should be performed daily until discharge from the hospital.
- Postdischarge office or clinic evaluation at 7–10 days to evaluate distal perfusion and to remove skin closure sutures or staples as needed.
- Duplex evaluation and ABIs at 1 month, 6 months, and then yearly for repair surveillance.

3.4 E-mail an Expert

- *E-mail address*: rmolnar8@att.net

REFERENCES

1. Diwan A, Sarkar R, Stanley JC, et al. Incidence of femoral and popliteal aneurysms in patients with abdominal aortic aneurysms. J Vasc Surg. 2000;31:863-9.
2. Dent TL, Lindenauer SM, Ernst CB, et al. Multiple arteriosclerotic arterial aneurysms. Arch Surg. 1972;105:338.
3. Cutler BS, Darling RC. Surgical management of arteriosclerotic femoral aneurysms. Surgery. 1973;74:764.
4. Graham LM, Zelenock GB, Whitehouse WM Jr, et al. Clinical significance of arteriosclerotic femoral artery aneurysms. Arch Surg. 1980;115:502.
5. Sapienza P, Mingoli A, Feldhaus RJ, et al. Femoral artery aneurysms: long-term follow-up and results of surgical treatment. Cardiovasc Surg. 1996;4:181.
6. Reddy DJ, Smith RF, Elliott JP, et al. Infected femoral artery false aneurysms in drug addicts: evolution of selective vascular reconstruction. J Vasc Surg. 1986;3:718-24.

CHAPTER

Popliteal Aneurysm Repair: Open

37

Giye Choe

1 PREOPERATIVE

1.1 Indications

Indications:
- Symptomatic popliteal aneurysms (thrombosis, pain, distal embolization, ischemic symptoms, etc.)
- Popliteal aneurysms >2 cm[1]
- For patients who are poor operative candidates, endovascular repair is an option; however, it has been shown to require more frequent reinterventions compared to open repairs.[2,3]

Contraindications:
- Inability to tolerate general anesthesia

1.2 Evidence

- Symptomatic popliteal aneurysms and those over 2 cm require surgical repair due to risk of critical limb ischemia and amputation untreated aneurysms.[4,5]
- Long-term patency rates of open repair are fairly good, with primary patency around 66–69%, secondary patency at 83.6–87%, and limb salvage rate at 86.7–87%.[5,6]
- Repair of asymptomatic aneurysms has better outcomes compared to symptomatic ones.[5,6] Absence of distal pulses is also associated with poorer surgical outcomes.
- In 2013, when compared to open repair, endovascular repair has comparable long-term patency results[7] but has high short-term reintervention rates.[2,3] The standard approach of repair is still open repair.

1.3 Materials Needed

- *For the vein harvest*: If using greater or lesser saphenous vein graft: #10 scalpel, electrocautery, self-retaining

retractors, fine tip metzenbaum scissors, 3-0 and 4-0 silk ties, papaverine saline solution, fine mosquito clamps, Gerald forceps, bulldog clamps. Ultrasound to locate vein preoperatively.
- *For the bypass*: #10, #11 scalpel, electrocautery, Adson forceps, two or more self-retaining retractors, two or more elastic vessel loops, umbilical tape, right angle clamps of various sizes, metzenbaum scissors, Potts scissors, vessel clamps of various sizes, 6-0 polypropylene suture, 3-0 Vicryl suture, regular diamond tipped needle holders, Debakey forceps, Castro needle holders, Gerald forceps, skin closure material of choice. Doppler probe. If not using vein graft synthetic graft of choice, usually PTFE or Dacron, sized appropriately.

1.4 Preoperative Risk Assessment

- Standard vascular preoperative risk assessment must include cardiovascular risk assessment related to general anesthesia.
- Should have screening for other aneurysms, especially abdominal aneurysms and contralateral limb evaluation.
- Should have had vein mapping to evaluate the greater or lesser saphenous vein for conduit.

1.5 Preoperative Checklist

- Surgical—laterality of procedure to be performed, approach and patient positioning
- Anesthesia—standard safety checklist including airway and blood product availability
- Nursing—availability of necessary equipment including synthetic graft, if needed. Surgical preparation should include the entire extremity, ideally including the foot.

Flowchart 37.1: Decision-making algorithm.

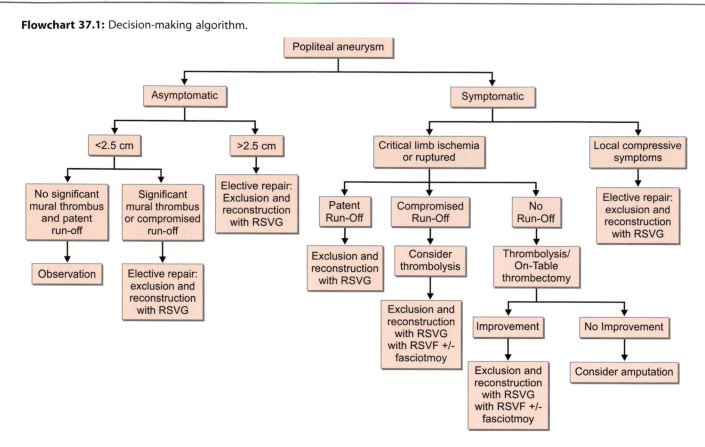

1.6 Decision-Making Algorithm

- Select the approach—if the aneurysm extends beyond the popliteal fossa into the adductor canal or distally into the gastrocnemius, select a medial approach identical to a femoropopliteal bypass or femorotibial bypass.
- Select the conduit—vein mapping should be done preoperatively to assess adequacy of veins. Vein graft generally has better outcomes compared to synthetic graft in this highly mobile area. If not adequate, select synthetic graft size-matched for the patient's normal arteries.
- Whether to excise aneurysm after exclusion—if the aneurysm is adherent to surrounding tissues, making it difficult to excise without injuring surrounding structures, it is better not to excise. It can also serve as a biologic encasing to protect the new graft (Flowchart 37.1).

1.7 Pearls and Pitfalls

Pearls:
- Under or overestimating the length of the aneurysm and choosing the wrong approach can make the case challenging.

- If the aneurysm sac is densely adherent to surrounding structures, it is acceptable to leave the sac in place, similar to an open abdominal aortic aneurysm (AAA) repair.

Pitfalls:
- Take care to avoid injuring the tibial and common peroneal nerve during dissection.

1.8 Surgical Anatomy

- The lazy S incision and the anatomy of the popliteal fossa, including the two head of the gastrocnemius, the semimembranosus and semitendinosus, biceps femoris and the tibial and common peroneal nerve in relation to the popliteal vein and artery (Fig. 37.1).

1.9 Positioning

- Prone with all pressure points well-padded for posterior approach. Medial approach can be done with the patient in supine position.

1.10 Anesthesia

- No major anesthetic concerns other than those related to patient's prior systemic health and airway management in prone.

2 PERIOPERATIVE

A medial approach is virtually identical to a femoropopliteal or femorotibial bypass, with ligation of the artery (Fig. 37.2B). Therefore, the approach detailed here is the posterior approach (Fig. 37.2A). Greater saphenous vein harvest is also identical to harvest techniques used in other procedures, and will not be discussed in depth other than to note that the vein is easily accessible with the patient lying prone.

2.1 Incision

Make a lazy S incision starting at the medial head of the gastrocnemius, crossing over the popliteal fossa and extending over the lesser saphenous vein. Carry the incision down to the aneurysm, placing self-retaining

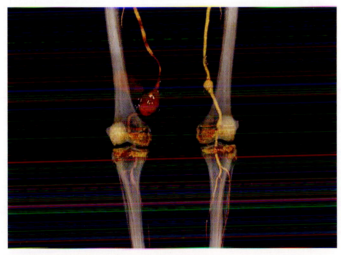

Fig. 37.1: Surgical anatomic illustration.

retractors in the surgical field to keep exposure. Take care to avoid injuring the common peroneal and tibial nerve.

2.2 Steps

- Identify the proximal extent of the aneurysm via palpation. Dissect around this and using a right angle clamp place a vessel loop around the proximal end.
- Expose the superficial aspect of the aneurysm—the aneurysm sac does not have to be circumferentially dissected out unless planning to remove it.
- Dissect down to the distal extent, down until you encounter normal healthy artery and place a vessel loop around this.
- Give IV heparin (usually 5,000 U).
- Place vessel clamps in the proximal and distal ends of the aneurysm, ideally in normal tissue with a healthy tissue cuff enough to allow sewing an anastomosis.
- Open the aneurysm sac using an 11 blade and Potts scissors. Control back bleeding branches of the geniculate arteries by oversewing from within the aneurysm sac. Usually, this can be done using a figure-of-eight suture.
- Perform the proximal anastomosis with the conduit of choice in an end-to-end fashion using a running 6-0 polypropylene suture. The proximal clamp can be released to check the anastomosis and fill the conduit to minimize air emboli. The bull dog clamp on the graft can be moved to ensure ideal length for sewing.
- Perform the distal anastomosis in the same fashion, taking care to avoid tension or kinking.
- Release the distal clamp and control any leaks.
- Check the distal pulses with a Doppler probe (Fig. 37.3).

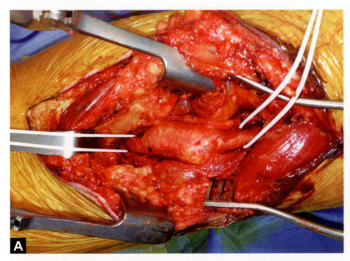
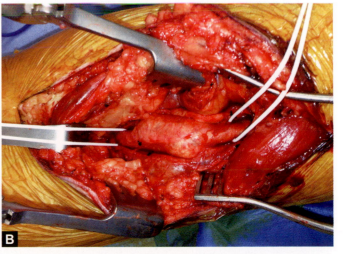

Figs. 37.2A and B: (A) Posterior approach and (B) medial approach.

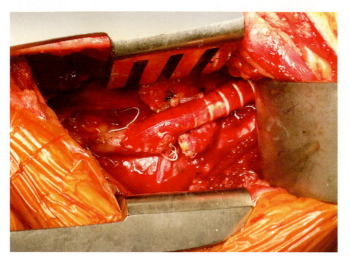

Fig. 37.3: Steps.

2.3 Closure

- Close the deeper fascial layer using 2-0 or 3-0 polyglactin suture, usually in a simple interrupted fashion.
- Close the dermal and skin layers in the usual fashion, most often simple interrupted sutures or a running "baseball" suture.

3 POSTOPERATIVE

3.1 Complications[6,8]

- Graft occlusion, early and late
- Surgical wound infection
- Hematoma formation
- Continued enlargement of aneurysm in cases where back bleeding was not controlled (similar to type 2 endoleaks)
- Amputation
- Death

3.2 Outcomes

- Five-year primary and secondary graft patency rate is around 66% and 85%, respectively.
- Outcomes are worse for symptomatic aneurysms compared to asymptomatic ones and also those patients who do not have distal pulses in the affected limb. Worse for elective cases. Patency of saphenous vein grafts is better than that of prosthetic grafts.

3.3 Follow-Up

Instructions:

- Arterial duplex and ankle-brachial index (ABIs) measured at the time of the first postoperative follow-up appointment.
- Thereafter up to the surgeon's discretion, usually every 3 months the first 6–12 months and then yearly thereafter, with duplex studies and ABIs.

3.4 E-mail an Expert

- *Email address*: choeg@ohsu.edu

REFERENCES

1. Cross JE, Galland RB, Hingorani A, et al. Nonoperative versus surgical management of small (less than 3 cm), asymptomatic popliteal artery aneurysms. J Vasc Surg. 2011;53:1145-1148.
2. Galiñanes EL, Dombrovskiy VY, Graham AM, et al. Endovascular versus open repair of popliteal artery aneurysms: outcomes in the US medicare population. Vasc Endovascular Surg. 2013;47:267-273.
3. Lovegrove RE, Javid M, Magee TR, et al. Endovascular and open approaches to non-thrombosed popliteal aneurysm repair: a meta-analysis. Eur J Vasc Endovasc Surg. 2008;36 (1):96-100.
4. Dawson I, Sie RB, van Bockel JH. Atherosclerotic popliteal aneurysm. Br J Surg. 1997;84:293-9.
5. Mahmood A, Salaman R, Sintler M, et al. Surgery of popliteal artery aneurysms: a 12-year experience. J Vasc Surg. 2003;37(3):586-93.
6. Pulli R, Dorigo W, Troisi N, et al. Surgical management of popliteal artery aneurysms: which factors affect outcomes? J Vasc Surg. 2006;43(3):481-7.
7. Antonello M, Frigatti P, Battocchio P, et al. Open repair versus endovascular treatment for asymptomatic popliteal artery aneurysm: results of a prospective randomized study. J Vasc Surg. 2005;42(2):185-93.
8. Dawson I, van Bockel JH, Brand R, Terpstra JL. Popliteal artery aneurysms. Long-term follow-up of aneurysmal disease and results of surgical treatment. J Vasc Surg. 1991; 13(3):398-407.

QUIZ

Question 1. In large single and multi-center reviews of management of popliteal aneurysms:
a. The posterior approach was preferred in the majority of cases.
b. Endovascular treatment was equivalent to open bypass.
c. Bypass with prosthetic material was superior to vein bypass.
d. The rate of amputation was higher with endovascular treatment.
e. Endovascular treatment was contraindicated in cases of acute limb ischemia.

Question 2. Popliteal aneurysms:
a. Are the second most common peripheral aneurysms.
b. Are associated with other aneurysms in less than 50% of cases.
c. Are bilateral in nearly 50% of cases.
d. Cannot be detected by physical examination.
e. Rarely are present with acute limb ischemia.

ANSWERS:
1. b   2. c

Popliteal Artery Aneurysm Repair: Endovascular

James R Ballard, Erica Mitchell

1 PREOPERATIVE

1.1 Indications

- Popliteal artery aneurysm >2 cm
- High-risk patient for open repair due to medical comorbidities and/or unsuitable conduit for open reconstruction
- *Contraindication*: Patient unable to take antiplatelet agent postprocedure
- *Contraindication*: Unable to establish vascular access to perform endovascular repair
- *Contraindication*: Aneurysm extends to <1 cm to the tibioperoneal trunk
- *Contraindication*: Aneurysm size requires resection due to mass effect
- *Contraindication*: Popliteal artery occlusion (Fig. 38.1).

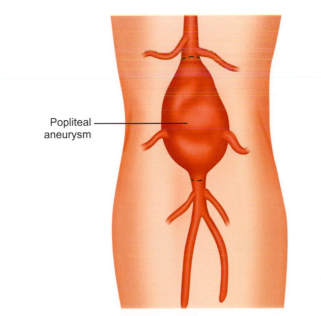

Popliteal aneurysm

Fig. 38.1: Popliteal artery aneurysm.

1.2 Evidence

- Endovascular popliteal artery aneurysm repair is an alternative to open aneurysm repair with reduced blood loss, quicker recovery, and shorter hospital stay.[1]
- Limb salvage rates appear to be similar between open and endovascular repair.[2–5]

1.3 Materials Needed

- Endovascular suite or operating room with imaging (fixed or portable C-arm)
- Duplex ultrasound for establishing access
- *Access*: micropuncture kit, arterial sheath (depends on stent size to be used) generally 7–12 Fr
- *Wires*: 0.35-in. system, access wire (micropuncture wire 0.18, Benson, J-Wire), glidewire, Storq wire, working length will depend on approach via antegrade or contralateral arterial access
- Flush catheter, guide catheter (Kumpe)
- *Stent graft*: Covered stent (Viabahn, WL Gore and Associates, Inc., Scottsdale, Flagstaff, AZ)
- Angioplasty balloons
- *Optional materials*: Contrast injector, angioplasty insufflators (Figs. 38.2A to D).

1.4 Preoperative Planning and Risk Assessment

Planning:
- *Vascular labs*: Arterial duplex of lower extremity with ankle-brachial index (ABI)
- Preoperative CTA or MRA with runoff or preoperative arteriogram
- Sizing and selection of stent grafts and sizing of access vessels based on preoperative imaging.
- Verify all necessary stents and or sheaths/catheters/wires are available for procedure (Figs. 38.3A and B)

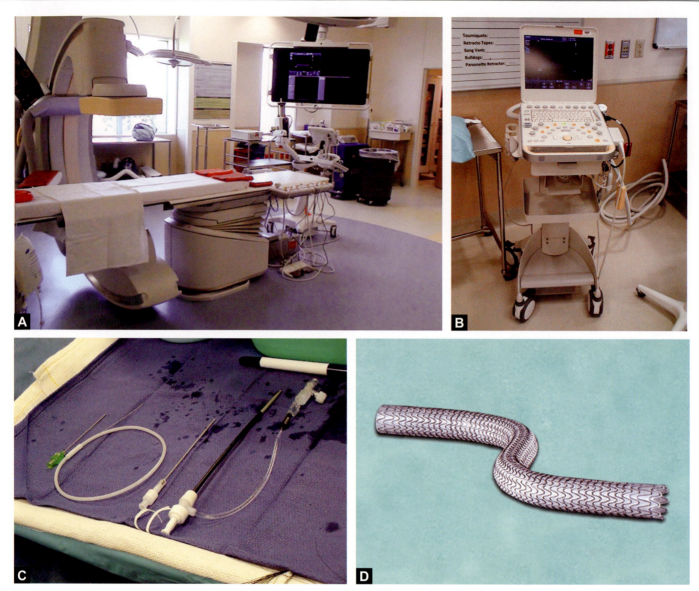

Figs. 38.2A to D: (A) Angiography suite. (B) Duplex Ultrasound. (C) Micropuncture kit. (D) Viabahn stent graft (WL Gore and Associates, Inc., Scottsdale, Flagstaff, AZ).

Risk assessment:
- *Low–intermediate risk*:
  - Absence of high-risk factors
- *High risk*:
  - Age > 80
  - Severe cardiac dysfunction
    - Left ventricle ejection fraction <25%
    - New York Heart Association (NYHA) class III or IV heart failure
    - Angina pectoris
    - Cardiac stress test positive for myocardial ischemia

- Severe renal insufficiency (creatinine > 3.0 mg/dL) or dialysis dependent

1.5 Preoperative Checklist

Sign in:
- Confirm patient identity, consent, site, and procedure to be performed
- Site marking visible
- Anesthesia equipment and medication check completed
- Equipment functioning

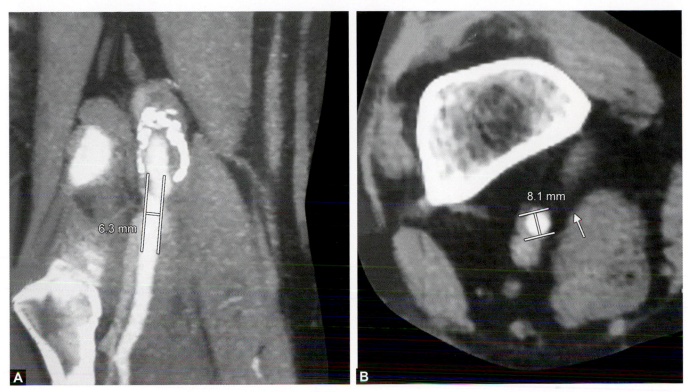

Figs. 38.3A and B: CTA with lower extremity runoff.

- Confirm known allergies
- Difficult airway/aspiration risk
- Risk of blood loss > 500 mL

Time out:

- Confirm all team members present and have introduced themselves by name and role
- Confirm patient name, site, and procedure
- Anticipated critical events
- Confirm preoperative antibiotic prophylaxis has been given within 60 minutes of incision
- Confirm all equipment needed is present
- Essential imaging displayed

Sign out:

- Name of procedure recorded
- Instrument, sponge, and needle counts correct
- Any specimen labeled
- Any equipment problems identified
- Any concerns for patient recovery
  - Preoperative clopidogrel 300 mg PO on morning of procedure or prior initiation of clopidogrel 75 mg daily
  - Preoperative and intraoperative blood pressure management.

1.6 Pearls and Pitfalls

Pearls:

- Aberrant anatomy involving tibioperoneal trunk or anterior tibial artery origin need to be identified prior to stent placement, which is especially critical in patients with limited tibial runoff.
- Open antegrade access eliminates need for percutaneous closure in diseased arteries.

Pitfalls:

- Avoid contralateral access in patients with steep aortic bifurcation or previous aortic surgery.
- Avoid percutaneous access in heavily diseased common femoral or superficial femoral arteries.

1.7 Positioning

- Supine
- If in operating room, ensure operating room table is compatible with angiography.
- *See* Figure 38.4.

1.8 Anesthesia

- Monitored anesthesia
- Local anesthesia with sedation
- General anesthesia in select cases

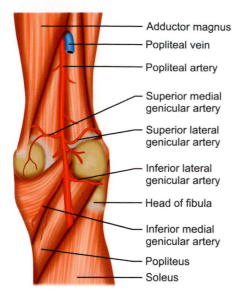

Labels on figure:
- Adductor magnus
- Popliteal vein
- Popliteal artery
- Superior medial genicular artery
- Superior lateral genicular artery
- Inferior lateral genicular artery
- Head of fibula
- Inferior medial genicular artery
- Popliteus
- Soleus

Fig. 38.4: Surgical anatomy of the popliteal artery.

2 PERIOPERATIVE

2.1 Access

- Open access of ipsilateral superficial femoral artery
- Percutaneous access of ipsilateral superficial femoral artery or contralateral common femoral artery with micropuncture access kit
- Placement of sheath.

2.2 Steps

- Arteriogram of superficial femoral artery (SFA)/popliteal artery and runoff
  - Size necessary stent
  - Obtain length of segment to be stented
- Gain wire access across aneurysm, typically initial wire access with guidewire or floppy tip wire, may require guiding catheter
- Secure working wire across lesion
- Arteriogram with wire and sheath in place for stent placement
- Deploy stent(s), stent should be sized to the vessel, oversizing by >10% may result in in-folding or fluting of graft material resulting in a type 1 endoleak
- Postdilation angioplasty with balloon sized to the artery
- Completion angiogram to include runoff (*see* Figs. 38.5 A to E).

2.3 Closure

Open access:
- Closure of common femoral or superficial femoral artery arteriotomy (transverse) with interrupted 5-0 or 6-0 Prolene sutures
- Incision closed in three layers, two layers of absorbable suture, and subcuticular skin suture with Dermabond skin glue.

Percutaneous access:
- Closure with percutaneous closure device of choice
- Alternative is manual pressure

3 POSTOPERATIVE

3.1 Complications

Most common complica1tions:
- Access site hematoma or bleeding
- Peri-incisional skin numbness or paresthesias

Least common complications:
- Early thrombosis of stent graft resulting in limb ischemia
- Lower extremity embolization or ischemia

3.2 Outcomes

- Primary patency varies widely at 1 year; in the literature it is between 47% and 93%.
- Primary-assisted patency at 1 and 3 years is 74% and 87%, respectively, which is comparable to open repair at 87% and 86%, respectively.
- Amputation rate at 1 and 3 years, 2% and 3%, respectively, which is comparable to elective open repair at 7% and 4%, respectively.

3.3 Follow-Up

- Arterial duplex prior to discharge from hospital to document evidence of endoleak and aneurysm sac size
- Arterial duplex every 3 months for first year then every 6 months
- X-ray every 6 months to evaluate for stent fracture.

3.4 E-mail an Expert

- *E-mail address*: mitcheer@@ohsu.edu

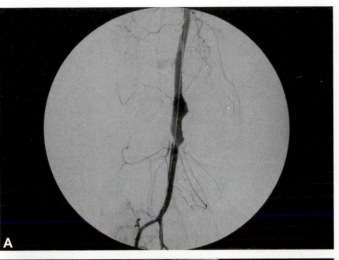

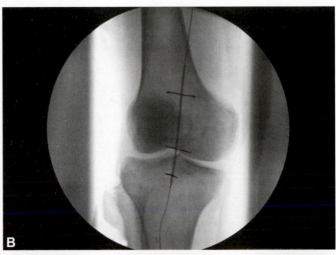

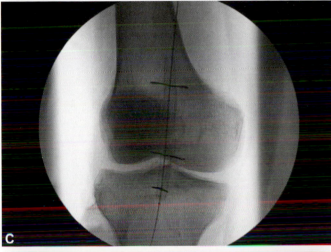

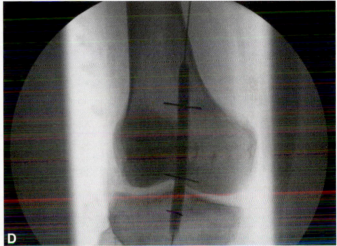

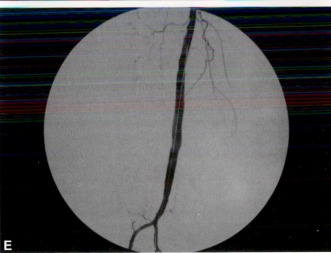

Figs. 38.5A to E: (A) Runoff with working wire in place across aneurysm. (B) Stent graft in place. (C) Stent graft deployed. Stent graft deployed but prior to dilation. (D) Balloon dilation of stent. Dilation of stent graft to diameter of native artery.

REFERENCES

1. Lovegrove RE, Javid M, Magee TR, et al. Endovascular and open approaches to non-thrombosed popliteal aneurysm repair: a meta-analysis. Eur J Vasc Endovasc Surg. 2008; 36:96-100.
2. Antonello M, Frigatti P, Battocchio P, et al. Open repair versus endovascular treatment for asymptomatic popliteal artery aneurysm repair: are the results comparable to open surgery? Eur J Vasc Endovasc Surg. 2006;32:149-54.
3. Liem TK, Landry GJ. Endovascular management of popliteal aneurysms. In: Moore WS (Ed). Endovascular Surgery, 4th edition. Saunders: Samuel Ahn; 2011. pp. 529-34.
4. Pulli R, Dorigo W, Fargion A, et al. Comparison of early and midterm results of open and endovascular treatment of popliteal artery aneurysms. Ann Vasc Surg. 2012;26:809-18.
5. Tsilimparis N, Dayama A, Ricotta JL. Open and endovascular repair of popliteal artery aneurysms: tabular review of the literature. Ann Vasc Surg. 2013;27(2):259-65.

CHAPTER 39

Femoropopliteal Bypass

Tina Chen, Peter Henke

1 PREOPERATIVE

1.1 Indications

Superficial femoral artery athero-occlusive disease resulting in:
- Lifestyle-limiting claudication
- Critical limb ischemia with rest pain or tissue loss

1.2 Evidence

- The most recent Cochrane review discussed two trials directly comparing above-knee reversed vein to synthetic bypass; both found a significant benefit in primary patency in using vein over synthetic materials by 5 years. No studies were evaluated directly comparing vein with other grafts.
- A 10-year, single center experience of 235 reversed greater saphenous vein bypasses to both above and below knee targets demonstrated a primary patency rate of 87% ± 4% at 3 years and 81% ± 6% at 5 years.

Compared to polytetrafluoroethylene (PTFE) bypasses at the same institution, the overall PTFE failure rate was three to four times that of saphenous vein bypasses.

1.3 Materials Needed

- *See* Figures 39.1 to 39.4.

1.4 Preoperative Planning and Risk Assessment

Planning:
- CT abdomen/pelvis with lower extremity runoffs
- Angiography of lower extremity
- Vein mapping and measurements

Risk assessment:
- Preoperative risk factors based on the PREVENT (Project of Ex Vivo vein graft Engineering via Transfection) III

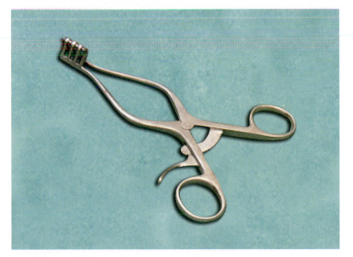

Fig. 39.1: Weitlaner retractors. Permits visualization of the superficial femoral artery and great saphenous vein.

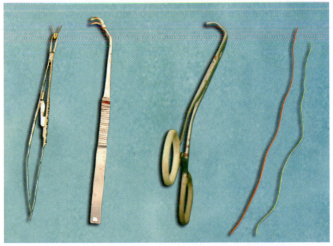

Fig. 39.2: Vascular clips, clamps, or vessel loops. Minimize blood loss and allow for vascular control during anastomosis.

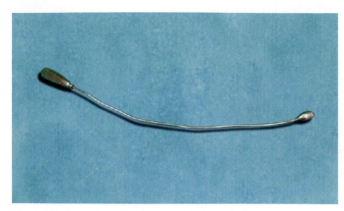

Fig. 39.3: Tunneler. Creation of path for vein bypass.

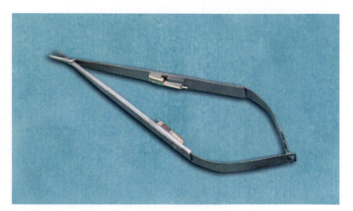

Fig. 39.4: Castroviejo's fine-needle drivers.

trial for prediction of amputation-free survival following surgical bypass:
- *Dialysis*:   4 points
- *Tissue loss*:   3 points
- *Age ≥ 75*:   2 points
- *Hct ≤ 30*:   2 points
- *CAD*:   1 point
• *Low risk*: ≤ 3 points
• *Intermediate risk*: 4–7 points
• *High risk*: ≥ 8 points

1.5 Preoperative Checklist

• Outpatient preoperative β-blocker, aspirin, and statin for cardiac risk reduction
• Imaging as needed to assess inflow and outflow targets
• Vein mapping with ultrasound and marking with permanent marker
• Ankle-brachial index and signals or pulses documented
• Cardiac evaluation including stress test and carotid duplex if high risk as appropriate
• Preoperative antibiotics against skin flora such as a first generation cephalosporin, or vancomycin in a penicillin-allergic patient
• Surgical clippers used to remove body hair in surgical field
• Skin prep wipes with chlorhexidine.

1.6 Decision-Making Algorithm

• *See* Flowchart 39.1.

1.7 Pearls and Pitfalls

Pearls:
• Alternative bypass origins must be kept in mind in the event of unanticipated arterial disease or plaque burden encountered at the proximal anastomotic site, or if vein quality and length are compromised.
• Both inflow and outflow play a large role in the long-term patency of bypasses. Pre- and intraoperative assessment of adequacy of inflow and outflow are critical.
• The suitability of an inflow site can be assessed intraoperatively with a direct intra-arterial pressure measurement compared to the radial arterial pressure; a resting gradient >10 mmHg is hemodynamically significant.
• If preoperative concerns exist regarding ipsilateral vein quality, it is advisable to prepare both extremities for harvest.
• Place the knee in 30° flexion during the procedure. When performing an above-knee bypass, place a stack of bundled towels under the proximal calf for elevation and exposure. When performing a below-knee bypass, place a stack of towels under the distal thigh.

Pitfalls:
• Avoid overdistension of the vein, which may result in endothelial injury.
• Avoid choosing a heavily calcified distal target if possible.
• Avoid twisting of conduit in tunneler by marking the anterior surface with methylene blue (do not use the same pen as used for the skin marker).

1.8 Surgical Anatomy

• *See* Figures 39.5 to 39.9.

1.9 Positioning

• *See* Figure 39.5.

1.10 Anesthesia

• General anesthesia versus epidural anesthesia
• Arterial line with easily accessible blood draws to monitor regularly intra-operative ACTs (activated clotting times)

Flowchart 39.1: Decision-making algorithm.

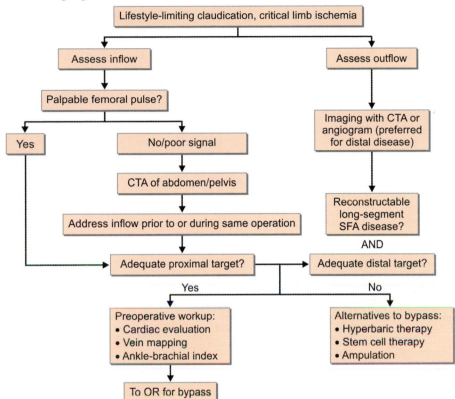

- Lifestyle-limiting claudication, critical limb ischemia
- Assess inflow
- Palpable femoral pulse?
- Yes
- No/poor signal
- CTA of abdomen/pelvis
- Address inflow prior to or during same operation
- Adequate proximal target?
- Yes
- Assess outflow
- Imaging with CTA or angiogram (preferred for distal disease)
- Reconstructable long-segment SFA disease?
- AND
- Adequate distal target?
- No
- Preoperative workup:
  - Cardiac evaluation
  - Vein mapping
  - Ankle-brachial index
- To OR for bypass
- Alternatives to bypass:
  - Hyperbaric therapy
  - Stem cell therapy
  - Ampulation

- Blood pressure stably maintained with SBP 100–160 mmHg; heart rate stably 60–100 bpm

2 PERIOPERATIVE

2.1 Incision

- *See* Figure 39.5.

2.2 Steps

See Figures 39.6 to 39.11.

Exposure of the above-knee popliteal artery along the distal third of the medial thigh requires posterior retraction of the sartorius muscle and anterior retraction of the vastus medialis muscle. The adductor hiatus may be further exposed by division of the adductor magnus tendon. Care must be taken to preserve geniculate arteries and the saphenous branch of the femoral nerve.

Medial exposure of the below knee popliteal artery (not pictured) is obtained by retracting the medial head of the gastrocnemius muscle posteriorly. As the popliteal vein is encountered first, vessel loops can be used to elevate the popliteal artery into the field.

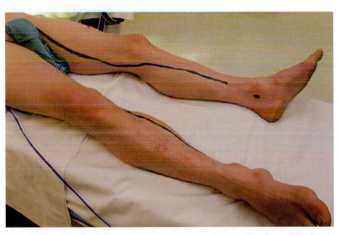

Fig. 39.5: Marked line spanning entire extremity (no skin bridges). Both legs marked and prepped for possible harvest.

2.3 Closure

- Closure of the groin involves closing the layers of the femoral sheath, scarpa's fascia, the subcutaneous tissue, and the skin.
- Closure of the leg below the knee does not include fascial closure to minimize risk of compartment syndrome.

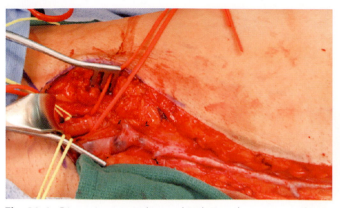

Fig. 39.6: Dissection carried to and isolating the common femoral, superficial femoral, and profunda femoris arteries. Isolate each of these and their major branches and control with vessel loops.

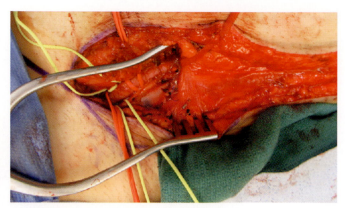

Fig. 39.7: Dissection and disconnect of the saphenofemoral junction. Oversew the femoral stump with Prolene in a running mattress fashion.

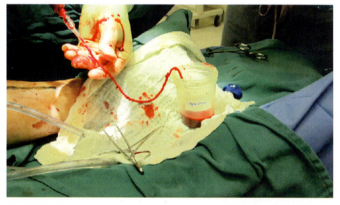

Fig. 39.8: Harvest of greater saphenous vein (GSV) with ligation of branches with silk ties. Meticulous handling of the vein is of utmost importance. Vein is briefly stored then dilated segmentally with a mixture of heparinized blood and papaverine. The vein is sutured to a blunt-tipped syringe, and dilation occurs with injection of the mixed solution against a pinched segment of vein between the fingers. The vein is sequentially dilated in this fashion.

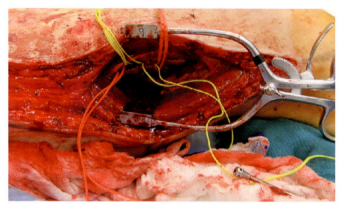

Fig. 39.9: Dissection of distal target. Medial exposure is the most common for both the above- and below-knee popliteal artery, as both are achieved by deepening the dissection through the previous saphenectomy incision.

3 POSTOPERATIVE

3.1 Complications

Most common complications:
- Graft occlusion
- Major wound complications

Least common complications:
- Graft infection
- Major amputation
- Graft hemorrhage
- Stroke/Transient ischemic attack (TIA)
- Myocardial infarction (MI)
- Death

3.2 Outcomes

Evaluation of all series published since 1981:
- *Patency of above-knee reversed greater saphenous vein (RGSV):* 1 month 99%, 6 months 91%, 1 year 84%, 2 years 82%, 4 years 69%
- *Patency of above-knee PTFE:* 6 months 89%, 1 year 79%, 2 years 74%, 4 years 60%
- *Patency of below-knee RGSV:* 1 month 98%, 6 months 90%, 1 year 84%, 2 years 79%, 4 years 77%

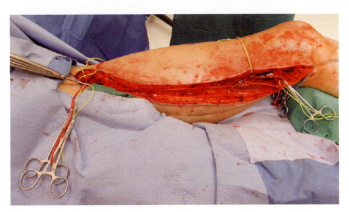

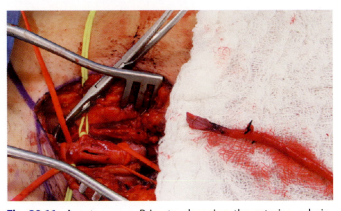

Fig. 39.10: Tunneling of vein graft. In a medial approach to the above-knee popliteal artery, tunneling the graft under the sartorius muscle provides a natural anatomic plane. Similarly, grafts to the below-knee popliteal artery (not pictured) are also tunneled under the sartorius; the tunneling then continues posterior to the knee between the femoral condyles to the exposed segment of the popliteal artery.

Fig. 39.11: Anastomoses. Prior to clamping the arteries, administer systemic heparin to the patient to achieve ACTs (activated clotting times) greater than 250 seconds. For both proximal and distal anastomoses, the target vessel is controlled with either vessel loops or vascular clamps. An arteriotomy is made in a plaque-free segment of the arteries with an 11-blade and extended with Potts scissors to the approximate size of the hooded vein graft. The vein is beveled at the end to allow for a hooded end to sew to the target vessel. The orientation is reversed so that the valves would no longer impede blood flow without requiring a valvulotomies. Sewing is performed with a running 5–0 or 6–0 Prolene, from heel to toe. Parachuting technique is also appropriate. Upon completion, perform a Doppler check at the anastomoses and the distal signals at the feet.

- Patency (secondary) of below-knee PTFE: 1 month 96%, 6 months 80%, 1 year 68%, 2 years 61%, 4 years 40%

3.3 Follow-Up

- Antiplatelet agent to be restarted postoperatively, with aspirin as the primary agent. Consider anticoagulation for high-risk bypasses (reoperation, poor distal target, poor conduit). Restart appropriate statin agent.
- Ankle brachial index (ABI) prior to discharge
- Follow-up in 4 weeks with ABI and graft scan
- Surveillance graft scans every 3 months, then every 6 months for 2 years, followed by annual scans.

3.4 E-mail an Expert

- *E-mail address*: henke@med.umich.edu

3.5 Web Resources/References

- www.vascularweb.org
- www.mdconsult.org
- Albers M, Battistella VM, Romiti M, et al. Meta-analysis of polytetrafluoroethylene bypass grafts to infrapopliteal arteries. J Vasc Surg. 2003;37:1263-9.
- Albers M, Romiti M, Braganca Pereira CA, et al. A meta-analysis of infrainguinal arterial reconstruction in patients with end-stage renal disease. Eur J Vasc Endovasc Surg. 2001;22:294-300.
- Archie JP Jr. Femoropopliteal bypass with either adequate ipsilateral reversed saphenous vein or obligatory polytetrafluoroethylene. Ann Vasc Surg. 1994;8(5): 475-84.
- Conte MS. Challenges of distal bypass surgery in patients with diabetes: patient selection, techniques, and outcomes. J Vasc Surg. 2010;52(3 Suppl):96S-103S.
- Dalman RL. Expected outcome: Early results, life table patency, limb salvage. In: Mills JL (Ed). Management of Chronic Lower Limb Ischemia. London: Arnold; 2000. pp. 106-12.
- Mills JL Sr. Infrainguinal disease: surgical treatment. In: Cronenwett JL, Johnston KW (Eds). Rutherford's Vascular Surgery, 7th edition. Philadelphia: Saunders; 2010. pp. 1682-703.
- Twine CP, McLain AD. Graft type for femoropopliteal bypass surgery. Cochrane Database Syst Rev. 2010;(5): CD001487.

QUIZ

Question 1: Based on the PREVENT III trial, all of the following are risk factors used for prediction of amputation-free survival following surgical bypass except:
a. Hct ≤ 30
b. Tissue loss
c. Platelets ≥ 500
d. Dialysis

Question 2: Which conduit has the highest patency rate for femoral to below-knee popliteal bypasses?
a. PTFE
b. Spliced arm vein
c. Dacron
d. Great saphenous vein

Question 3: Cardiac risk reduction has been demonstrated in patients taking all of the following preoperatively except:
a. Cilostazol
b. β-Blocker
c. Aspirin
d. Statin

Question 4: What is the approximate primary patency of a femoral to below-knee reversed great saphenous vein bypass at 2 years?
a. 60%
b. 70%
c. 80%
d. 95%

Question 5: During the bypass operation, which of the following is tested to insure adequate systemic heparinization?
a. PTT
b. INR
c. Factor Xa
d. ACT

Femoropopliteal Bypass, Reversed Vein

Jean Marie Ruddy, Luke P Brewster

1 PREOPERATIVE

1.1 Indications

- Femoropopliteal bypass is most commonly performed for symptomatic atherosclerotic disease of the superficial femoral and/or popliteal artery, including intermittent claudication, rest pain, nonhealing ischemic ulcers, or gangrene.
- Less frequent indications for elective femoropopliteal bypass include femoral or popliteal artery aneurysms and nonatherosclerotic occlusive disease such as popliteal entrapment syndrome or cystic adventitial disease.
- Patients with mild intermittent claudication symptoms that are not lifestyle-limiting are seldom treated with bypass, as the natural history of this condition infrequently progresses to threaten the limb and a failed bypass can significantly worsen ischemic symptoms and may jeopardize the extremity.
- The use of reversed saphenous vein graft cannot be advised when the vein diameter is <2.5 mm or if vein mapping identifies long segments of sclerotic changes. A notable, however, would be in the setting of limb salvage where disadvantaged vein has proven improved patency over prosthetic graft.

1.2 Evidence

- Single segment autogenous greater saphenous vein (in either a reversed or in situ) is the best available conduit for lower extremity bypass grafting.
- Failure of autogenous vein grafts occurs in a multimodal pattern. Acute thrombosis within the first month may be attributed to technical defect or inadequate inflow or outflow.
- Approximately 10–35% of patients will suffer graft thrombosis within the first 2 years following bypass.

During this time point, myointimal hyperplasia is the most likely cause, and it may be due to stenosis within the vein or at the anastomoses.

- At >2 years, graft failure is generally attributable to progression of atherosclerotic disease.
- Bypass failure usually presents as a return of preoperative symptoms, and these symptoms may be worse than the initial presenting symptoms. Prior to failure, failing bypass grafts are usually asymptomatic and may not be detected simply by physical examination or the measurement of ankle pressures.
- Given the excellent secondary patency results obtained when intervention precedes failure, routine surveillance of the autogenous lower extremity bypass graft is imperative.
- Thrombotic occlusion of a bypass graft may occur suddenly, with an acute onset of symptoms. Such patients may develop a profoundly ischemic limb if the bypass had been performed for limb salvage, or may have a return of their preoperative claudication symptoms.[1-3]

1.3 Materials Needed

- Major vascular instrument set
- Vein tunneler
- Prolene suture, 5-0 and 6-0
- Doppler probe

1.4 Preoperative Risk Assessment

High risk—considered one of the four deadliest operations in NEJM article:
- Coronary artery disease (CAD)
- Diabetes mellitus (DM)
- Chronic obstructive pulmonary disease (COPD)
- Acute limb ischemia
- Contralateral amputation

- Small vein (<2.5 mm)
- Poor arterial outflow below the knee

1.5 Preoperative Checklist

Sign in:
- Site marked
- Consent signed

Time out:
- Site verified
- Define inflow
- Define outflow
- Define conduit

Sign out:
- Verify and mark distal arterial signals.
- Plan to monitor postoperative cardiovascular function.

1.6 Decision-Making Checklist

Lifestyle limiting claudication:
- Exercise and maximal medical therapy
- Ankle branchial index (ABI) and pulse volume recording (PVR) measurements
- Contrasted imaging
- Vein mapping
- Operative cardiovascular risk factors

Distal rest pain and tissue loss:
- Wound care
- Contrasted imaging
- Vein mapping
- Operative cardiovascular risk factors

1.7 Pearls and Pitfalls

Pearls:
- Great saphenous vein diameter >2.5 mm, harvest extra length, secure branches, ultrasound preoperative in OR and mark vein
- Utilize adjuncts such as common femoral artery endarterectomy or iliac angioplasty/stenting if necessary to maximize inflow.
- Target vessel with adequate runoff.
- Tunnel anatomically, minimize graft tension.

Pitfalls:
- Minimize closing suture tension to decrease skin necrosis and wound infection.

1.8 Surgical Anatomy

- The external iliac artery transitions into the common femoral artery, as it passes under the inguinal ligament (Fig. 40.1A).

- Superficial femoral artery atherosclerotic disease often begins at the origin and may extend its entire length, but it is also common for the stenosis/occlusion to begin at the outlet of the adductor canal. Beyond this landmark, the superficial femoral artery becomes the popliteal artery and depending on its plaque burden this vessel may be a bypass target above or below the knee.
- In the medial thigh, the greater saphenous vein may be harvested from its origin near the medial malleolus proximally to the saphenofemoral junction (Fig. 40.1B).

1.9 Positioning

- Supine position
- Prep from umbilicus to toes on target limb and conduit limb if separate
- Cover operative field with Ioban
- Groin exposure with leg externally rotated and abducted (Fig. 40.2)
- Knee frog-legged and supported on a bump for popliteal exposure

1.10 Anesthesia

- General anesthesia
- Aggressive pulmonary care to ensure immediate postoperative extubation
- Antibiotic therapy initiated within one hour of incision
- Normothermia
- Minimize OR time

2. PERIOPERATIVE

2.1 Incision

- *See* Figures 40.3A to C.

2.2 Steps

- *See* Figures 40.4A to F.

2.3 Closure

- The groin incision should be closed in several layers. Three layers of deep Vicryl suture can effectively reapproximate the femoral sheath and adipose tissues of the groin. The skin can then be closed with interrupted vertical mattress sutures to provide additional strength.

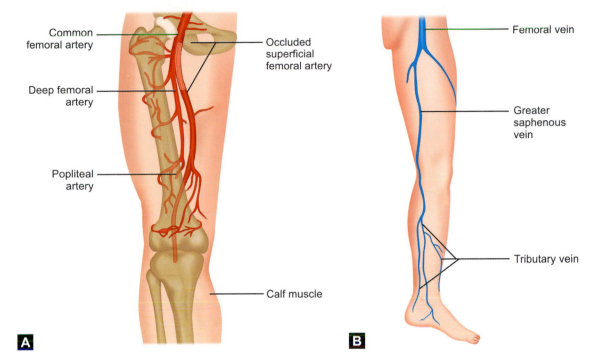

Figs. 40.1A and B: Surgical anaomy of lower extremity vasculature.

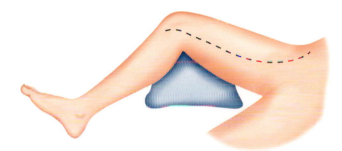

Fig. 40.2: Lower extremity positioning for femoro-polited bypass.

- Vein harvest and distal target incisions should also be closed with a deep layer of Vicryl suture and the skin may be treated with staples.

3. POSTOPERATIVE

3.1 Complications

Most common complications postoperative:
- Bleeding
- Myocardial infarction
- Wound infection
- *Graft occlusion*: have plan before leaving the OR whether would re-explore.

Most common complications long term:
- Leg edema
- Graft stenosis and thrombosis.

3.2 Expected Outcomes

- The use of saphenous vein graft for femoral to above-knee popliteal artery bypass can produce 5-year patency up to 75% and secondary patency of 65%.
- When saphenous vein is utilized as conduit to the below-knee popliteal artery, primary and secondary patency rates of 65% have been reported.

3.3 Follow-Up

Clinic visits at 3-month intervals for first 18 months and every 6 months thereafter to include:
- Discussion of clinical symptoms
- Graft surveillance ultrasound
- ABIs

3.4 E-mail an Expert

- *E-mail address*: j.m.ruddy@emory.edu; lukebrewst@aol.com.

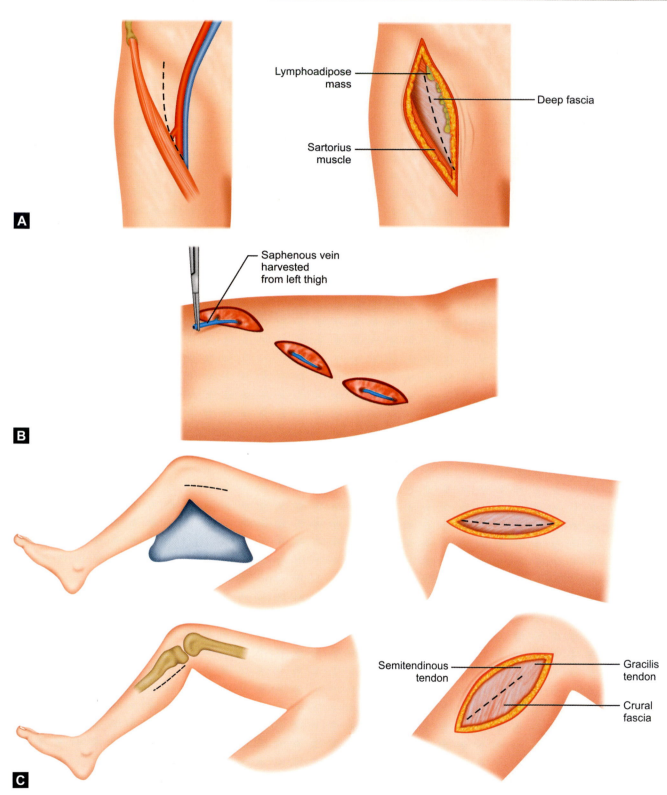

Figs. 40.3A to C: (A) Longitudinal groin incision allows access to common femoral artery and saphenofemoral venous junction. The incision may be displaced laterally to avoid scar tissue and optimize common femoral artery exposure in the setting of a repeat procedure. (B) Distal target incision should be positioned for above (a) or below (b) knee popliteal artery exposure. (C) Medial thigh incisions for vein harvest.

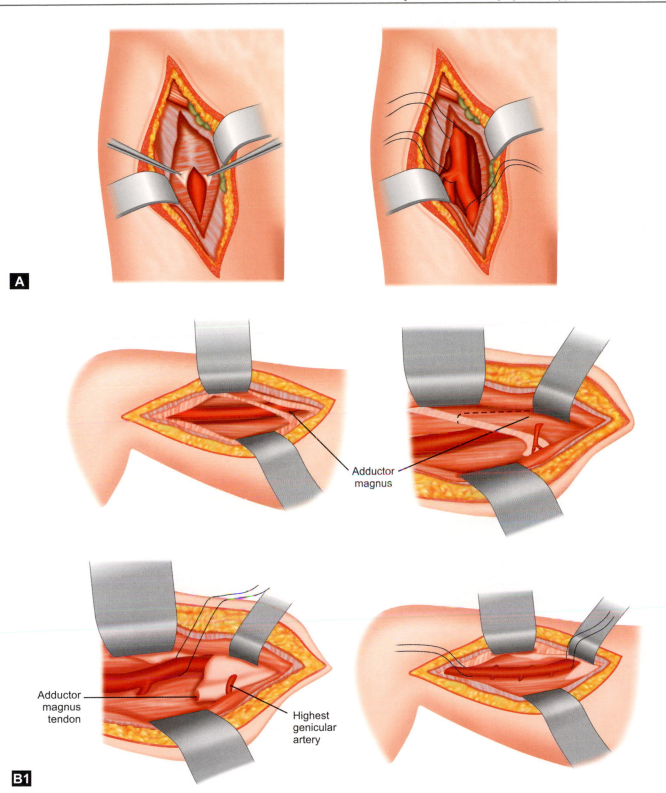

Figs. 40.4A and B1: (A) Proximal arterial exposure. Longitudinal groin incision allows exposure of common femoral, superficial femoral, and profunda femoris arteries. (B1) Distal exposure, above-knee popliteal artery. Distal superficial femoral or above-knee popliteal artery exposed by retracting adductor magnus muscles and entering the adductor canal. Distal exposure may extend into popliteal fossa where the popliteal artery is located medial to the vein and encountered first. The distal target is often dissected first.

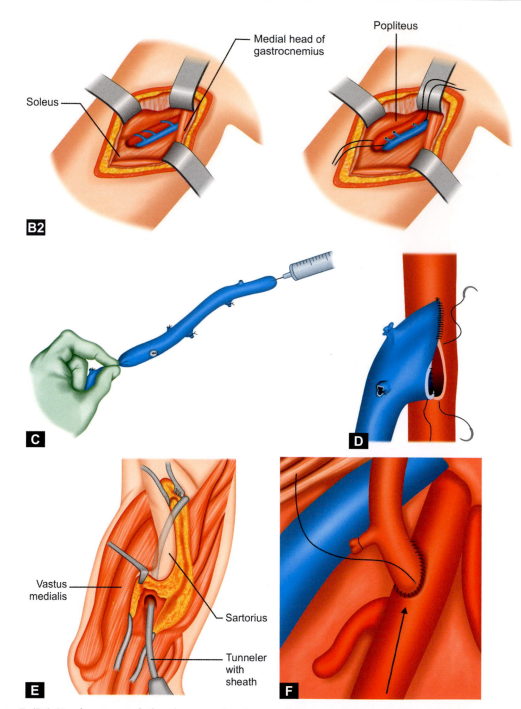

Figs. 40.4B2 to F: (B2) Distal exposure, below-knee popliteal artery. Exposure of the below-knee popliteal artery involves retraction of gastrocnemius and soleus muscles inferiorly. The popliteal vein is located medially in this location and must be carefully dissected away from the artery for adequate exposure. (C) Vein preparation. Following harvest, the saphenous vein is prepared by injecting with heparinized saline with pressurized sequential compression to dilate the vein and identify leaks. (D) Proximal anastomosis. The proximal anastomosis may be constructed with circumferential running 5-0 Prolene suture. (E) Tunnel vein anatomically. Following proximal anastomosis, the vein is distended with inflow and tunneled anatomically toward the target vessel. Care should be taken to avoid twisting of the vein in the tunnel. Additionally, it is advisable to tunnel in two steps to avoid extrinsic compression due to accidental intramural tunneling. (F) Distal anastomosis. The vein is measured and trimmed to minimize tension and the distal anastomosis may be constructed with 6-0 Prolene suture in a circumferential running fashion. Yasorgil clips are often used for proximal and distal occlusion of the target vessel to minimize vessel injury.

3.5 Web Resources

- http://www.webmd.com/a-to-z-guides/femoropopliteal-bypass-fem-pop-bypass-for-peripheral-arterial-disease
- http://www.hopkinsmedicine.org/healthlibrary/test_procedures/cardiovascular/femoral_popliteal_bypass_surgery_92,P08294/
- http://www.urmc.rochester.edu/encyclopedia/content.aspx?ContentTypeID=92&ContentID=P08294
- http://www.keckmedicalcenterofusc.org/condition/document/14810

SUGGESTED READING

Conte MS, Bandyk DF, Clowes AW, et al. Risk factors, medical therapies and perioperative events in limb salvage surgery: observations from the PREVENT III multicenter trial. J Vasc Surg. 2005;43:456-64.

Klinkert P, Post PN, Breslau PJ, et al. Saphenous vein versus PTFE for above-knee femoropopliteal bypass. A review of the literature. Eur J Vasc Endovasc Surg. 2004;27(4):357-62.

Pereira CE, Albers M, Romiti M, et al. Meta-analysis of femoropopliteal bypass grafts for lower extremity arterial insufficiency. J Vasc Surg. 2006;44(3):510-17.

Veith FJ, Gupta SK, Ascer E, et al. Six-year prospective multicenter randomized comparison of autologous saphenous vein and expanded polytetrafluoroethylene grafts in infrainguinal arterial reconstructions. J Vasc Surg. 1986;3:104-14.

REFERENCES

1. Johnson WC, Lee KK. A comparative evaluation of polytetrafluoroethylene, umbilical vein, and saphenous vein bypass grafts for femoral-popliteal above-knee revascularization: a prospective randomized Department of Veterans Affairs cooperative study. J Vasc Surg. 2000; 32(2):268-77.
2. Landry GJ, Moneta GL, Taylor L M Jr, et al. Long-term outcome of revised lower-extremity bypass grafts. J Vasc Surg. 2002;35(1):56-62.
3. Mills JL Sr, Wixon CL, James DC, et al. The natural history of intermediate and critical vein graft stenosis: recommendations for continued surveillance or repair. J Vasc Surg. 2001;33(2):273-8.

QUIZ

Question 1. A 54-year-old male patient with atherosclerotic disease of the right distal superficial femoral artery may require femoropopliteal bypass with reversed saphenous vein graft if he suffers from any of the following EXCEPT:
a. Mild claudication at 1 mile
b. Rest pain
c. Tissue loss
d. Gangrene

Question 2. When exposing the below-knee popliteal artery, the first vessel encountered is:
a. Anterior tibial artery
b. Suprageniculate artery
c. Popliteal vein
d. Peroneal artery

Question 3. After performing a femoral–popliteal bypass with reversed saphenous vein, you note the ankle brachial index to be lower than you would expect. Which is not a likely cause of this finding:
a. Tunneling inadvertently traversed a fascial plane
b. Tunneling impinged upon the biceps femoris tendons
c. During tunneling the vein graft was twisted
d. Vein stenosis due to retained valve

Question 4. During examination of the venous conduit on the back table, you notice a stenotic portion that does not dilate. The best next step is to:
a. Throw away the vein and use a prosthetic
b. Manually pressure dilate the stenotic portion until it dilates or bursts.
c. Resect this portion and perform a venovenostomy
d. Patch this stenotic portion with a synthetic arterial patch.

Question 5. During a follow-up visit 2 years after bypass grafting, you note that the patient's ankle brachial index has decreased by 0.1 each visit and the distal graft's velocity is now under 40 cm/s. Which is probably not a reasonable next step:
a. Add dual antiplatelet therapy
b. Schedule for an arteriogram
c. Schedule for a computed tomography arteriogram
d. Recommend a therapeutic plan for salvage of the vein graft

ANSWERS: 1. a 2. c 3. d 4. c 5. a

In Situ Venous Femoropopliteal Bypass

chapter 41

Domenic R Robinson, Barend ME Mees

1 PREOPERATIVE

1.1 Indications

- Life-style limiting claudication
- Critical limb ischemia (CLI)
- Popliteal aneurysm
- Popliteal entrapment
- Trauma

Contraindication:

- Great saphenous vein (GSV) absent or unsuitable (<2.5 mm)

1.2 Evidence

- Open surgery for revascularization is appropriate in patients with claudication and failed medical treatment or with critical limb ischemia due to TASC C and D lesions of the femoropopliteal segment.[1]
- Open surgery for revascularization should be preferred over endovascular surgery if the life expectancy of the patient is more than 2 years.[2]

- Infrainguinal bypass surgery using autologous vein as conduit has significant better patency than using prosthetic.[3]
- There is no difference in patency or limb salvage between reversed GSV or in situ GSV bypass surgery.[3]

1.3 Materials Needed

- Valvulotome (Mills, Lemaitre) (Figs. 41.1 and 41.2)
- Hand-held Doppler (Fig. 41.3)
- Angiography equipment (needle, tubing, contrast, image intensifier) (Fig. 41.4)

1.4 Preoperative Planning and Risk Assessment

Planning:

- Imaging of adequate inflow and patent target vessels (angiography, CTA, MRA)
- Duplex GSV mapping (and marking)

Risk assessment:

- Peripheral bypass surgery is high-risk surgery.

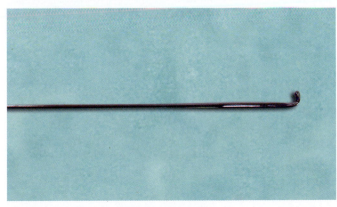

Figs. 41.1: Mills valvulotome (close-up).

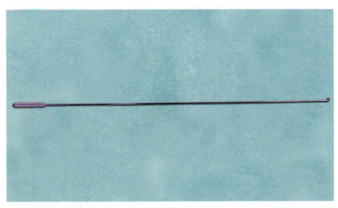

Fig. 41.2: Mills valvulotome.

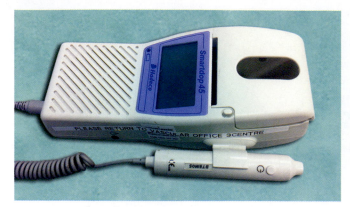

Fig. 41.3: Hand-held Doppler.

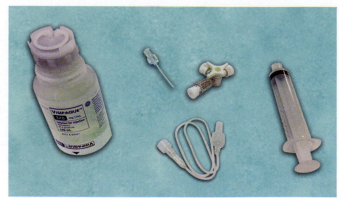

Fig. 41.4: Angiography equipment: Cannula, tubing, contrast.

- All patients planned for peripheral bypass surgery need complete preoperative cardiovascular/pulmonary/renal assessment.
- Perioperative risk should be lowered by starting patients preoperatively on statin, aspirin and possibly also on a beta-blocker.
- *High risk factors*:
  - *Cardiac*:
    - Ischemic heart disease
    - Critical aorta stenosis
    - Age > 70
    - Emergency operation
  - *Pulmonary*:
    - COPD
    - Smoking
  - Hypertension
  - Diabetes
  - Obesity

1.5 Preoperative Checklist

Sign in:
- Is correct leg marked?
- Is GSV marked?

Time out:
- Anesthetist to give prophylactic antibiotics
- Anesthetist to administrate intraoperative heparin before clamping
- Discuss possible critical moments (difficult proximal clamping, etc.)
- Expected duration of operation 2–3 hours
- Confirm presence of necessary equipment (valvulotome, etc.)

Sign out:
- Postoperative normotension

- Postoperative anticoagulation
- Vascular observations (pulses)

1.6 Decision-Making Algorithm

- *See* Flowchart 41.1.

1.7 Pearls and Pitfalls

Pearls:
- Preoperative ultrasound marking of GSV allows easy identification of vein and prevents creation of large skin flaps prone to necrosis.
- Putting a calibrating sticker on thigh before angiogram for marking tributaries.
- In case of a short common femoral artery (CFA) or insufficient proximal GSV length, perform proximal anastomosis on profunda femoris artery (PFA) or (endarterectomized) superficial femoral artery (SFA).
- Leave a small patent AV fistula just proximal from distal anastomosis to preserve proximal graft flow in case of graft occlusion.
- If possible, extend venotomy for proximal and distal anastomosis through a suitable side-branch to create a broad hood and prevent narrowing at heel of the anastomosis.
- Leave a proximal tributary of the GSV long for easy access for completion angiogram.

Pitfalls:
- Cut terminal valves of GSV with Pott's scissors before making proximal anastomosis.
- Beware of double GSV system.
- Avoid distal kinking of the graft by releasing surrounding soft tissue.
- Avoid damage to saphenous nerve during dissection of the above-knee popliteal artery.
- Failure to ligate a large tributary may lead to a symptomatic AV fistula.
- Early graft occlusion due to residual valve in GSV bypass.
- Risk of graft infection with wound complications.

Flowchart 41.1: Decision-making algorithm.

1.8 Surgical Anatomy

- *See* Figures 41.5 to 41.8.

1.9 Positioning

Drawing:
- Entire leg shaved with a clipper in anesthetic bay.
- Urine catheter deviated underneath contralateral leg.
- Supine position with gel pad positioned at foot of operating table to facilitate external rotation and 30° of flexion of knee.
- Sterile preparation of ipsilateral lower abdomen and entire leg, with foot in sterile clear plastic bag.

1.10 Anesthesia

Prophylactic antibiotics:
- General or spinal anesthesia
- Invasive arterial blood pressure monitoring

2 PERIOPERATIVE

2.1 Incision

Distal Incision

Above-knee popliteal:
- Longitudinal incision distal third medial thigh over preoperatively marked GSV.
- Dissect GSV and confirm >3 mm diameter.
- Open fascia over sartorius muscle.

- Retract sartorius muscle posteriorly and adductor muscles anteriorly and dissect in horizontal plane to expose vascular sheath.
- Avoid injury to crossing saphenous nerve.
- Expose target (soft) above-knee popliteal artery and dissect from vein.

See Figures 41.9 and 41.10.

Below-knee popliteal:
- Longitudinal incision proximal third medial calf over preoperatively marked GSV.
- Dissect GSV and confirm >3 mm diameter.
- Open crural fascia.
- Retract gastrocnemius muscle posteriorly and if distal exposure needed, divide soleus muscle fibers from tibia.
- If more proximal exposure required, divide tendons of sartorius, gracilis, and semitendinosus muscle.
- Dissect in horizontal plane posterior from tibia and expose vascular sheath.
- Dissect target (soft) below-knee popliteal artery, usually behind accompanying vein.

See Figures 41.11 and 41.12.

Proximal Incision

- Oblique or longitudinal incision in the groin.
- Oblique incision is performed parallel to inguinal ligament just above groin crease.
- Longitudinal incision is made directly over the femoral pulse (one third above and two thirds below inguinal

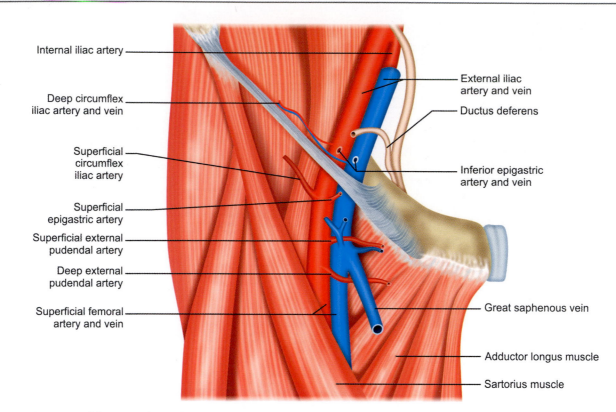

Fig. 41.5: Anatomy of ilioinguinal vessels.

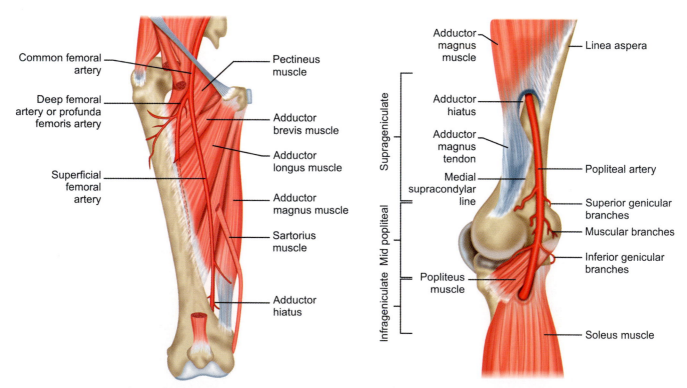

Fig. 41.6: Anatomy of superficial femoral artery.

Fig. 41.7: Anatomy of above-knee popliteal artery, posterior view.

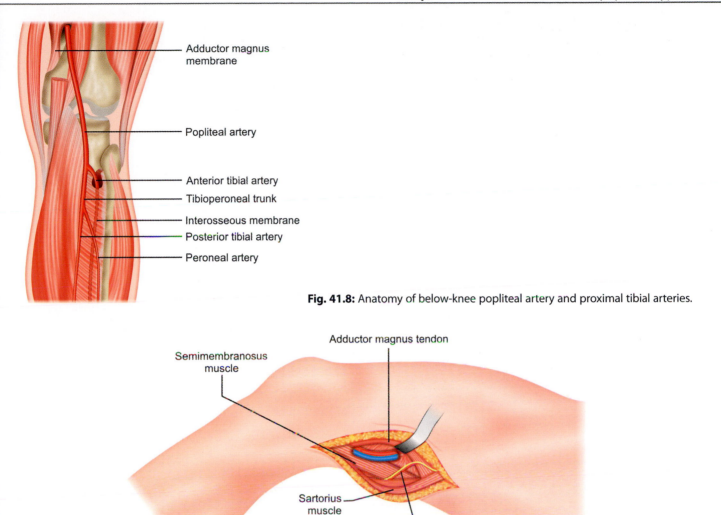

Adductor magnus membrane

Popliteal artery

Anterior tibial artery

Tibioperoneal trunk

Interosseous membrane

Posterior tibial artery

Peroneal artery

Fig. 41.8: Anatomy of below-knee popliteal artery and proximal tibial arteries.

Adductor magnus tendon

Semimembranosus muscle

Sartorius muscle

Saphenous nerve and superior genicular artery

Fig. 41.9: Incision to above-knee popliteal artery.

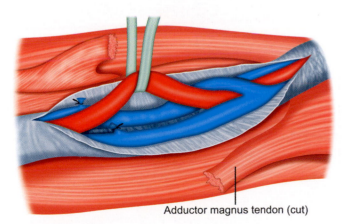

Adductor magnus tendon (cut)

Fig. 41.10: Isolation of above-knee popliteal artery.

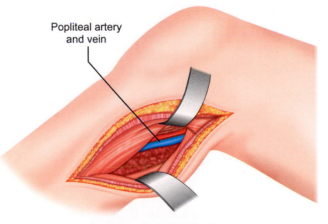

Popliteal artery and vein

Fig. 41.11: Incision to below-knee popliteal artery.

ligament) and curved medially over marked saphenofemoral junction and GSV.

- Dissect through superficial tissue containing inguinal lymph nodes. Ligate superficial branches of femoral vessels.
- Open fascia lata and retract sartorius muscle laterally (Figs. 41.13 and 41.14)

- Dissect saphenofemoral junction and proximal GSV and confirm >3 mm diameter.
- Open femoral sheath and dissect common femoral artery (CFA) and origins profunda femoris artery or deep femoral artery (PFA) and superficial femoral artery (SFA) (Fig. 41.15).

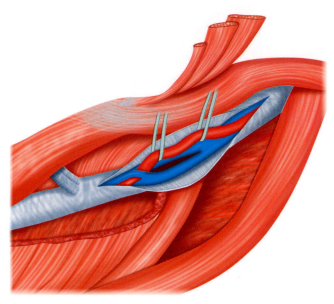

Fig. 41.12: Isolation of below-knee popliteal artery.

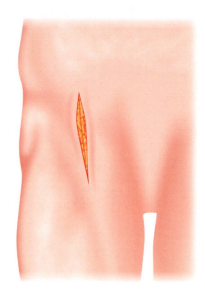

Fig. 41.13: Longitudinal incision in groin, extending medially over great saphenous vein.

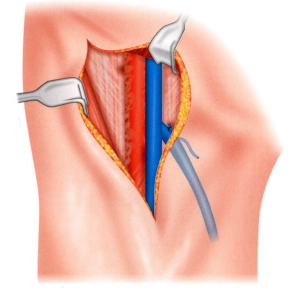

Fig. 41.14: Exposure of femoral sheath and saphenofemoral junction.

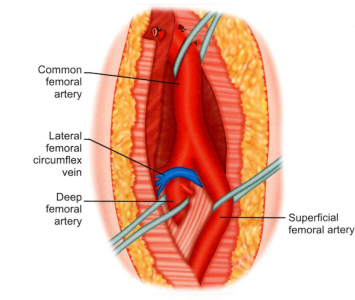

Common femoral artery

Lateral femoral circumflex vein

Deep femoral artery

Superficial femoral artery

Fig. 41.15: Isolation of femoral arteries.

2.2 Steps

- Administer 70–100 units/kg bolus of heparin intravenously.
- *Harvesting GSV*:
  - Ligate and divide tributaries to saphenofemoral junction (leave one long).
  - Clip proximal tributaries from GSV in thigh.

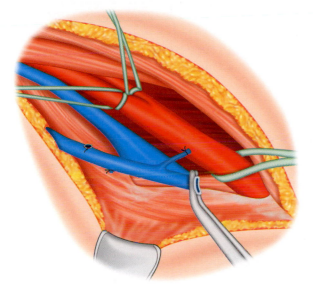

Fig. 41.16: GSV is divided from SFJ with one tributary left long. (GSV: great saphenous vein; SFJ: Saphenofemoral junction).

- Divide saphenofemoral junction with small cuff of common femoral vein over Satinsky clamp (Fig. 41.16).
- Close venotomy of common femoral vein with continuous running 5-0 Prolene.
- *Proximal anastomosis*:
  - Prepare GSV for anastomosis by excising terminal valves with Pott's scissors and extending venotomy into suitable side-branch.
  - Clamp CFA, SFA, and PFA.
  - Determine site of anastomosis according to length of GSV.
  - Additional length can be gained by further dissecting GSV.
  - Open CFA and confirm adequate inflow, perform endarterectomy if necessary.
  - Match venotomy with arteriotomy (Figs. 41.17A and B).
  - Perform cobra-hood end-to-side anastomosis with continuous 5-0 Prolene (Fig. 41.18)
  - Remove clamps.
- *Preparing GSV*:
  - Ligate and divide distal GSV ensuring sufficient length to swing onto target popliteal artery.
  - Introduce valvulotome in distal GSV and disrupt all valves.
  - Beware not to feed valvulotome into proximal anastomosis.
- *Distal anastomosis*:
  - Confirm adequate pulsatile inflow through GSV.

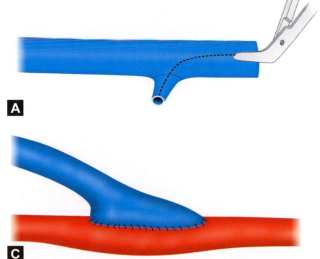

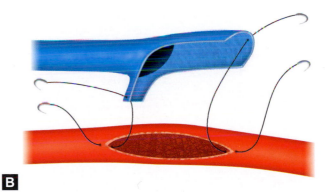

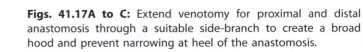

Figs. 41.17A to C: Extend venotomy for proximal and distal anastomosis through a suitable side-branch to create a broad hood and prevent narrowing at heel of the anastomosis.

- Soft clamp on distal GSV after flushing with heparanized saline.
- Clamp popliteal artery.
- Perform arteriotomy in disease-free segment of popliteal artery.
- Match venotomy with arteriotomy.
- Confirm presence of backflow.
- Avoid kinking or torsion of GSV.
- Perform cobra-hood end-to-side anastomosis with continuous 6-0 Prolene.
- Flush graft and popliteal artery prior to completing anastomosis.
- *Ligation of arteriovenous fistulae (AVFs)*:
  - Use hand-held sterile Doppler to locate AVFs by manual compression on bypass (Fig. 41.19).

- Clip or tie AVFs using small incisions (Fig. 41.20).
- Perform a check angiogram through proximal GSV tributary to identify residual AVFs and confirm anastomosis patency and satisfactory outflow (Fig. 41.21).
- Clip or tie remaining AVFs.

2.3 Closure

- Perform groin closure with a minimum of two subcutaneous layers.
- Close superficial fascia in distal incisions over the GSV graft.
- Close skin with subcuticular absorbable sutures.
- Optionally leave drains adjacent to proximal and distal anastomosis.

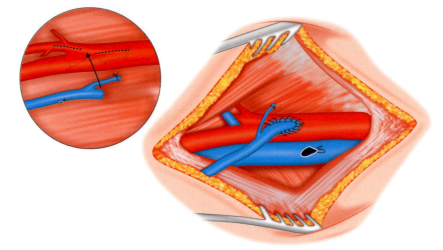

Fig. 41.18: Proximal anastomosis of GSV on CFA. If insufficient length of GSV, anastomosis can be performed onto PFA. (GSV: Great saphenous vein; CFA: Common femoral artery; PFA: Profunda femoris artery).

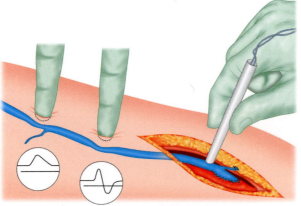

Fig. 41.19: Location of arteriovenous fistulae with Doppler, note different waveforms.

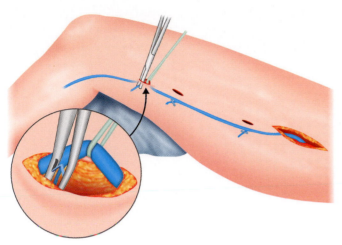

Fig. 41.20: Clipping of arteriovenous fistulae.

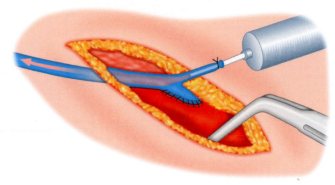

Fig. 41.21: Angiogram performed through proximal GSV tributary. (GSV: Great saphenous vein).

3. POSTOPERATIVE

3.1 Complications

General:
- Mortality (2.5%)
- Cardiac (myocardial infarct, atrial fibrillation; 5%)
- Respiratory (chest infection, pulmonary embolus)
- Urinary tract infection

Specific:
- Wound infection/dehiscence (beware superficial location of in situ bypass; 5%)
- Hematoma
- Lymph leakage
- Early graft occlusion (5%)
- Major amputation (2%)
- Neuralgia (femoral/saphenous)

3.2 Outcomes

- Above-knee femoropopliteal bypass
- Five-year primary patency 70%
- Five-year limb salvage 75%
- Below-knee femoropopliteal bypass
  - Five-year primary patency 75%
  - Five-year limb salvage 80%

3.3 Follow-Up

- Antiplatelet and statin therapy.
- Review 4–6 weeks postoperatively with graft surveillance duplex.
- Subsequently 3–6 monthly duplex for graft surveillance.

3.4 E-mail an Expert

- *E-mail addresses*: domenicrobinson@gmail.com or barend.mees@mumc.nl

SUGGESTED READINGS

Cronenwett JL, Johnston KW. Rutherford's Vascular Surgery. Philadelphia: Elsevier; 2010.

Kenneth O, Robert BR. Atlas of Vascular Surgery; Operative Procedures. Philadelphia: W.B. Saunders; 1998.

Valentine RJ, Wind GG. Anatomic exposures in Vascular Surgery. Philadelphia: Lippincott Williams & Wilkins; 2003.

REFERENCES

1. Norgren L, Hiatt WR, Dormandy JA, et al. TASC II Working Group. Inter-society consensus for the management of peripheral arterial disease (TASC II). J Vasc Surg. 2007; 45(Suppl S):S5-S61.
2. Bradberry AW. Bypass versus angioplasty in severe ischemia of the leg (BASIL): multicenter, randomized controlled trial. BASIL trial participants. Lancet. 2005;366:1925-34.
3. Twine CP, McLain AD. Graft type for femoro-popliteal bypass surgery. Cochrane Database Syst Rev. 2010;12(5):CD001487.

chapter 42

Femoropopliteal Bypass, Prosthetic and Vein Cuff

Niten Singh

1. PREOPERATIVE

1.1 Indications

- Severe claudication
- Critical limb ischemia (rest pain or tissue loss)

1.2 Evidence

- The gold standard of lower extremity arterial reconstruction is femoropopliteal bypass with autogenous vein.
- Prosthetic femoropopliteal bypass fares worse than autogenous conduits in all infrainguinal reconstructions.
- When vein is not available prosthetic bypass [PTFE (polytetrafluoroethylene) and Dacron] to the above-knee popliteal artery is a viable option.
- Below-knee popliteal artery bypass with prosthetic alone has poor results and requires adjunctive maneuvers such as anticoagulation and anastomotic modification (vein patch or cuff).
- Adjunctive maneuvers such as distal vein patch for below-knee bypass has better limb salvage than without adjunctive maneuvers.[1-4]

1.3 Materials Needed

- Self-retaining retractor system (Fig. 42.1)
- Scanlon tunneling system (Fig. 42.2)
- Vascular needle driver and suture (6-0 and 7-0 polypropylene suture) (Figs. 42.3A and B)
- Vascular graft—either PTFE or Dacron (PTFE pictured here) usually 6 mm (Fig. 42.4)

1.4 Preoperative Risk Assessment

Planning:

- Coronary risk assessment particularly in those with claudication symptoms

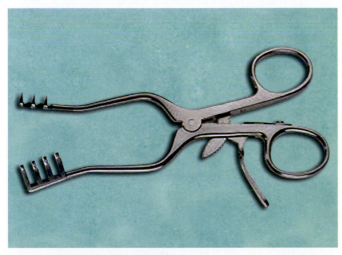

Fig. 42.1: Self-retaining retractor.

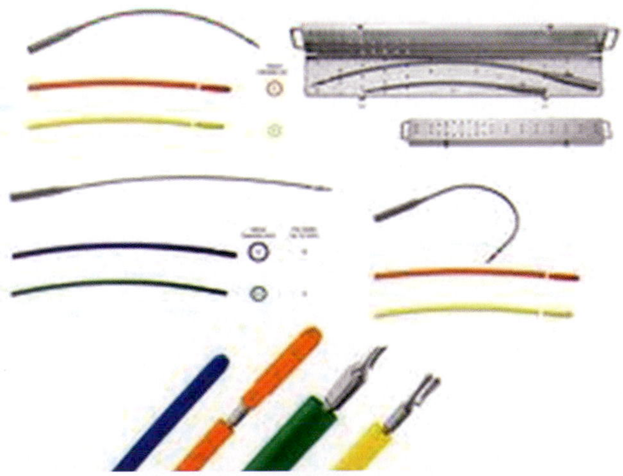

Fig. 42.2: Tunneling device.

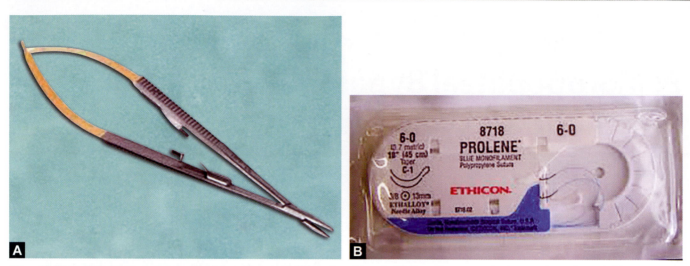

Figs. 42.3A and B: (A) Vascular needle driver (Castro-Viejo depicted here). (B) Vascular suture (polypropylene depicted here).

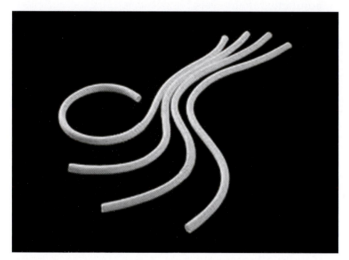

Fig. 42.4: Prosthetic vascular graft—PTFE graft depicted here. (PTFE: Polytetrafluoroethylene).

- In patients with critical limb ischemia optimal medical management of cardiac factors along with expeditious repair
- Preoperative noninvasive studies (ankle brachial index [ABI], tissue perfusion [TcPO$_2$])
- Arteriogram clearly identifying distal target (above- or below-knee popliteal artery) as well identifying any disease in the inflow femoral artery (Figs. 42.5A and B)

Risk assessment:
- *Low risk*:
  - Most patients would not be considered low risk as they all have associated coronary disease.

- *Intermediate risk*:
  - Patients with stable coronary and pulmonary comorbid conditions.
- *High risk*:
  - Unstable cardiac disease
  - Unstable pulmonary disease
  - Lower extremity contractures preventing exposure.

1.5 Preoperative Checklist

- Preoperative control of medical issues to include β-blockers, statin, and antiplatelet regimen.
- Ensuring that correct prosthetic graft is available.
- Preoperative vein mapping even in the case of inadequate vein as a short segment of superficial vein will be required for the vein patch for infrapopliteal bypass.

1.6 Decision-Making Algorithm

- *See* Flowchart 42.1.

1.7 Pearls and Pitfalls

Pearls:
- Always approach any bypass by exposing the distal (outflow) target first as it will be more variable than the proximal (inflow) site.
- The approach to the above-knee popliteal artery and below-knee popliteal artery is avascular not through muscle.
- Feel for the groove between the sartorius and the vastus medialis muscles for the above-knee popliteal artery exposure and always push the sartorius inferiorly.

- Dividing the semimembranosus and semitendinosus tendons within the superior portion of the below-knee incision will greatly assist in exposure of the popliteal artery.
- The proximal soleus fibers do not have to be incised unless more distal exposure of the popliteal artery is necessary.
- When constructing a vein patch a 2–3 cm segment of vein is required and a segment of vein can usually be found in the thigh near the greater saphenous vein (GSV) even if the GSV was harvested.
- A tunnel beneath the sartorius muscle allows for a more protected location of the graft than the subcutaneous location.
- When tunneling to the below-knee popliteal artery, a graft placed between the two heads of the gastrocnemius muscle will allow for a less steep angle versus a tunnel in the subcutaneous location.
- Always heparinize after the exposure and tunnel has been created.
- An externally supported (ringed) graft has not been demonstrated to improve patency but is often employed when crossing points of flexure.
- Placing a sterile 6-in. ACE wrap around the thigh after the tunneling device has been placed can decrease bleeding from this site after the patient is anticoagulated.

Pitfalls:

- Incising the soleus without discretion can lead to postoperative hematoma.
- Too short of vein patch will not allow a proper graft interface with the artery.
- If you are dividing muscle during the popliteal exposure you are in the wrong plane.

- A tunnel placed in the subcutaneous plane is more vulnerable than in the normal anatomic plane.

1.8 Surgical Anatomy

- *See* Figure 42.6.

1.9 Positioning

- Place the patient in the supine position and utilize "bumps" (sterile towels) to elevate the leg.
- Place the bump under the *calf* for above-knee exposure.
- Place the bump under the *thigh* for below-knee exposures.

1.10 Anesthesia

- Regional anesthesia with an epidural or spinal is associated with better outcomes.
- Do not use spinal anesthesia if the case is expected to be long.
- General anesthesia must always be used with caution in this patient population.[5]

2 PERIOPERATIVE

2.1 Incision

See Figures 42.7A to C.

Flowchart 42.1: Decision-making algorithm.

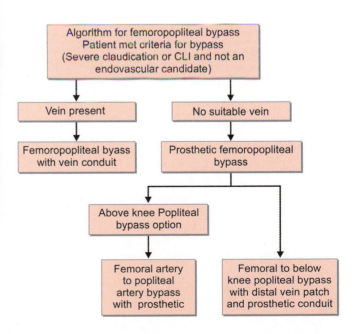

Figs. 42.5A and B: (A) Arteriogram of left lower extremity illustrating the inflow vessel, the common femoral artery. Note the occlusion of the profunda femoris artery as well as the occluded superficial femoral artery with a proximal stent in place. (B) Arteriogram of the same patient with outflow site of the bypass (the above-knee popliteal artery).

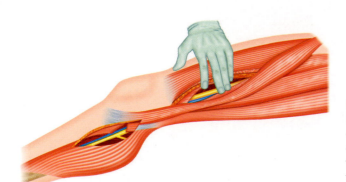

Fig. 42.6: The lower extremity is depicted here with the above-knee and below-knee exposure. A classic medial approach is employed to reach these regions. With dissection in the thigh occurring between the Sartorius and vastus medialis muscle and the dissection for the below-knee popliteal artery occurring medial to the edge of the tibia. Note the proximity of both incisions to the knee.

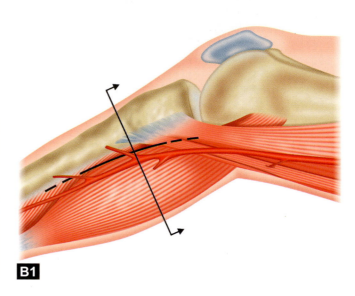

A

B1

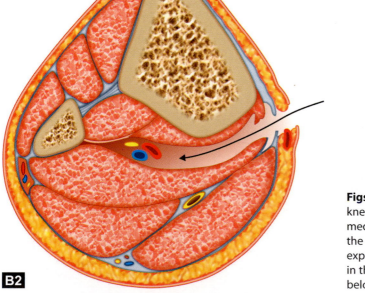

B2

Figs. 42.7A and B: (A) Incision for the exposure of the above-knee popliteal artery exposure. The incision is placed low on the medial aspect of the thigh between the groove created between the vastus medialis and sartorius muscle. (B) Incision for the exposure of the below-knee popliteal artery. The incision placed in the medial aspect of the calf just distal to the knee immediately below the tibia.

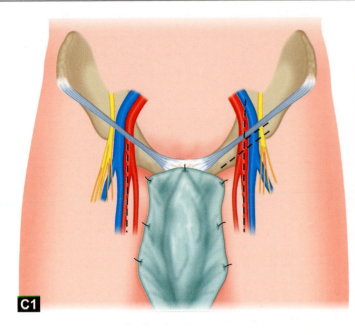

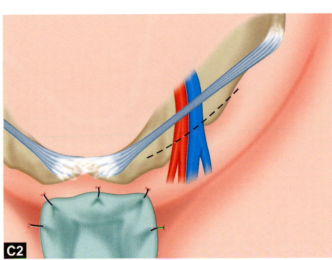

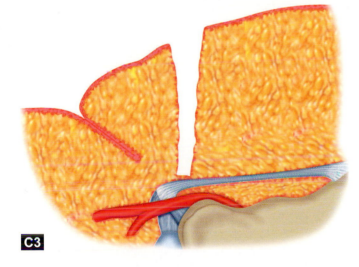

Figs. 42.7C: The femoral artery incision is placed either longitudinally or in an oblique fashion. The anterior superior iliac spine and pubic tubercle are palpated and a line between these depicts the inguinal ligament. Often in patients a calcified femoral artery can be palpated if there is not palpable pulse or the patient is obese.

2.2 Steps

- *Above-knee femoropopliteal bypass*:
  - Incision placed in groove between vastus medialis and sartorius muscles.
  - Fascia incised and sartorius muscle pushed inferiorly.
  - Identify vein and dissect it away from the artery.
  - Identify soft portion suitable for bypass.

See Figures 42.8A to E.

- *Below-knee bypass*:
  - Incision placed medially close to the knee
  - Incision into superficial fascia and push gastrocnemius muscle inferiorly

  - Divide the tendons of the semimembranosus and the semitendonosus in the superior portion of the incision.
  - Dissect popliteal vein away from artery.
  - Identify suitable portion of artery for bypass.
  - May need to divide portion of soleus muscle if popliteal artery does not appear suitable for bypass.

See Figures 42.9A to D.

- *Identify femoral artery*:
  - Incision—either longitudinal or oblique
  - Identify common femoral artery; superficial femoral artery, and profunda femoris artery and control with vessel loops

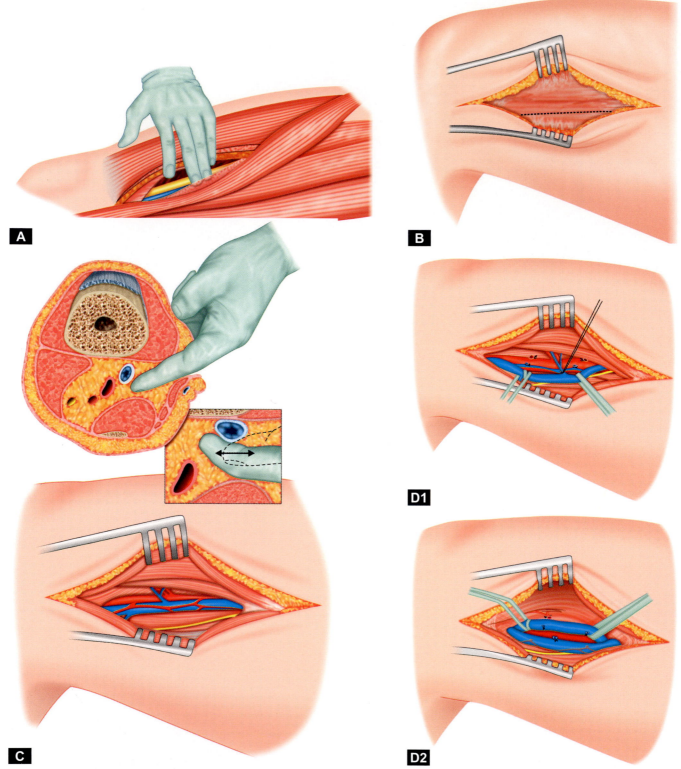

Figs. 42.8A to D: (A) The above-knee popliteal artery incision is carried out deeper into the subcutaneous tissue and the fascia between the sartorius and vastus medialis is opened (B). The vessels can be palpated immediately beneath the femur (C) and the popliteal artery is than controlled with vessel loops (D).

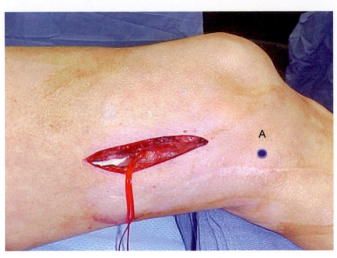

Fig. 42.8E: Intraoperative photo of the above-knee incision.

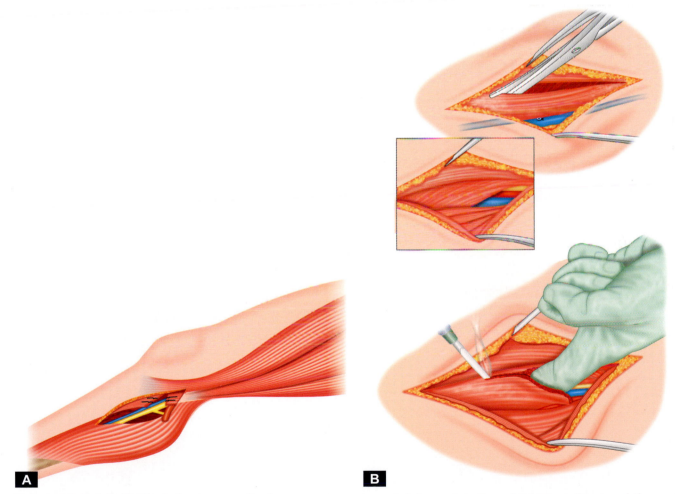

Figs. 42.9A and B: (A) The below-knee popliteal artery exposure is carried deeper into the subcutaneous tissue and the medial head of the gastrocnemius is pushed inferiorly. Note that with division of the semimembranosus and semitendinosus tendons in the proximal aspect of the incision, the exposure can be facilitated. If more distal exposure the popliteal artery is required than division of the proximal soleus fibers can be performed (B).

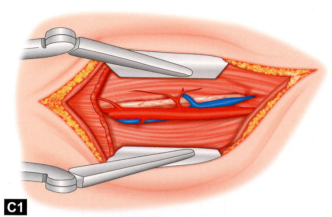

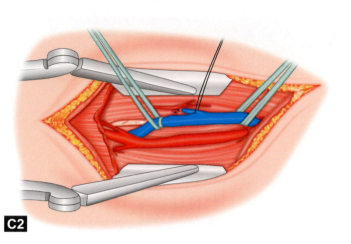

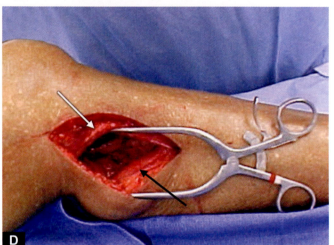

Figs. 42.9C and D: After dissecting the popliteal vein away from the artery, vessel loops can be employed to control the vessel (C). Intraoperative photo of the below-knee exposure (D).

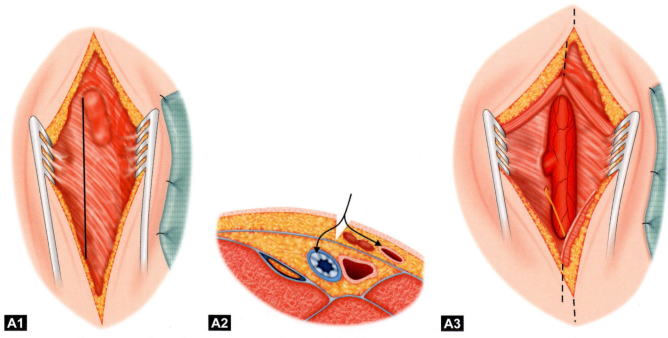

Figs. 42.10A: The common femoral artery incision is deepened directly over the artery to avoid creating skin flaps.

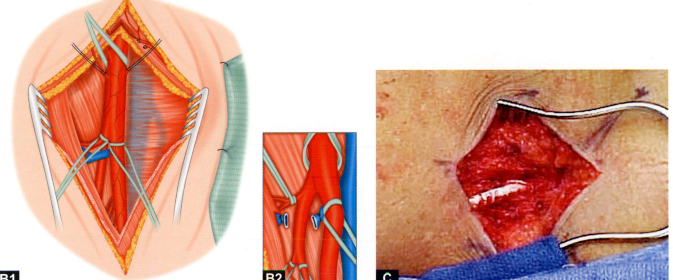

Figs. 42.10B and C: The common femoral, superficial femoral, and profunda femoris arteries are controlled with vessel loops and can be clamped if necessary (B). Intraoperative photo of the common femoral exposure (C).

- May need to divide portion of the inguinal ligament to obtain a softer area of the common femoral artery.

See Figures 42.10A to C.

- *Tunneling*:
  - For an above-knee bypass the graft is tunneled from the distal incision to the proximal incision below the sartorius muscle to the proximal incision.
  - Ensure the line is in the same position of the graft to avoid twisting of the graft.
  - When tunneling to the below-knee popliteal artery an incision above the knee (same as above-knee popliteal artery exposure) will allow for easier placement of the graft between the two heads of the gastrocnemius muscle.

See Figures 42.11A to C.

- *Anastomosis*:
  - The graft is beveled for the proximal anastomosis with the common femoral artery.
  - Similarly the graft is beveled for the distal anastomosis.

See Figure 42.12.

- *For below-knee popliteal artery bypass*:
  - Creation of 2–3 cm vein patch (Fig. 42.13)
  - Incision of proximal two thirds of vein patch (Fig. 42.14)
  - Creation of bypass to vein patch/popliteal artery (Figs. 42.15A and B)

2.3 Closure

- The groin wound is closed and approximated in layers with either a running absorbable suture or interrupted sutures.
- The distal incision is closed with approximation of the subcutaneous fascia and skin.

3 POSTOPERATIVE

3.1 Complications

Most common complications:
- Postoperative hematoma/seroma
- Graft thrombosis
- Cardiac complications.

Least common complications:
- Immediate wound issues
- Cardiac and pulmonary complications especially if utilizing regional anesthesia

3.2 Outcomes

- Primary patency of above-knee prosthetic bypass is 66% at 3 years.
- Primary patency of below-knee bypass with vein patch is approximately 50% at 2 years.

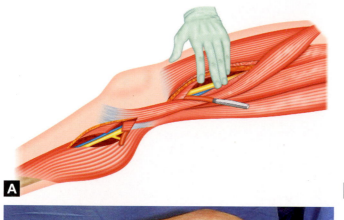

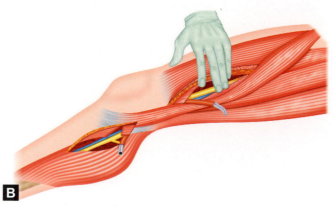

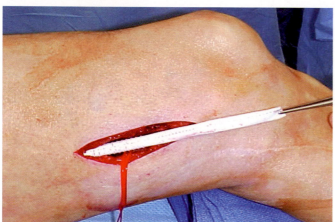

Figs. 42.11A to C: (A) If a below-knee popliteal artery anastomosis is required a thigh incision depicted in Figure 42.8 should be performed to facilitate creation of a tunnel between the two heads of the gastrocnemius muscle into the thigh. Once the distal tunnel is created the graft can be tunneled more proximally to the femoral site in a subsartorius muscle plane (B). This plane is the same that would be required for a femoral to above-knee popliteal artery bypass. Intraoperative photo of the tunnel from the above-knee popliteal exposure to the femoral exposure (C).

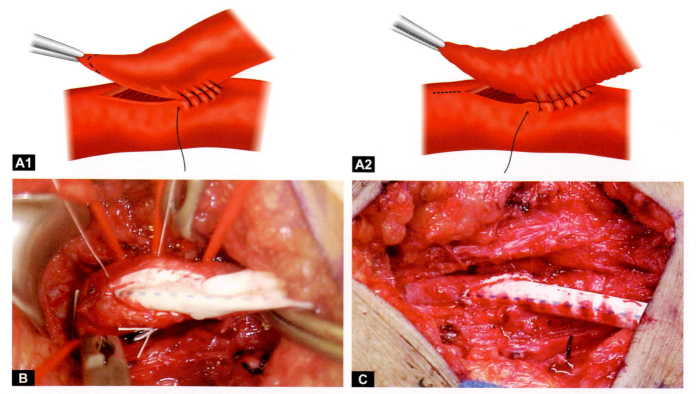

Figs. 42.12A to C: (A) A standard anastomosis performed proximally and distally with 6-0 polypropylene or polytetrafluoroethylene suture. Intraoperative photo of the femoral anastomosis (B) and (C).

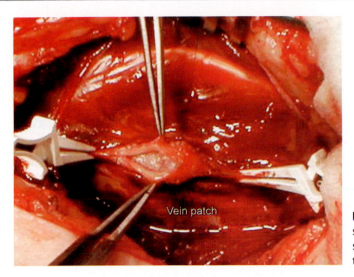

Vein patch

Fig. 42.13: If a below-knee popliteal artery bypass is to be constructed a 2–3 cm vein patch is sewn to the popliteal artery. The suitable vein segment can generally be found in the thigh even if the greater saphenous vein has been previously harvested.

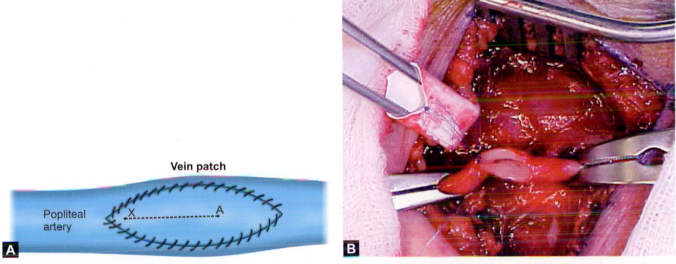

Figs. 42.14A and B: (A) After the vein patch is sewn to the artery the proximal two thirds is incised for the graft anastomosis. Intraoperative photo of the graft to vein patch anastomosis (B).

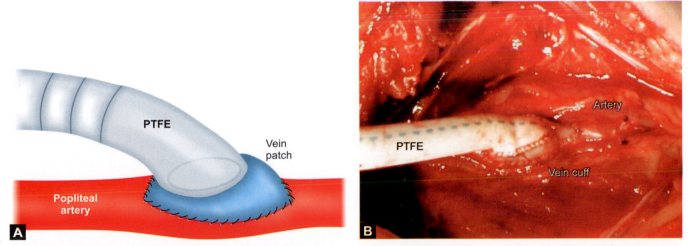

Figs. 42.15A and B: (A) The 6-mm PTFE graft is sewn to the vein patch on the popliteal artery to create the distal anastomosis. (B) Intraoperative photo depicting the graft to popliteal artery-vein patch anastomosis.

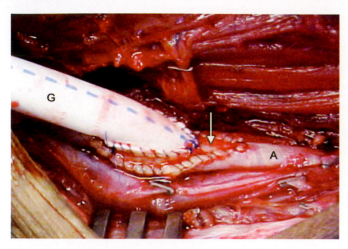

Figs. 42.15C: Magnified photo revealing the graft–to-vein patch anastomosis. Note g is graft; white arrow is vein patch; and A is artery (C). (PTFE: Polytetrafluoroethylene).

Expected outcomes:
- Resolution of claudication symptoms.
- Healing of ischemic tissue loss or healing of amputation if tissue loss is extensive.
- Patients with claudication symptoms alone should be ambulating on POD#1.

3.3 Follow-Up

- Graft surveillance of prosthetic grafts has not been shown to be beneficial.

- When a vein patch is employed simple surveillance of the distal anastomosis is sufficient.
- ABI and toe pressures are a sound method to follow these grafts along with symptom resolution.
- If a below-knee popliteal bypass was employed with a vein patch, anticoagulation should be instituted.

REFERENCES

1. Veith FJ, Gupta SK, Ascer E, et al. Six year prospective multicenter randomized comparison of autologous saphenous vein and expanded polytetrafluoroethylene grafts in infrainguinal arterial reconstructions. J Vasc Surg. 1986; 3:104-14.
2. Stonebridge PA, Prescott RJ, Ruckley CV. Randomized trial comparing infrainguinal polytetrafluoroethylene bypass grafting with and without vein interposition cuff at the distal anastomosis. The Joint Vascular Research Group. J Vasc Surg. 1997;26:543-50.
3. Neville RF, Attinger C, Sidawy AN. Prosthetic bypass with a distal vein patch for limb salvage. Am J Surg. 1997;174: 173-6.
4. Neville RF, Lidsky M, Capone A, et al. An expanded series of distal bypass using the distal vein patch technique to improve prosthetic graft performance in critical limb ischemia. Eur J Vasc Surg. 2012;44:177-82.
5. Singh N, Sidawy AN, DeZee K, et al. Factors predictive of acute failure of infrainguinal lower extremity arterial bypass. J Vasc Surg. 2008;47:556-61.

QUIZ

Question 1. When considering infrainguinal bypass which of the following statements are true?
a. Utilizing a prosthetic bypass to the above-knee popliteal artery is as durable as autogenous conduits.
b. Adjunctive maneuvers for a below-knee popliteal artery bypass have been shown to improve patency.
c. Surveillance of prosthetic grafts is the same as for autogenous grafts and helps maintain primary or primary assisted patency.
d. The use of externally supported PTFE grafts has been demonstrated to improve primary patency.

Question 2. Regarding the above-knee popliteal artery exposure which of the following are true?
a. The plane of dissection is in the groove created above the vastus medialis muscle.
b. The plane of dissection is between the vastus medialis and Sartorius muscles.

c. The plane of dissection is easily obtained by dividing the sartorius muscle.
d. The plane of dissection is created by dissecting below the sartorius muscle.

Question 3. When constructing a bypass graft to the below-knee popliteal artery which of the following statements is true?
a. The operation proceeds with identification of proximal (inflow) site first and the exposure of the distal (outflow) site second.
b. The graft is tunneled in the subcutaneous tissue from the distal (outflow site) to the proximal (inflow) site to facilitate the distal graft to artery angle.
c. A 7–8 mm length vein patch is required to facilitate the distal anastomosis.
d. An incision in the distal thigh often facilitates tunneling of the graft in an anatomic plane.

1. b 2. b 3. d

ANSWERS:

Tibial Artery Bypass

Amir Azarbal

1 PREOPERATIVE

1.1 Indications

Indications:
- Rest pain
- Tissue loss

Contraindications:
- Unacceptable surgical risk
- Lack of venous conduit (relative)
- Unsuitable anatomy—lack of adequate target vessel or poor outflow

1.2 Evidence

- Patency rates[1-5]
- *Great saphenous veins (GSV)*

	Great saphenous veins (GSV) (5 years)	Alternate vein (2 years)	ePTFE (2 years)
– Primary patency	63–67%	64%	46%
– Secondary patency	70–78%	70%	58%
– Foot preservation	78%	75%	64%

1.3 Materials Needed

- Inflow—generally the most distal disease-free vessel is chosen

- Outflow—Inadequate outflow will result in reduced flows through bypass and reduced patency
- Venous conduit
- Tunneler (Fig. 43.1)
- Self-retaining retractors (Fig. 43.2)
- Vessel loops
- Embolectomy catheters (for possible control of tibial vessels) (Fig. 43.3)
- Vein table for preparation of venous conduit (Fig. 43.4)

1.4 Preoperative Risk Assessment

- Peripheral vascular surgery classified as a high-risk procedure per ACC/AHA guidelines[6]
- *Patients without acute limb threatening ischemia can proceed with preoperative cardiac testing as follows*:
  - *Conditions requiring preoperative cardiac evaluation and treatment*:
    - Unstable coronary syndromes (unstable angina)
    - New congestive heart failure (CHF)
    - New York Heart Association (NYHA) Class IV CHF
    - *Significant arrhythmias*:
      - Mobitz II anterio-venous (AV) block
      - Third degree AV block

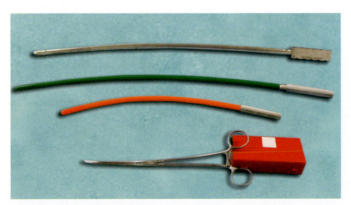

Fig. 43.1: Tunneling devices.

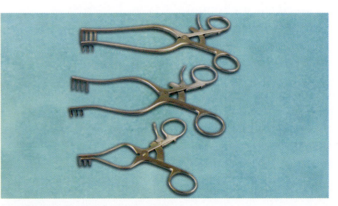

Fig. 43.2: Self-retaining retractors.

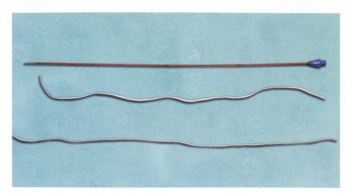

Fig. 43.3: Vessel loops and embolectomy catheters can be used for control of distal vessels.

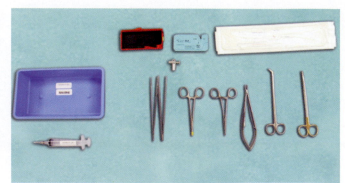

Fig. 43.4: Vein table set-up for preparation of vein graft.

- Symptomatic ventricular arrhythmias
- New ventricular tachycardia
- Supraventricular tachycardia (SVT), not rate controlled
  - *Severe valvular disease*:
    - Aortic stenosis (pressure gradient > 40 mm Hg, Valve area < 1 cm)
    - Symptomatic mitral stenosis

Patients with functional capacity of >4 metabolic equivalent (METS): Proceed with surgery

Patients with functional capacity of < 4 METS and

- *< 3 clinical risk factors*: Proceed with surgery with heart rate control.
- *> 3 clinical risk factors*: Consider further cardiac testing if it will change management.

1.5 Preoperative Checklist

- Aspirin
- Statin
- Perioperative β-blockade (if indicated)
- Blood glucose control
- Review of angiogram
- Vein mapping

1.6 Decision-Making Checklist

Assessment of patient's functional status, anatomy, extent of critical limb ischemia, and the likelihood of successful outcome are the factors that must be considered to determine the appropriate therapy:

- Endovascular therapy
- Bypass
- Primary amputation

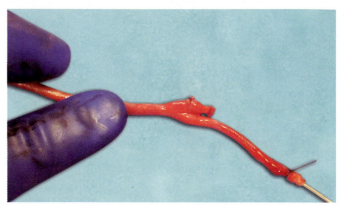

Fig. 43.5: Preparation of vein graft for proximal anastomosis.

Selection of inflow vessels and distal target vessels- designed to keep bypass as short as possible.
Selection of conduit:

- GSV
- Multisegment GSV
- Arm vein
- Prosthetic
- Selection of artery exposure and conduit tunnel

1.7 Pearls and Pitfalls

Pearls:

- "No touch" vein harvest technique—minimal handling of the vein with forceps to prevent injury
- Spatulation of proximal anastomosis (*see* Fig. 43.5)
- *Maneuvers for control of distal vessels*:
  - Vessel loops
  - Embolectomy catheters
  - Tourniquet
- Choosing suitable profunda femoral, superficial femoral or popliteal arteries as the inflow sites will help shorten the length of bypass and may avoid reoperation in previously dissected groins

Pitfalls:
- Performing tibial bypass for claudication—Tibial bypass does not reliably improve claudication symptoms as the bypass is distal to the geniculate branches that supply the calf musculature
- Lack of outflow

1.8 Surgical Anatomy

- Exposure of common inflow sites (*see* Chapter 42).
- *Exposure of distal targets*:
  - Anterior tibial   anterior incision
  - Posterior tibial   medial calf incision
  - Proximal peroneal   medial calf incision
  - Distal peroneal   lateral calf incision and fibulectomy (not covered)

See Figure 43.6.

1.9 Surgical Anatomy

- Understanding of the anatomy of the calf compartments is essential (Fig. 43.6).
- The posterior tibial and proximal peroneal are within the deep posterior compartment and are approached through the a medial incision.

- The anterior tibial artery is in the anterior compartment.

1.10 Positioning

- Supine
- Hair removed with clippers
- Groin towel
- Prep cranial enough to expose saphenofemoral junction and common femoral artery if needed
- Sterile bump under distal thigh

1.11 Anesthesia

- Padding of pressure points is essential for these lengthy procedures.
- Seatbelt should be placed high enough so as to not interfere with access or femoral vessels.
- Heparin: 80–100 IU/kg 3 minutes prior to clamping of arteries and 1000 IU redosed every hour while vessels are clamped.
- Protamine reversal of heparin (up to 1 mg protamine/1,000 IU of heparin) may be indicated for coagulopathic bleeding.

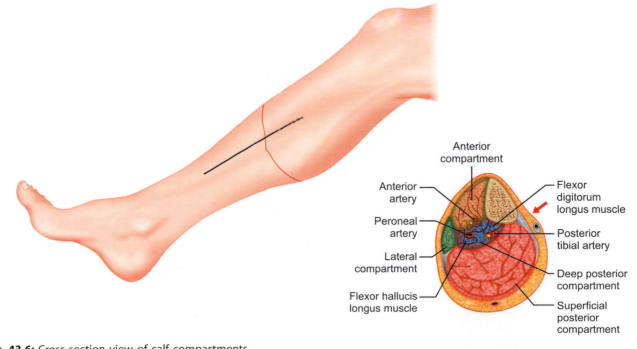

Fig. 43.6: Cross-section view of calf compartments.

2 PERIOPERATIVE

2.1 Incision

- Anterior tibial artery
  - Over anterior compartment
- PT/peroneal
  - Medial calf incision posterior to tibia (*see* Fig. 43.7)

2.2 Steps

Anterior tibial artery
- *Dissection*:
  - Subcutaneous tissue divided with electrocautery
  - The extensor digitorum longus muscle and tibialis anterior muscle are separated bluntly
  - The anterior tibial artery is found anterior to the interosseous membrane, usually surrounded by paired anterior tibial veins
- *Tunnel*:
  - Anatomic (*see* Figs. 43.8 and 43.9)
    - Vein graft tunneled to popliteal fossa by making a medial calf incision
    - Proximal soleal muscle attachments to tibia are divided to expose the interosseous membrane

- A large defect is made in the interosseous membrane to connect the deep posterior and anterior calf compartments
  - Subcutaneous (*see* Fig. 43.10)
    - Lateral or medial to knee

PT/Peroneal:
- Dissection (*see* Figs. 43.11A and B)
- Medial calf incision
- Divide subcutaneous layer (avoid injury to saphenous vein)
- Gastrocnemius muscle is retracted posterior
- Attachment of soleus muscle to tibia is divided (any encountered soleal veins are ligated and divided (*see* Fig. 43.12)
- Posterior tibial artery is encountered and is surrounded by paired posterior tibial veins (*see* Fig. 43.13)
- Peroneal artery is encountered by retracting PTA and PTV posterior and dissecting more lateral in the deep posterior compartment
- *Tunnel*:
  - *Anatomic tunnel to popliteal fossa*:
    - Must be between the medial and lateral head of the gastrocnemius muscle
    - *See* Figures 43.14 and 43.15

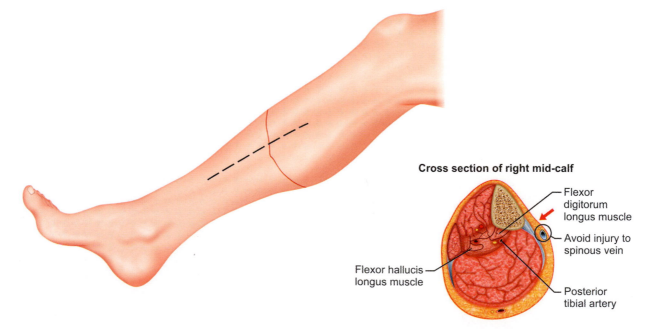

Cross section of right mid-calf

Flexor digitorum longus muscle

Avoid injury to spinous vein

Flexor hallucis longus muscle

Posterior tibial artery

Fig. 43.7: Medial calf incision for exposure of posterior tibial and peroneal arteries.

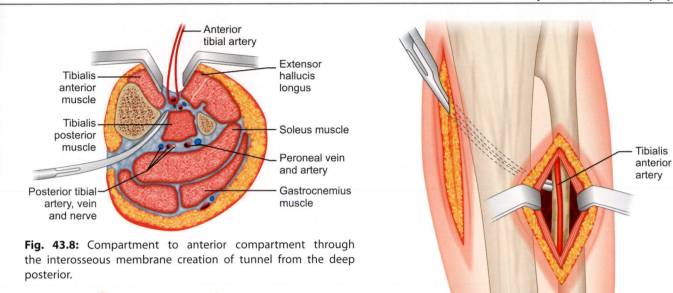

Anterior
tibial artery

Extensor
hallucis
longus

Tibialis
anterior
muscle

Tibialis
posterior
muscle

Soleus muscle

Peroneal vein
and artery

Posterior tibial
artery, vein
and nerve

Gastrocnemius
muscle

Tibialis
anterior
artery

Fig. 43.8: Compartment to anterior compartment through the interosseous membrane creation of tunnel from the deep posterior.

Lateral subcutaneous tunnel

Medial subcutaneous tunnel

Anterior compartment

Fig. 43.9: A curved aortic clamp can be used to create a tunnel through the interosseous membrane.

Fig. 43.10: Bypass grafts to the anterior tibial artery can also be tunneled in the subcutaneous plane from either the medial or lateral direction.

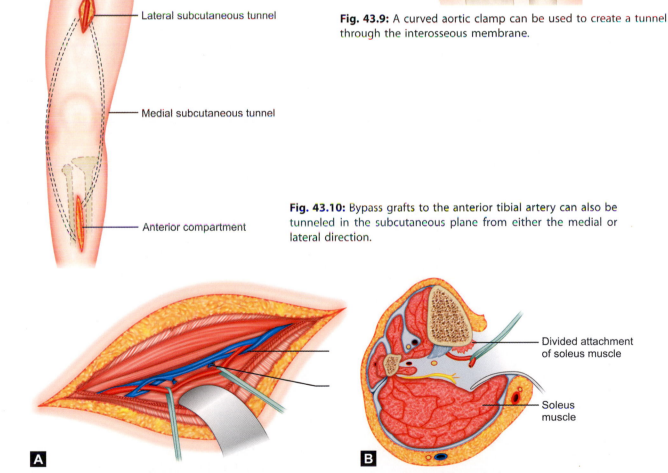

Divided attachment
of soleus muscle

Soleus
muscle

A

B

Figs. 43.11A and B: (A) Crossing veins anterior to the tibial arteries can be ligated to expose a suitable segment for distal anastomosis. (B) The deep posterior compartment is exposed by dividing the tibial attachments of the soleus m. and retracting soleus m. posteriorly.

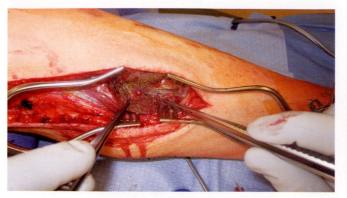

Figs. 43.12: The attachment of the soleus m. to the tibia is divided to expose the deep posterior calf compartment.

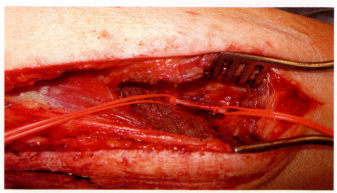

Fig. 43.13: Posterior tibial artery.

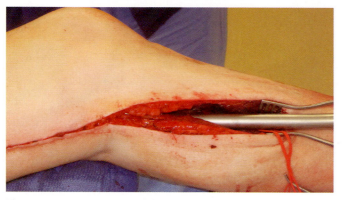

Fig. 43.14: Anatomic tunnel through popliteal fossa for a femoral-posterior tibial artery bypass graft.

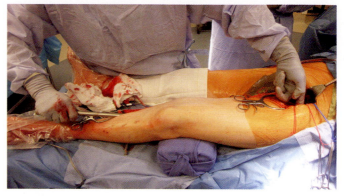

Fig. 43.15: Anatomic tunnel through popliteal fossa for a femoral-posterior tibial artery bypass graft.

2.3 Closure

- *Closure*:
  - Absorbable 2-0 suture for subcutaneous layer
  - Skin with interrupted vertical mattress nylon suture.

3 POSTOPERATIVE

3.1 Complications

Most common complications:
- Wound complications
- Cardiac complications
- Thrombosis of graft

3.2 Outcomes

Expected outcomes:
- *See* patency table

3.3 Follow-Up

Follow-Up:
- *Surveillance US*:
  - Baseline surveillance US is performed.
  - Surveillance US are performed every three month in the first year after bypass and then every 6–12 months
- *Angiogram is performed for*:
  - Graft velocity >350 cm/s
  - *Proximal graft velocity*: graft lesion velocity ratio of >3.5
  - Decrease in ankle-brachial index > 0.15.

3.4 E-mail an Expert

- *E-mail address*: azarbala@ohsu.edu

3.5 Web Resources/References

- Rutherford R. Vascular Surgery. Philadelphia: Elsevier. 2010
- Rutherford's Vascular Surgery online: www.expertconsultbook.com.
- Valentine J, Wind G. Anatomic Exposures in Vascular Surgery. Philadelphia: Lippincott Williams & Wilkins; 2003

- Zarins C, Gewertz B. Atlas of Vascular Surgery. Philadelphia: Elsevier; 2005

REFERENCES

1. Taylor LM Jr, Edwards JM, Porter JM. Present status of reversed vein bypass grafting: five-year results of a modern series. J Vasc Surg. 1990;11(2):193-205; discussion 205-6.
2. Donaldson MC, Mannick JA, Whittemore AD. Femoral-distal bypass with in situ greater saphenous vein. Long-term results using the Mills valvulotome. Ann Surg. 1991;213 (5):457-64; discussion 64-5.
3. Mortality results for randomised controlled trial of early elective surgery or ultrasonographic surveillance for small abdominal aortic aneurysms. The UK Small Aneurysm Trial Participants. Lancet. 1998;352(9141):1649-55.
4. Albers M, Romiti M, Brochado-Neto FC, et al. Meta-analysis of alternate autologous vein bypass grafts to infrapopliteal arteries. J Vasc Surg. 2005;42(3):449-55.
5. Dorigo W, Pulli R, Castelli P, et al. A multicenter comparison between autologous saphenous vein and heparin-bonded expanded polytetrafluoroethylene (ePTFE) graft in the treatment of critical limb ischemia in diabetics. J Vasc Surg. 2011;54(5):1332-8.
6. Fleisher LA, Beckman JA, Brown KA, et al. ACC/AHA 2007 guidelines on perioperative cardiovascular evaluation and care for noncardiac surgery: a report of the American College of Cardiology/American Heart Association Task Force on Practice Guidelines (Writing Committee to Revise the 2002 Guidelines on Perioperative Cardiovascular Evaluation for Noncardiac Surgery): developed in collaboration with the American Society of Echocardiography, American Society of Nuclear Cardiology, Heart Rhythm Society, Society of Cardiovascular Anesthesiologists, Society for Cardiovascular Angiography and Interventions, Society for Vascular Medicine and Biology, and Society for Vascular Surgery. Circulation. 2007;116(17):e418-99.

QUIZ

Instructions: Include three to five brief questions that test the reader's understanding of the key concepts covered within the chapter each with multiple choice answers (A to D).

Question 1. Which of the following is not an indication for a tibial artery bypass?
a. Rest pain
b. Nonhealing ulcer
c. 1 block claudication
d. Gangrene

Question 2. Least acceptable conduit for a tibial bypass is:
a. Single greater saphenous vein
b. Multisegment greater saphenous vein
c. Multisegment arm vein
d. Heparin bonded ePTFE

Question 3. Which tibial vessel is not approached through a medial calf incision?
a. AT
b. Proximal PT
c. Distal PT
d. Proximal peroneal

Question 4. Which structure is found in the anterior compartment?
a. Soleus muscle
b. Posterior tibial artery
c. Saphenous vein
d. Extensor digitorum longus muscle

Question 5. Which preoperative condition(s) generally required cardiac evaluation prior to nonemergent peripheral vascular surgery?
a. Aortic stenosis, pressure gradient >40 mm Hg
b. Atrial fibrillation, heart rate 80
c. Type I AV block
d. Stable, reduced ejection (45%), and 4MET functional capacity

ANSWERS:
1. c   2. d   3. a   4. d   5. a

Arterial Thrombolysis and Mechanical Lysis

Barend ME Mees, Ramon L Varcoe

1 PREOPERATIVE

1.1 Indication

Acute limb ischemia or acute onset/deterioration of claudication as result of:

- Thrombosis of arterial segment secondary to ruptured atherosclerotic plaque
- Embolic occlusion
- Bypass graft thrombosis
- Popliteal aneurysm occlusion
- Thrombosis associated with extrinsic arterial compression (popliteal entrapment, cystic adventitial disease)

Contraindications:

- *Absolute:*
  - Established cerebrovascular event (including TIA; <2 months)
  - Active bleeding disorder
  - Recent gastrointestinal bleeding (<10 days)
  - Neurosurgery (<3 months)
  - Intracranial trauma (<3 months)
- *Relative:*
  - *Major:*
    - Cardiopulmonary resuscitation (<10 days)
    - Major surgery or trauma (<10 days)
    - Uncontrolled hypertension (>180 mm Hg systolic or >110 mm Hg diastolic)
    - Puncture of noncompressible vessel
    - Intracranial tumor
    - Recent eye surgery
  - *Minor:*
    - Hepatic failure
    - Bacterial endocarditis
    - Pregnancy
    - Diabetic hemorrhagic retinopathy

1.2 Evidence

- Limb salvage and mortality rates were equivalent for catheter directed thrombolysis and surgical revascularization in the three major randomized trials to evaluate thrombolytic therapy (Rochester, TOPAS, STILE).[1-3]
- Due to the less invasive nature and potential for lower morbidity, thrombolytic therapy is the first-line treatment of choice in patients with acute limb ischemia grades I and IIa (TASC II consensus).[4]
- Preoperative thrombolysis of acutely thrombosed popliteal artery aneurysms improves limb salvage rate when compared with surgical revascularization alone (Swedish Vascular Registry).[5]

1.3 Materials Needed

- Basic angiographic equipment
- Ultrasound
- Thrombolysis infusion catheter (different lengths) (Figs. 44.1 to 44.3)
- Thrombolytic agent [Urokinase, Alteplase (rt-PA), Tenecteplase (TNK-tPA)]
- Mechanical thrombectomy devices (Possis, Trellis; *see* Section 2.3)

1.4 Preoperative Planning and Risk Assessment

Planning:

- Arterial imaging of the ischemic limb and its inflow should the clinical urgency not preclude this delay to definitive treatment (Duplex ultrasound, CT Angiography, MR Angiography) (Figs. 44.4A to C).

Risk assessment:

- Elderly patients (>75 years) have a significantly higher risk of hemorrhagic complications.

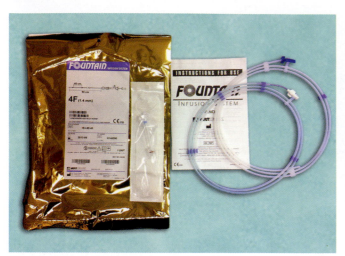

Fig. 44.1: Thrombolysis catheter, 4 Fr, 90 cm, 40-cm side holes; occluding wire; hemostasis valve.

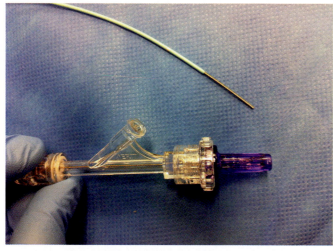

Fig. 44.3: Thrombolysis catheter setup with occluding wire through hemostasis valve, occluding distal end hole of catheter.

1.5 Preoperative Checklist

Sign in:
- Is the correct puncture site marked?

Time out:
- Prophylactic antibiotics
- Heparin infusion
- Discuss possible critical scenarios such as bleeding and embolization
- Expected duration of operation 1 hour
- Confirm presence of necessary equipment (sheaths, wires, catheters, infusion catheters, thrombolytic agent, mechanical thrombectomy devices, etc.)

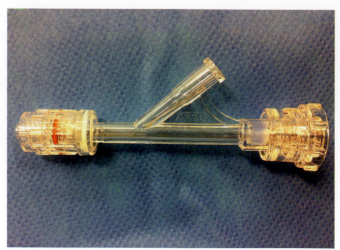

Fig. 44.2: Hemostasis valve with infusion port as well as valve for occluding wire.

Sign out:
- High-dependency unit/intensive care unit monitoring
- Neurological observations
- Vascular observations

1.6 Decision-Making Algorithm

- *See* Flowchart 44.1.

1.7 Pearls and Pitfalls

Pearls:
- Use a contralateral retrograde common femoral access approach.
- Use ultrasound guidance to avoid traumatic, glancing or high puncture.
- If a skin incision is used keep it small so that the sheath tamponades any skin edge bleeding.
- If bleeding does occur upsize the sheath one French size.
- Run the background heparin infusion at a subtherapeutic rate.
- When securing the catheter to the skin using adhesive dressings leave a redundant loop in case of inadvertent traction.
- Use a closure device at the completion of the infusion (repeat local anesthetic infiltration).

Pitfalls:
- Avoid a high puncture above the inguinal ligament.
- Avoid traumatic or multiple punctures of the access artery.
- Avoid angioplasty or other vessel trauma prior to the thrombolysis infusion.
- Avoid ipsilateral antegrade puncture as kinking of the sheath is a common problem.

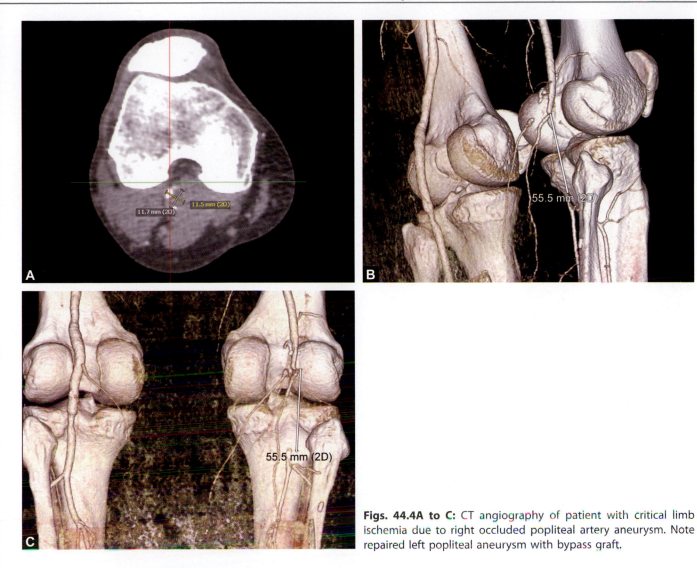

Figs. 44.4A to C: CT angiography of patient with critical limb ischemia due to right occluded popliteal artery aneurysm. Note repaired left popliteal aneurysm with bypass graft.

Flowchart 44.1: Algorithm delineating suggested imaging and management strategy for patients with acute limb ischemia based on Rutherford category.

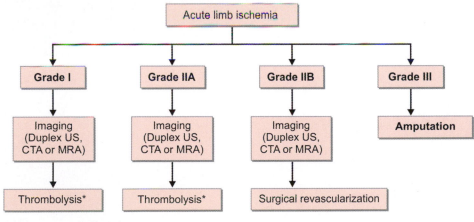

1.8 Surgical Anatomy

- *See* Figure 44.5.

1.9 Positioning

Supine position on the X-ray table

1.10 Anesthesia

- Prophylactic antibiotics
- Local anesthetic infiltration with sedation if required

2 PERIOPERATIVE

2.1 Puncture

Sterile preparation of both groins:
- Local anesthesia
- Contralateral retrograde CFA puncture
- Perform angiogram of affected limb of interest, including inflow and run-off arteries (Fig. 44.6)

2.2 Steps

- Cannulate occluded segment using glidewire and shaped catheter.
- Select an infusion catheter with the appropriate length of side holes.

- Position thrombolysis infusion catheter within the occluded segment of artery/bypass through a long sheath (Figs. 44.7 and 44.8).
- Initiate thrombolysis with bolus of thrombolytic agent (i.e. 200,000 units of urokinase).
- Start subtherapeutic heparin infusion (i.e. 500 units per hour) through sheath to prevent sheath thrombosis.
- If indicated use mechanical thrombectomy device (*see* Section 2.3).
- Completion angiogram

2.3 Mechanical Thrombectomy Devices

AngioJet (Possis):
- The AngioJet's innovative design is based on the Bernoulli principle which found that high velocity fluid creates a local low pressure zone. The AngioJet pumps saline through the catheter where it creates fine jets of saline that are focused backwards from the tip of the catheter to create a negative pressure zone. The AngioJet draws thrombus into the catheter where it is fragmented and evacuated to a waste bag (Figs. 44.9 and 44.10).

Trellis:
- The Trellis system utilizes two compliant balloons to isolate thrombus and deliver targeted lytic therapy. The system consists of a sinusoidal wire attached to a

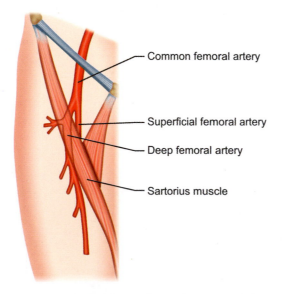

Fig. 44.5: Anatomy of common femoral artery with landmarks (anterior iliac crest, pubic bone, inguinal ligament).

- Common femoral artery
- Superficial femoral artery
- Deep femoral artery
- Sartorius muscle

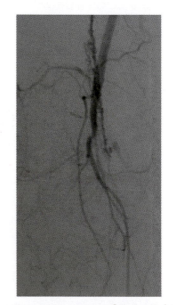

Fig. 44.6: Subtraction angiogram confirming right popliteal artery occlusion.

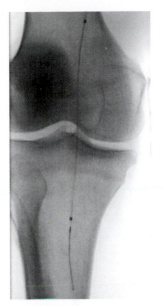

Fig. 44.7: Advance thrombolysis catheter over guidewire after crossing occlusion.

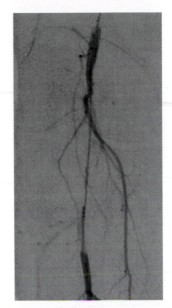

Fig. 44.8: Thrombolysis catheter (10-cm side holes) positioned in occluded popliteal artery.

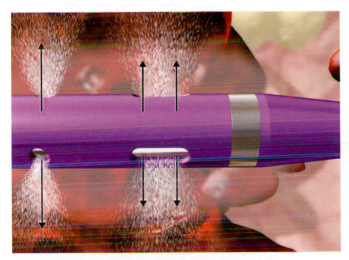

Fig. 44.9: Pulse spray AngioJet catheter tip.

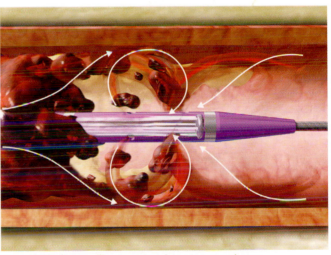

Fig. 44.10: Bernoulli principle of AngioJet catheter.

battery powered drive unit, which is inserted through the backend of the catheter. The wire oscilates between 500 and 3,000 rpm, working to further expose thrombus to the thrombolytic to enhance thrombolysis. Documented use of the Trellis system has shown greatest procedural success by running the device for approximately 10 minutes per treatment segment. When treatment is complete, residual lytic and/or liquefied thrombus may be aspirated through the integrated aspiration port on the Trellis system (Figs. 44.11 and 44.12).

2.4 Dressings

- Leave sheath and infusion catheter in situ and stick the catheter to the thigh with layered adhesive dressings, such as the IV3000 by 3M.
- Connect sterile tubing on infusion catheter and thrombolysis pump (dosage urokinase 80,000 units per hour).

2.5 Relook

- Reposition patient on X-ray table 8–12 hours after start of thrombolysis.

- Perform an angiogram through the indwelling femoral sheath.
- Continue thrombolysis for another session if dissolution of thrombus is incomplete (max 48 hours).
- If there is increasing pain or unsatisfactory dissolution of thrombus, increase the dosage of thrombolytic infusion (e.g. urokinase 100,000 units per hour).
- When there is satisfactory thrombus resolution and revascularization has been achieved, treat any underlying arterial stenosis with balloon angioplasty ± stent (Figs. 44.13 to 44.16).

2.6 Closure

- Remove sheath and use an arterial closure device.
- Alternatively leave sheath in place for 4 hours of observation prior to removal and manual compression as per normal protocols.

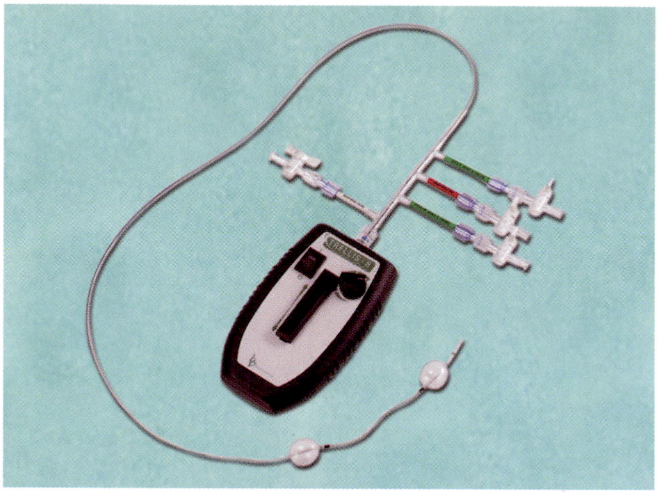

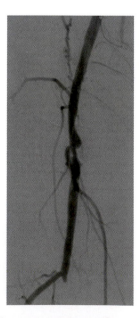

Fig. 44.11: Trellis system and oscillation drive unit and integrated dispersion wire.

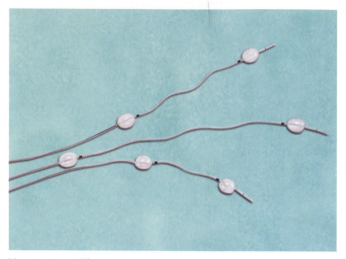

Fig. 44.12: Different length Trellis infusion catheters with two occluding balloons and drug infusion holes between the balloons.

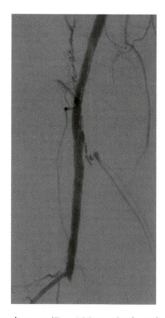

Fig. 44.13: Follow-up angiogram after 24 hours of thrombolysis (urokinase 200,000 units bolus and 80,000 units per hour and heparin 500 units per hour) demonstrating resolution of the thrombus in the occluded popliteal artery and an irregular popliteal artery aneurysm segment.

Fig. 44.14: Covered stent (7 × 100 mm) placed to exclude popliteal artery aneurysm.

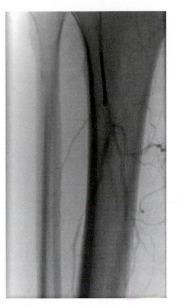

Fig. 44.15: Suction thrombectomy of residual thrombus in tibi-operoneal trunk.

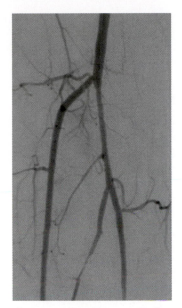

Fig. 44.16: Completion angiogram.

3 POSTOPERATIVE

3.1 Complications

- Death (3–5%)
- Major hemorrhage (5%)
- Minor hemorrhage (15%)
- Embolization (1–5%)
- Compartment syndrome (1–10%)

3.2 Outcomes

- One-year limb salvage (80%)
- One-year mortality (15%)

3.3 Follow-Up

- Consider oral anticoagulation for postoperative period (6–12 weeks determined by likelihood of recurrence/ underlying cause).
- Review 4–6 weeks postoperatively with duplex of treated limb/graft.

3.4 Video Clips 📹

- Infusion catheter
- AngioJet
- Trellis

3.5 E-mail an Expert

- *E-mail address*: r.varcoe@unsw.edu.au; barend.mees @mumc.nl

SUGGESTED READING

Cronenwett JL, Johnston KW. Rutherford's Vascular Surgery. Philadelphia: Elsevier, 2010.

Thompson MM, Morgan RA, Matsumura JS, et al. Endovascular Intervention for Vascular Disease. New York: Informa Healthcare, 2008.

REFERENCES

1. Ouriel K, Shortell CK, DeWeese JA, et al. A comparison of thrombolytic therapy with operative revascularization in the initial treatment of acute peripheral arterial ischemia. Journal of Vascular Surgery 1994;19(6):1021-30.
2. Weaver FA, Comerota AJ, Youngblood M, et al. Surgical revascularization versus thrombolysis for nonembolic lower extremity native artery occlusions: results of a prospective randomized trial. The STILE Investigators. Surgery versus Thrombolysis for Ischemia of the Lower Extremity. Journal Vascular Surgery 1996;24(4):513-21; discussion 521-3.
3. Ouriel K, Veith FJ, Sasahara AA. A comparison of recombinant urokinase with vascular surgery as initial treatment for acute arterial occlusion of the legs. Thrombolysis or peripheral arterial surgery (TOPAS Investigators). New England Journal of Medicine 1998;338(16):1105-11.
4. Norgren L, Hiatt WR, Dormandy JA, et al. TASC II Working Group. Inter-Society Consensus for the Management of Peripheral Arterial Disease (TASC II). J Vasc Surg. 2007; 45(Suppl S):S5-67.
5. Ravn H, Bergqvist D, Björck M. Swedish Vascular Registry. Nationwide study of the outcome of popliteal artery aneurysms treated surgically. Br J Surg. 2007; 94(8):970-7.

chapter 45

Femorofemoral Bypass

Elliot Stephenson, Greg Moneta

1 PREOPERATIVE

1.1 Indications

Indications:
- Iliac occlusive disease
- In conjunction with endovascular aorto-uni fem stent grafts
- Aortofemoral graft limb occlusion or graft infection
- In conjunction with axillary to femoral artery bypass for aortoiliac occlusive disease

Contraindications:
- Inadequate inflow or donor artery
- Inadequate outflow

1.2 Evidence

- Two-year patency of >80% and 5-year patency of 49–82% mean value of 65%
- No difference in patency between Dacron and PTFE[1,2]

1.3 Materials Needed

- Vascular instruments including vascular clamps for clamping femoral arteries (profunda, subclavian, Debakey, and Fogarty Mush clamps)

See Figures 45.1 and 45.2.
- Large straight aortic vascular clamp for tunneling

See Figure 45.3
- Suture Prolene (5-0, 6-0, 7-0) or PTFE CV-6, CV-7
- *Conduit*: most commonly externally supported PTFE, but Dacron, cryopreserved femoral vein or autologous femoral vein can be used)
- Weitlaner self-retractors, hand-held retractors

See Figure 45.4
- Iron intern or other self-retractor device can be helpful, particularly with obese patients
- A tunneling device (Scanlon or Oregon Tunneler) may also be helpful to assist in tunneling

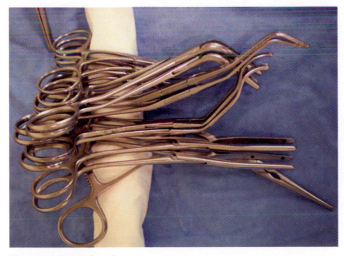

Fig. 45.1: Vascular clamps.

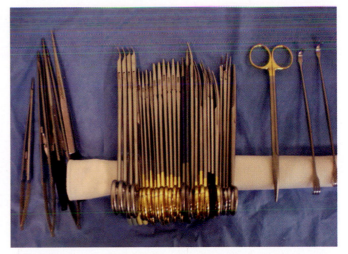

Fig. 45.2: Vascular instruments, including Pott's scissors, Castroviejo needle drivers, and clip appliers.

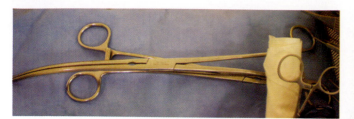

Fig. 45.3: Straight aortic clamps for tunneling.

- Loupe magnification
- Vessel loops
- Doppler box and sterile Doppler probe
- Heparin saline solution (10 units heparin/mL)

1.4 Preoperative Planning

Planning:
History and physical examination including careful pulse examination:
- Electrocardiogram (EKG or ECG)
- Chest X-ray (CXR)
- Baseline laboratories complete blood count (CBC), chemistry, coagulation panel and type and screen)

Where applicable:
- Cardiopulmonary clearance
- Echocardiogram
- Stress test
- Pulmonary functions tests

Imaging:
- Angiogram
- CT angiogram

Risk assessment:
- This (as with all peripheral vascular interventions) is a high-risk procedure.
- Relative increases in risk:
  - Advancing age
  - Cardiac disease
  - Chronic obstructive pulmonary disease
  - Reoperative surgery
  - Previous femoral access

1.5 Preoperative Checklist

Preinduction—Sign in:
- Patient has confirmed:
  - Identity
  - Site
  - Procedure
  - Consent

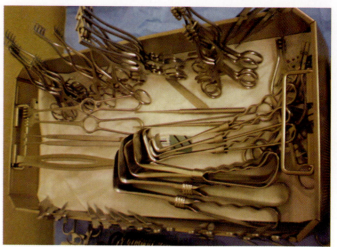

Fig. 45.4: Assorted retractors (handheld and self-retaining).

- The surgical site is marked (both groins for femoro-femoral bypass).
- Anesthesia checklist completed
- Pulse oximeter is in place and functioning.
- Verbalize patient allergies
- Are there any concerns for a difficult airway or risk of aspiration?
- Are there adequate fluids and/or blood products as there is chance for significant (>500 mL) of blood loss?

Before Incision—time out:
- All members introduce themselves and their roles in the surgery.
- Surgeon, anesthesia professional and nurse verbally confirm:
  - Patient
  - Site
  - Procedure
- Review of critical steps from the surgeon including:
  - Systemic heparin 3 minutes prior to clamping femoral arteries
  - Hourly redosing of heparin or checking serial activated clotting times
  - Clamping both femoral arteries
  - Unclamping the clamped femoral arteries
- Anesthesia team reviews any patient specific concerns.
- Nursing team reviews all equipment is sterile and available.
- Antibiotic prophylaxis confirmed to be given within 1 hour of skin incision.
- Angiograms or CT angiograms should be displayed.

Before patient leaves room—sign out:
- Nurse verbally confirms with team:

– the procedure
– sponge and instrument count
– any equipment issues needing to be addressed

1.6 Decision-Making Algorithm

• *See* Flowchart 45.1.

1.7 Pearls and Pitfalls

Pearls:

• Need adequate inflow and outflow, use of preoperative angiogram to assess inflow and potentially intervene with angioplasty or stenting of donor iliac artery to improve inflow.
• Adequate exposure of inguinal ligament to allow tunneling along the anterior fascia.
• Ensure adequate length and orientation to avoid kinking the graft.
• Tunnel the graft cephalad initially so it has an inverted U configuration.

Pitfalls:

• Graft kinking
• Tunneling graft too superficial where it will be more mobile and have higher propensity to kink.
• Inadequate inflow to keep Femorofemoral bypass open.
• Inadequate outflow.

1.8 Surgical Anatomy

The relevant surgical anatomy is familiar to most vascular surgeons. The inguinal ligament should be exposed at the superior portion of the wound for tunneling. The common femoral artery (CFA), superficial femoral artery (SFA), and profunda femoral artery (profunda) are the main arteries that need to be dissected and controlled inferior to the inguinal ligament. Additionally circumflex branches frequently are present and should be controlled with care taken to avoid injury or ligation as they may provide valuable collateral pathways. The femoral nerve and vein are in close proximity lateral and medial to the CFA respectively. Lastly, the sartorius muscle overlies the profunda artery and may be needed to be mobilized laterally to expose the more distal profunda if that is the only artery available for anastomosis (Fig. 45.5).

1.9 Positioning

Patient should be positioned in supine position with arms out stretched. Care should be taken to ensure adequate padding to avoid nerve injury. An upper body warmer may be used. The abdomen from the umbilicus to the knees should be available for prepping. Sequential compression devices and a urinary catheter should be in place. Retention straps should be either placed across the chest or below the knees (Fig. 45.6). This model is representative of the area to prep.

Flowchart 45.1: Decision-making algorithm.

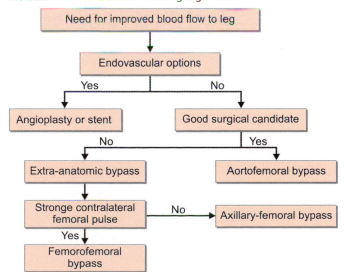

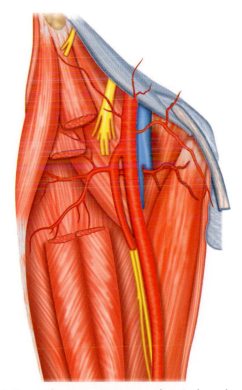

Fig. 45.5: Femoral artery anatomy and main branches and the relation to the inguinal ligament.

The field is then squared off with sterile drapes or towels. A groin towel is also placed and stapled in place. Two split sheets are used to complete the sterile draping (Fig. 45.7).

Lastly the area is covered with Ioban.

1.9 Anesthesia

* Systemic Heparin (80–100 units/kg) for administration prior to clamping femoral arteries.
* Protamine (1 mg to reverse 100 units of heparin) for possible use following completion of anastomosis.
* Adequate IV access in case of significant bleeding.
* Adequate blood pressure monitoring with arterial line when applicable.
* Sodium bicarbonate and vasopressors should be available at time of unclamping of legs as this may have effect on BP or have washout of potassium and lactic acid.

2 PERIOPERATIVE

The incision will depend in part on the planned artery (CFA, SFA, or profunda) for each anastomosis, but in general will be similar. *See* Figure 45.8.

For access to the CFA a transverse incision can be made in order to avoid crossing the groin crease. If the profunda artery is to be used then a longer longitudinal incision may be necessary.

See Figure 45.9.

The skin and subcutaneous tissues are divided. The dissection is carried medial to the sartorius muscle. On the donor side a femoral pulse should be present to assist with localizing the artery. Care should be taken to dissect directly to the artery as this area is rich in lymphatics and more extensive dissection increases the risk of postoperative lymphatic leak and lymphocele. Any lymphatic tissues should be ligated or clipped on both sides before dividing.

See Figure 45.10.

The femoral sheath is opened to expose the femoral artery. The dissection is usually carried out to expose the profunda, SFA, and CFA and circumferentially dissect each in order to control each.

See Figure 45.11.

An adequate place for the anastomosis on both the donor and recipient artery must be chosen. Ideally this is a segment that can be easily controlled with clamps and vessel loops. Additionally the chosen segment should

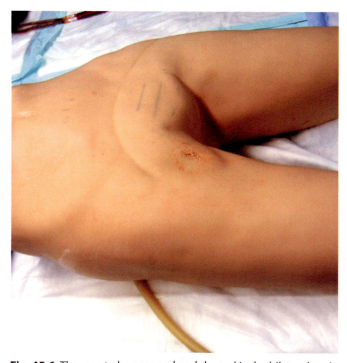

Fig. 45.6: The area to be prepped and draped is the bilateral groin regions, including the proximal anterior thighs, with extension of the surgical field to the level of the umbilicus.

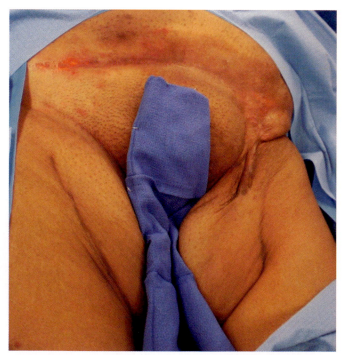

Fig. 45.7: Image of prepped field prior to placement of Ioban.

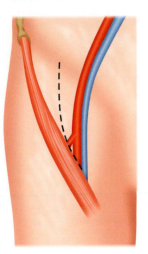

Fig. 45.8: Incision in relation to sartorius muscle and anterior superior iliac spine.

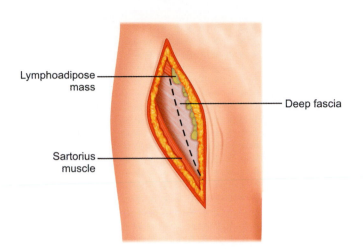

Fig. 45.9: Following incision, subcutaneous tissue divided to expose deep fascia (femoral sheath).

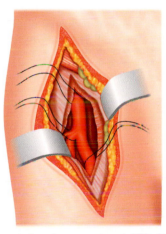

Fig. 45.10: Femoral sheath opened and CFA, SFA, and profunda dissected and encircled with vessel loops.

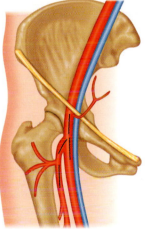

Fig. 45.11: Potential arteriotomy locations on the CFA, SFA, and profunda. The location should be based on the arteries and degree of disease. Placing the arteriotomy too proximal on the CFA can lead to kinking, particularly in obese patients.

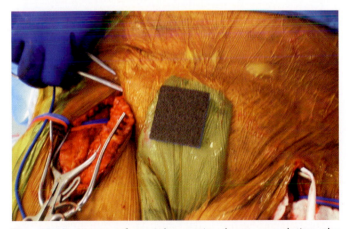

Fig. 45.12: Image of straight aortic clamp completing the subcutaneous tunnel. Note the cephalad location of the tunnel to minimize chance of graft kinking.

have minimal disease, although it is frequently necessary to sew to a diseased segment. Black lines on the figure represent different locations for arteriotomy.

See Figures 45.12 to 45.14.

A tunnel is made. This process is best facilitated by exposing the inguinal ligament and the anterior abdominal fascia. Blunt dissection with a finger along the anterior abdominal fascia from both the left and right groin incisions creates the beginning of the tunnel. A straight aorta clamp is then advanced from one of the incisions and used to pull the graft through the tunnel.

See Figure 45.15.

Heparin is administered intravenously and the clamp vessels used. After three minutes the arteriotomy in the donor vessel is made and the graft beveled to fit the

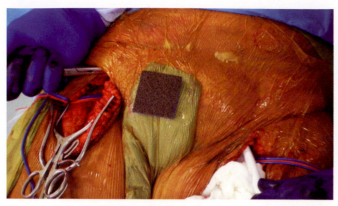

Fig. 45.13: The graft is pulled through the tunnel, with care being taken to maintain orientation, with dotted lines facing anteriorly.

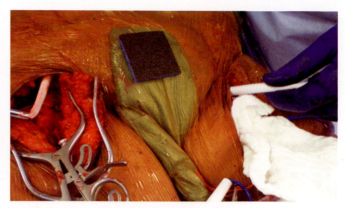

Fig. 45.14: The completed tunnel with graft in proper orientation.

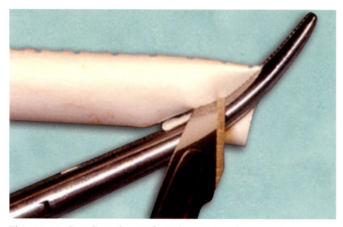

Fig. 45.15: Beveling the graft with a Metzenbaum scissors.

arteriotomy. A femoral endarterectomy can sometimes be of assistance at this time if the artery is severely diseased.

See Figure 45.16.

Complete anastomosis using monofilament running suture: Use Prolene suture for CryoVein, Dacron or autologous femoral vein. When using PTFE graft, PTFE sutures are recommended.

The completed femorofemoral bypass graft. *See* Figures 45.17 to 19. It is important to ensure that there is no kinking in the graft and there is good flow, both with palpation of a pulse and assessing intraoperative doppler signals. Additionally, it is important to remove retractors and ensure that this does not lead to any new kinking as the tissue may shift, particularly in obese patients.

Completed Anastomoses

Following completion of the anastomosis there is frequently suture hole bleeding from the graft. Usually pressure with or without a topical hemostatic agent is sufficient for hemostasis. The suture line should be carefully probed to ensure there are no areas of bleeding requiring suture repair. If bleeding is still moderate, Protamine (1 mg/100 units of circulating heparin) can be administered to counter the effects of the heparin

After hemostasis, both incisions are thoroughly irrigated and the incisions are closed in layers with absorbable sutures. The skin is closed with a subcuticular monofilament absorbable suture. Skin glue is then used to seal the incisions.

3 POSTOPERATIVE

3.1 Complications

Most common complications:
- Bleeding or hematoma
- Lymphocele
- Infection
- Graft kinking or thrombosis

Least common complications:
- Graft infection
- Pseudoaneurysm

3.2 Outcomes

Expected outcomes:
- Long-term patency of 80% at 2 years and 60% at 5 years.
- May need revision or assisted patency with iliac stenting of iliac donor artery.
- May need to be thrombectomized or revised surgically.
- Wound complications should be aggressively managed to the relative high risk from two groin incisions and use of synthetic material, seromas should be drained and sartorius flaps used to cover graft.

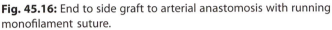
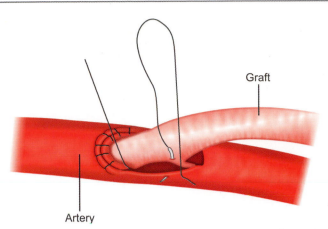

Fig. 45.16: End to side graft to arterial anastomosis with running monofilament suture.

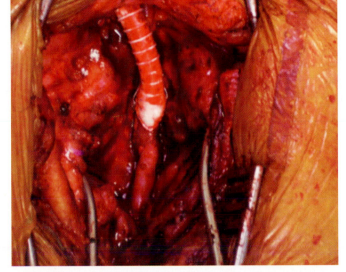

Fig. 45.17: Completed left end to side graft to CFA anastomosis. Note there is a left femoral to popliteal graft just distal to the femorofemoral bypass anastomosis.

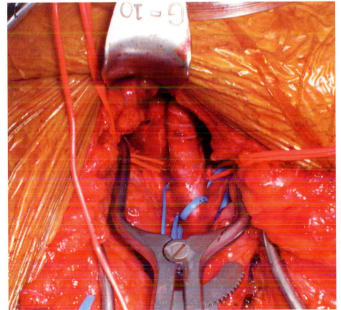

Fig. 45.18: Completed right end to side graft to CFA anastomosis.

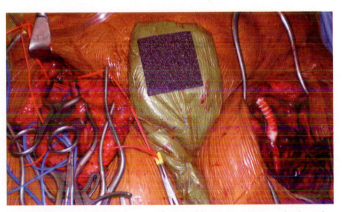

Fig. 45.19: Completed femorofemoral bypass prior to closing the groin incisions.

3.3 Follow-Up

- Follow up in 2 weeks to ensure adequate healing of groin incisions.
- Follow up in 3 months with a graft flow study.
- Follow up surveillance for the life time of the graft with surveillance graft flow duplex examinations every 3 months for the first year, every 6 months for the second year and yearly following two years if no concerning findings on surveillance.

3.4 E-mail an Expert

- *E-mail address*: stepheel@ohsu.edu

REFERENCES

1. Ricco JB, Probst H. on behalf of the French University Surgeons Association (AURC). Long-term results of a multicenter randomized study on direct versus crossover bypass for unilateral iliac artery occlusive disease J Vasc Surg. 2008;47:45-54.
2. Eiberg JP, Roder O, Stahl-Madsen M, et al. Fluoropolymer-coated Dacron versus PTFE grafts for femorofemoral crossover bypass: a randomized trial. Eur J Vasc Endovasc Surg. 2006;32:431-8.

QUIZ

Question 1: All of the following can be used for conduit for a femorofemoral bypass EXCEPT?
a. Externally supported PTFE
b. Dacron
c. Cryopreserved saphenous vein
d. Saphenous vein
e. None of the above

Question 2: The two year patency for a femorofemoral bypass is approximately what percent?
a. 20%
b. 40%
c. 60%
d. 80%

Question 3: The most important landmark for tunneling the graft during a femorofemoral bypass:
a. The femoral vein
b. The profunda femoral artery
c. The inguinal ligament
d. The sartorius muscle

Question 4: The following factors should be considered prior to deciding on Femorofemoral bypass for revascularization except?
a. A presence of autologous conduit
b. B adequacy of contralateral femoral pulse
c. C endovascular stenting candidacy
d. D surgical candidacy

Coiling Peripheral Pseudoaneurysms

Ashley K Vavra, Mark K Eskandari

1 PREOPERATIVE

1.1 Indications and Contraindications

Indications:
- Large or enlarging asymptomatic and symptomatic pseudoaneurysms of the visceral, lower extremity, upper extremity, and cervical arteries

Relative contraindications:
- Need to maintain patency of the feeding vessel
- Small vessel size or severe angulation/tortuosity

1.2 Evidence

- Given the rare incidence of visceral or peripheral arterial pseudoaneurysms, there are limited large reviews of outcomes with long-term follow-up after treatment using endovascular techniques including coiling. However, based on the current literature, coiling of pseudoaneurysms is associated with decreased morbidity when compared to open repair with between 80% and 100% long-term success rate.[1]
- Compared to true aneurysms, pseudoaneurysms of visceral arteries have a high risk of rupture and early intervention is indicated.[2,3]

1.3 Materials Needed

- Ultrasound
- Fluoroscopy with fixed imaging, fidelity unit (Fig. 46.1)
- Coaxial catheter system with varying catheter sizes dependent on target vessel size
- Appropriate sheath size for catheter placement and coil delivery
- Coils (retrievable and nonretrievable)
- Potential adjuvant materials
- Covered stent (e.g. GORE Viabahn, Atrium iCAST)

- Absorbable bioprosthetic material (Gelfoam, Oxycel)
- Nonabsorbable particles (Polyvinyl alcohol, Embospheres)
- Polymers (Onyx)

1.4 Preoperative Risk Assessment

Planning:
- Noninvasive testing (ultrasound, CT angiography, MR angiography)
- Invasive testing with percutaneous angiography is the gold standard for diagnosis

Low risk:
- Asymptomatic
- Small pseudoaneurysm size
- Narrow neck

Intermediate risk:
- Wide neck
- Increased vessel tortuosity

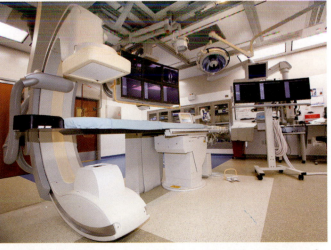

Fig. 46.1: An angiography suite is an essential component for advanced endovascular procedures.

High risk:

- Advanced age
- Multiple comorbidities
- Associated rupture or hemorrhage

1.5 Preoperative Checklist

Sign in:

- Identify any allergy to contrast dye and confirm appropriate prophylaxis
- Confirm appropriate blood type and cross-match if bleeding is a concern
- Confirm planned access site and route (percutaneous or open)
- Confirm presence and working order of equipment required

Time out:

- Confirm that appropriate antibiotic prophylaxis has been given
- Identify any anesthetic concerns

Sign out:

- Confirm final procedure
- Confirm plans for postoperative disposition and monitoring

1.6 Decision-Making Algorithm (Flowchart 46.1)

- Depending on the location of the pseudoaneurysm, access via the femoral or brachial arteries is utilized.
- In the setting of trauma and potentially unstable patient, treatment of a pseudoaneurysm that will require highly selective angiogram may not be amenable to endovascular intervention given the time required for the procedure.
- Once anatomy is established, evaluate whether the feeding vessels should be spared or if they can be sacrificed.
- If essential, evaluate neck size to determine whether amenable to coiling or if coverage with a stent is required.
- If nonessential and high collateral flow, embolization of distal in addition to proximal feeding vessels may be required.

1.7 Pearls and Pitfalls

Pearls:

- To ensure adequate occlusion, the coil should form a dense, tight configuration and not an elongated open configuration, which decreases thrombus formation.

Flowchart 46.1: Decision-making algorithm.

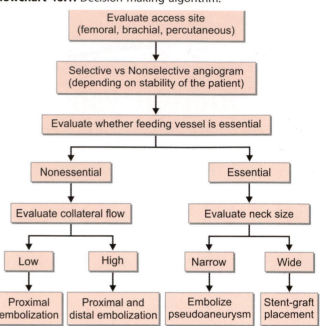

- Coils that are too small are at risk for distal embolization. An anchoring coil, which is oversized by 1–2 mm, can be placed initially to prevent embolization of subsequently placed coils.
- Catheter and coil diameter must be concordant. Avoid use of side-hole catheters that can prevent adequate deployment of the coils and polyurethane catheters due to high friction during coil delivery.

Pitfalls:

- Vessel occlusion after coil embolization can be prolonged in patients with underlying coagulopathy.

1.8 Surgical Anatomy

- For femoral artery access, puncture site should be in the common femoral artery over the femoral head and well above the origin of the profunda femoris artery (Fig. 46.2).
- For brachial artery access, the left brachial artery often provides a more direct route to the descending thoracic and abdominal aorta. Left-sided access also avoids any wire or catheter manipulation across the origin of the innominate and carotid artery, thus reducing the periprocedural stroke risk. A puncture site ~1 cm above the antecubital crease allows for post-procedure compression against the humeral head (Fig. 46.3).
- Knowledge of potential collaterals that could lead to revascularization of the pseudoaneurysm is key to

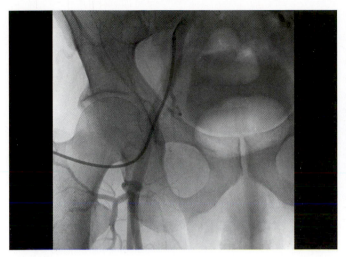

Fig. 46.2: Access of the common right common femoral artery over the femoral head confirmed with angiogram for embolization of a left internal iliac artery pseudoaneurysm.

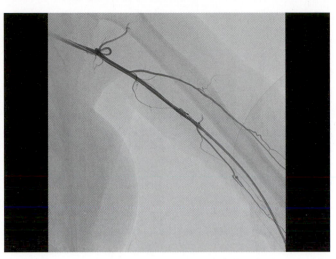

Fig. 46.3: Percutaneous access to the left brachial artery for embolization of splenic artery aneurysm.

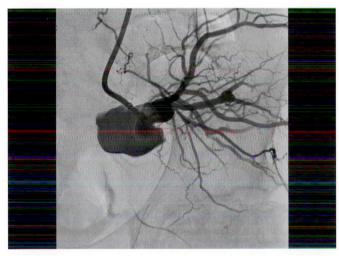

Fig. 46.4: Aneurysm of a branch of the internal iliac artery demonstrating multiple arterial branches in the outflow of the aneurysm.

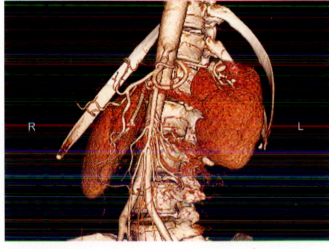

Fig. 46.5: Tortuous splenic artery with associated aneurysm.

determine appropriateness of both proximal and distal embolization (Fig. 46.4).
- Increased tortuosity and angulation of the affected vessel can make difficult the selection of the vessel to be embolized and catheter stabilization during the procedure (Fig. 46.5).
- If the pseudoaneurysm has a wide neck, adjuncts such as a covered stent may be employed to prevent distal embolization of coils or thrombosing agents used in the pseudoaneurysm (Figs. 46.6A and B)

1.9 Positioning

- Supine position

- Arm position varies depending on area visualized and access site

1.10 Anesthesia

- Consider local or regional block with monitored anesthesia care for patients with multiple comorbidities.
- General anesthesia may be required for prolonged cases.

2 PERIOPERATIVE

2.1 Incision

- An ultrasound may be used to assist in percutaneous access of the common femoral or brachial artery.

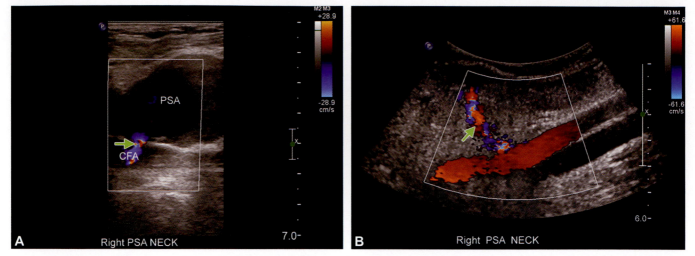

Figs. 46.6A and B: Ultrasound of common femoral artery pseudoaneurysms with both wide/short (A) and narrow/long (B) pseudoaneurysm neck anatomy.

- Alternatively a cut down may be employed for insertion of the access sheath under direct visualization, particularly for large sheaths placed in small brachial arteries.

2.2 Steps

- After access is obtained and a sheath of the appropriate size inserted, a nonselective angiogram is performed to identify collateral flow and any source of bleeding if performed for trauma (Fig. 46.7).
- Combination of small caliber hydrophilic wire and angled catheter can be used to access the inflow artery to perform a selective angiogram (Fig. 46.8).
- Treatment of the pseudoaneurysm or aneurysm is performed based on the algorithm listed above (Figs. 46.9A and B).
- Completion angiogram is performed to ensure adequate exclusion of the pseudoaneurysm or aneurysm from the circulation (Fig. 46.10).

2.3 Closure

- Sheath size of 6 Fr can often be employed and manual pressure applied for hemostasis following removal.
- If a closure device is employed, there are a variety of options including:
  - Boomerang device
  - Collagen plug device (ex. Angioseal)
  - Clip device (ex. Starclose)
  - Suture device (ex. Perclose)

3 POSTOPERATIVE

3.1 Complications

Most Common Complications:
- Access site complications
  - Pain
  - Hematoma (femoral or brachial sheath with associated neurologic compression requiring evacuation)
  - Pseudoaneurysm
- Postembolization syndrome (pain, fever, nausea, vomiting, leukocytosis) from end-organ ischemia with visceral artery pseudoaneurysms

Least common complications:
- Recanalization of the embolized vessel
- Coil migration or embolization
- Intraprocedural rupture
- Severe ischemia of end-organ requiring resection

3.2 Outcomes

- Primary exclusion of the aneurysm is expected in 80% to 90% of cases, with up to 100% success rate after second intervention, if required.
- Erosion and recanalization with or without secondary bleed or rupture may occur more frequently in the setting of associated infection or inflammation such as seen with splenic artery pseudoaneurysms associated with pancreatitis.

3.3 Follow-Up

- Follow-up imaging is required to ensure adequate exclusion from the circulation.

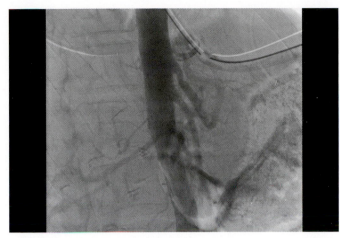

Fig. 46.7: Celiac artery angiogram demonstrating a distal splenic artery aneurysm.

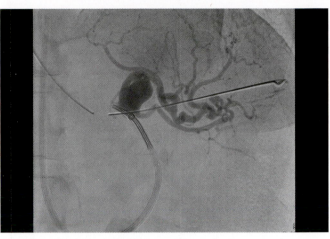

Fig. 46.8: Selective angiogram of the splenic artery that demonstrates the aneurysm and its outflow.

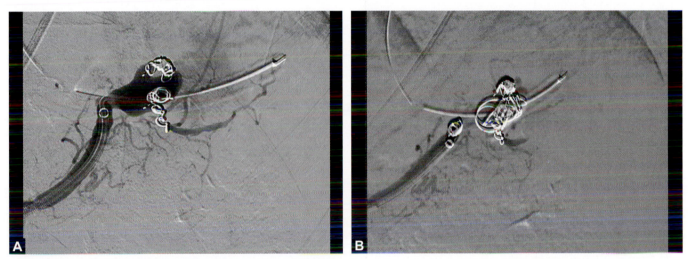

Figs. 46.9A and B: Placement of detachable coils in the proximal and distal feeding vessels of the splenic artery aneurysm.

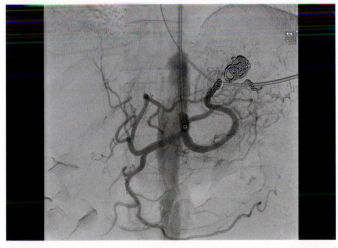

Fig. 46.10: Completion angiogram demonstrating exclusion of the aneurysm from the circulation.

- Imaging is usually performed via non-invasive modalities such as CTA, MRA, or ultrasound.
- Timing of follow-up imaging is dependent on the presentation and postoperative course of the patient, but a minimum of 30-day follow-up is recommended.

3.4 E-mail an Expert

- *E-mail address*: ashleyvavra@yahoo.com

3.5 Web Resources/References

- www.vascularweb.org Society of Vascular Surgeons

REFERENCES

1. Frankhauser GT, Stone WM, Naidu SG, et al. The minimally invasive management of visceral artery aneurysms and pseudoaneurysms. J Vasc Surg. 53:966-70.

2. Guillon R, Garcier JM, Abergel A, et al. Management of splenic artery aneurysms and false aneurysms with endovascular treatment in 12 patients. Cardiovasc Int Radiol. 2003;26:256-60.

3. Tessier DJ, Stone WM, Fowl RJ, et al. Clinical features and management of splenic artery pseudoaneurysm: case series and review of the literature. J Vasc Surg. 2003;35(5): 969-74

QUIZ

Question 1: What is the gold standard imaging modality for the diagnosis of arterial pseudoaneurysm:
a. CT angiography
b. MR angiography
c. Percutaneous angiography
d. Ultrasound

Question 2: What is the optimal approach to a pseudoaneurysm with multiple outflow branches:
a. Covered stent use
b. Embolization of the pseudoaneurysm only
c. Embolization of both proximal and distal vessels
d. Injection with thrombin

Question 3: Which factors may influence the appropriateness of endovascular approach for use of coil embolization in the treatment of a pseudoaneurysm:

a. Need to preserve the patency of the involved vessel
b. Severe tortuosity or angulation of the involved vessel
c. Severe aortoiliac atherosclerotic disease
d. All of the above

Question 4: A 34-year-old woman undergoes coil embolization of a splenic artery aneurysm via left brachial artery access. She subsequently develops complaints of numbness and tingling in the thumb and first finger. The most likely diagnosis is:
a. Brachial sheath hematoma
b. Direct injury to the median nerve
c. Brachial artery thrombosis
d. Embolization from brachial artery access site

ANSWERS:

1. c   2. c   3. d   4. a

Coiling Endoleak

LeAnn A Chavez, John G Carson

1 PREOPERATIVE

1.1 Indications

- Endoleak defined as persistent blood flow in aneurysm sac
- *Types of endoleaks*:
  - *I*: Proximal and distal graft attachment zones
  - *II*: Patent braches vessels with flow into aneurysm sac
  - *III*: Mid-graft fabric tear or disassociation of graft limbs
  - *IV*: Graft wall fabric porosity or suture hole.
- *Indications for repair*:
  - Presence of type I or III endoleak
  - Persistent type II endoleak with sac expansion.
- *Contraindications*:
  - Renal failure/renal insufficiency
  - Bacteremia
  - Contrast allergy

1.2 Evidence

Incidence of a type II endoleak is approximately 10–25%[1,2]:
- Most type II endoleaks resolve spontaneously.[3]
- Persistent type II endoleaks may cause aneurysm sac enlargement.[4]
- Success rate of secondary intervention for endoleak repair is about 43%.[5]

1.3 Materials Needed

- Prior imaging studies or arteriogram
- Fluoroscopy
- Contrast media
- Injectable heparinized saline
- 5 French micropuncture catheter
- Ultrasound 4–7 mHz liner transducer
- 0.035 J-Wire
- 0.035 Rosen
- 5-Fr sheath
- 5-Fr pigtail
- 5-Fr hydrophilic catheter
- 2.8-Fr microcatheter
- 0.014 Hydrophilic guidewire
- Coils/polymer
- Closure device (optional)

See Figures 47.1A to C.

1.4 Preoperative Risk Assessment

American Society of Anesthesiologist Physical Status Classification System[6]:
- *Low risk*:
  - *I*: A normal healthy patient
  - *II*: A patient with mild systemic disease
- *Intermediate risk*:
  - *III*: A patient with severe systemic disease
- *High risk (must have anesthesiologist present)*:
  - *IV*: A patient with severe systemic disease that is a constant threat to life.
  - *V*: A moribund patient who is not expected to survive without the operation.
  - *VI*: A declared brain-dead patient whose organs are being removed for donor purposes

Arterial access:
- *Low risk*:
  - None to minimal plaque in iliac and femoral vessels
- *Intermediate risk*:
  - Moderate plaque in iliac and femoral vessels
  - Tortuous iliac arteries
- *High risk*:
- Severe plaque in iliac and femoral vessels
- Severe tortuosity of iliac vessels

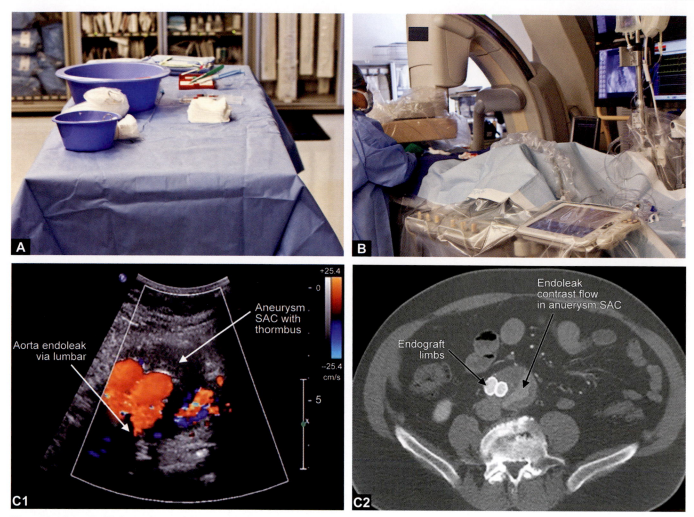

Figs. 47.1A to C: (A) Procedure Table A sterile back table is setup with materials. Additional materials are readily available in storage units. (B) Fluoroscopy procedure room standard setup for room allows physician access to right femoral sheath and ability to visualize monitors without difficulty. Notice fluoroscopy control panel is included in sterile drape. (C) Preoperative imaging studies may include ultrasound or CT images.

- Associated iliac aneurysm
- Lower extremity outflow obstruction

1.5 Preoperative Checklist

Sign in:
- All materials available and in-stock prior to procedure.
- Available preprocedure imaging studies
- Patient laboratory studies; Complete blood count (CBC), creatinine, electrolytes, coagulation panel
- Appropriate X-ray shielding for patient and staff
- Mark potential sites of access

Time out:
- Identify patient by two or more identifiers (i.e. medical record number [MRN] and date of birth [DOB])

- State planned procedure
- State access sites
- Patient allergy status
- Confirm preoperative antibiotics given.
- Confirm necessary equipment available.

Sign out:
- Procedure end time
- Total fluoroscopy time and total dose area product
- Type and total contrast injected
- Documentation of products used

1.6 Decision-Making Algorithm[7]

- Surveillance images are recommended. Duration depends on extent of endoleak, clinical suspicion, and/or

Flowchart 47.1: Decision-making algorithm.

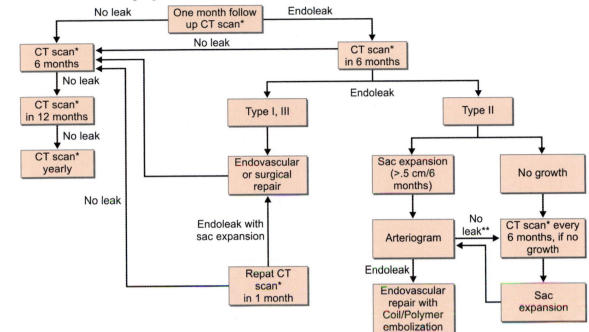

*Surveillance imaging may include ultrasound duplex and/or CT scan.
** No endoleak identified after arteriogram, may consider repeat imaging surveillance or surgical repair.

predicted response to observation verses treatment.
• If endoleak persists after intravascular embolization repair may consider:
  – *Percutaneous reintervention*:
    ▪ Transperitoneal
    ▪ Translumbar
  – *Surgical options*:
  – Laparoscopic clips
  – Open repair
See Flowchart 47.1

1.7 Pearls and Pitfalls

Pearl:
• Appropriate preprocedural imaging
• Variety of embolization product readily available
• Appropriate fluoroscopy imaging techniques are necessary to visualize source of endoleak (i.e. magnification and angulation).

Pitfall:
• Inadequate preprocedural imaging may prolong procedure, require more contrast, and increase radiation exposure.
• Inadequate product supply may lead to unnecessary additional procedures and patient exposure.
• Improper visualization may lead to lack of identification of endoleak source.

1.8 Surgical Anatomy[8]

• Abdominal aorta has multiple branches.
• Pelvic collaterals provide intravascular access to source of endoleak.
• Location of forearm bifurcation may vary 2–4 centimeters above or below the antecubital crease. Examination with ultrasound will help prevent unnecessary injury.
See Figures 47.2A and B.

1.9 Positioning

• Supine
• Appropriate fluoroscopy shields
• Groins exposed and prepped
• Upper extremity access available, if needed. Prefer left upper extremity to limit catheter crossing thoracic aortic arch.

1.10 Anesthesia

• Awake with local 1% lidocaine
• Conscious moderate sedation with local 1% lidocaine
• Monitoring:
  – Noninvasive blood pressure cuff
  – Pulse oximetry

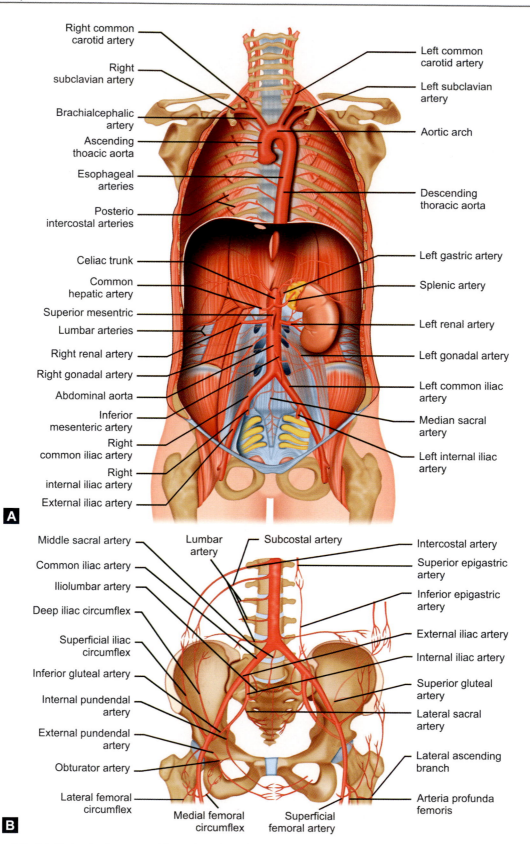

Right common carotid artery
Right subclavian artery
Brachialcephalic artery
Ascending thoacic aorta
Esophageal arteries
Posterio intercostal arteries
Celiac trunk
Common hepatic artery
Superior mesentric
Lumbar arteries
Right renal artery
Right gonadal artery
Abdominal aorta
Inferior mesenteric artery
Right common iliac artery
Right internal iliac artery
External iliac artery

Left common carotid artery
Left subclavian artery
Aortic arch
Descending thoracic aorta
Left gastric artery
Splenic artery
Left renal artery
Left gonadal artery
Left common iliac artery
Median sacral artery
Left internal iliac artery

A

Middle sacral artery
Common iliac artery
Iliolumbar artery
Deep iliac circumflex
Superficial iliac circumflex
Inferior gluteal artery
Internal pundendal artery
External pundendal artery
Obturator artery
Lateral femoral circumflex
Medial femoral circumflex

Lumbar artery
Subcostal artery
Superficial femoral artery

Intercostal artery
Superior epigastric artery
Inferior epigastric artery
External iliac artery
Internal iliac artery
Superior gluteal artery
Lateral sacral artery
Lateral ascending branch
Arteria profunda femoris

B

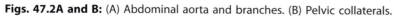

Figs. 47.2A and B: (A) Abdominal aorta and branches. (B) Pelvic collaterals.

- Telemetry
- Oxygen provided via nasal cannula

2 PERIOPERATIVE[9]

2.1 Arterial Access

- Ultrasound guidance helps to identify access vessel patency and atherosclerotic disease.
- Bony landmarks of anterior iliac spine and pubic symphysis can help to locate appropriate position of common femoral artery.
- Brachial artery access two finger breaths above the antecubital crease. Beware of possible high bifurcation of radial and ulnar arteries.

See Figures 47.3A and B.

2.2 Steps

- *See* Figures 47.4A to H.

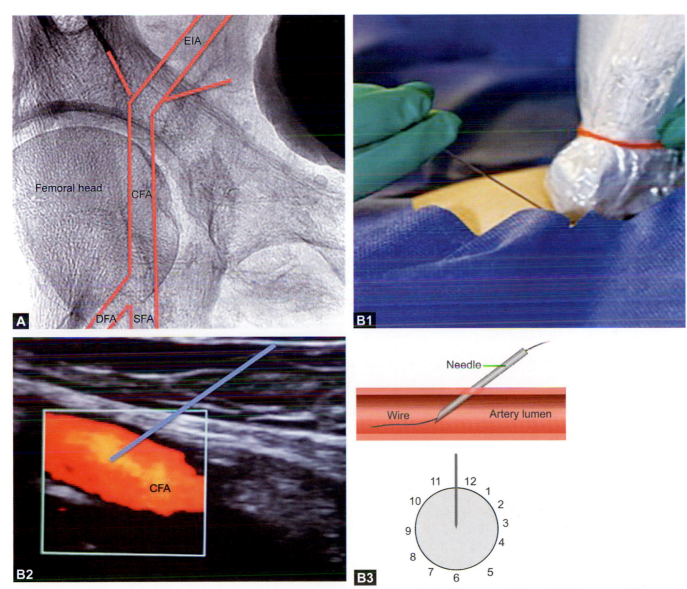

Figs. 47.3A and B: (A) Femoral access fluoroscopic image shows landmarks in relationship to arterial vessels. EIA, external iliac artery; CFA, common femoral artery; DFA, deep femoral artery; SFA, superficial femoral artery. (B1, 2, 3) Ultrasound of femoral vessels External view of ultrasound transducer against right groin in longitudinal orientation. Blue line is trajectory of access needle on ultrasound image. In transverse view needle should access artery at the 12 o'clock position. CFA, common femoral artery.

- Access arm if needed to access inferior mesenteric artery via superior mesenteric artery, or common femoral artery for internal iliac artery access.
- Arteriogram and selection of access vessel (superior mesenteric artery or internal iliac artery) using 0.035 hydrophilic wire and selective catheter.
- Advancement of microcatheter and 0.014 wire into the aneurysm sac.
- Catheter directed injection of polymer or coils
- Completion arteriogram
- Closure (*see* below)

2.3 Closure

If anticoagulation utilized:
- Recommend activated clotting time (ACT) prior to sheath removal.

- Safe to remove sheath when ACT <180.
- Pain medications administration may improve patient cooperation with sheath removal.

Femoral access:
- Supine position with bed flat
- Pressure is applied one to two finger breaths proximal to the skin puncture site.
- Expose ipsilateral foot so the color can be observed.
- May use Doppler to monitor presence of distal signal.
- 5–6 Fr sheath, hold pressure for 20 minutes.
- Larger sheaths pressure is held for up to 30 minutes.
- After sheath removal patient should remain flat for 6 hours.
- May raise head in reverse trendelenburg.

Brachial access:
- Similar process as explained for femoral sheath.

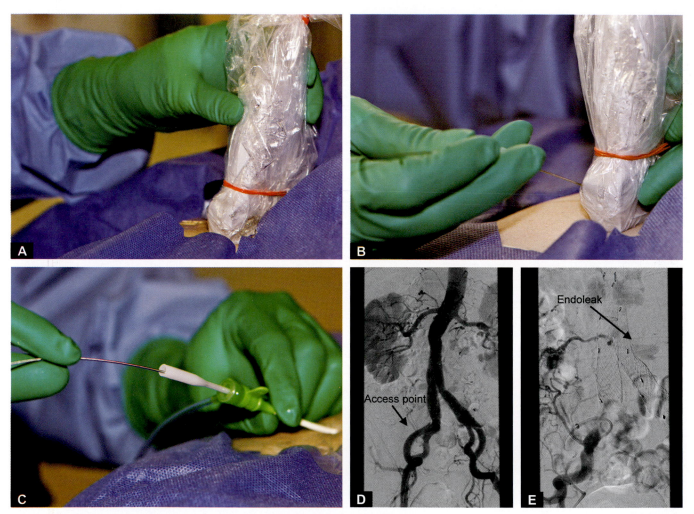

Figs. 47.4A to E: (A) Use ultrasound to identify artery. (B) Ultrasound guidance access with 22-gauge needle after infiltration with 1% lidocaine in subcutaneous tissue. (C) Modified Seldinger technique place wire and identify course with fluoroscopy. Place sheath over wire. Flush sheath with heparinized saline. (D) Longer length wire followed with pigtail catheter. Anterior-posterior aortogram to identify source of endoleak. May consider systemic anticoagulation. (E) Additional views in right axial orientation (RAO) view endoleak source.

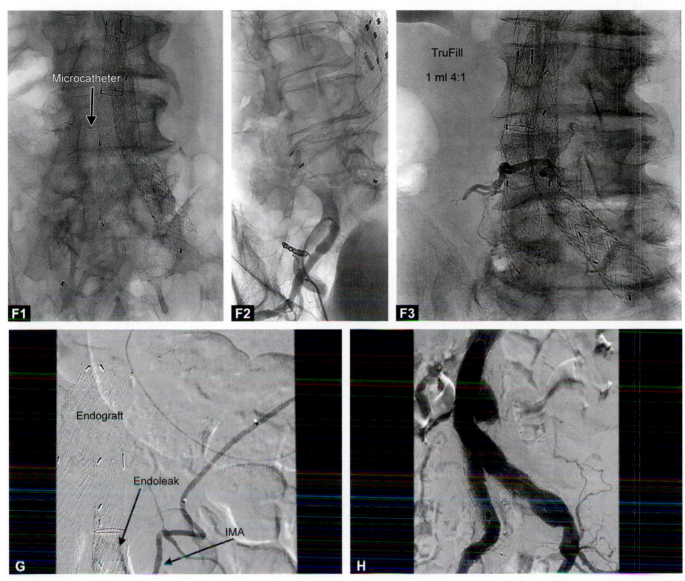

Figs. 47.4F to H: (F) 1,2,3 Catheter directed intravascular embolization of source. May also inject coil or polymer into aneurysm sac. A completion arteriogram confirms successful embolization of endoleak. (G) Arteriogram showing inferior mesenteric artery (IMA) as endoleak source. (H) Type III endoleak angiographic image.

- Monitoring of distal pulse and absence of neurological deficits in the ipsilateral hand are important.

3 POSTOPERATIVE

3.1 Complications

Most common:
- Persistent flow through endoleak/recurrence of endoleak.
- Access site complication (i.e. hematoma, pseudoanuerysm, arteriovenous (AV) fistula, and infection)
- Retroperitoneal hematoma

- Vasovagal response with sheath exchange or removal

Least common complications:
- Renal failure
- Paralysis
- Nerve injury
- Graft infection

3.2 Expected Outcomes

- Embolization of sac aneurysm source.
- Sac thrombosis confirmed with follow-up imaging.
- Resolution of endoleak and decreased size of aneurysm sac.
- Discharge patient same day

3.3 Follow-Up

Surveillance imaging at 1 month, 6 months, then yearly:
- CT scan with IV contrast
- Ultrasound duplex[10,11]

3.4 E-mail an Expert

- *E-mail address*: john.carson@ucdmc.ucdavis.edu

3.5 Web/Other Resources

- www.depuy.com
- www.terumomedical.com
- www.cook.com
- www.vascularweb.org
- Rutherford Vascular Surgery 7th Edition
- *Ultrasound for Surgeons*: A Basic Course, 2nd Edition CD, http://www.facs.org/education/ultrasound/course.html

REFERENCES

1. Rhee SJ, Ohki T, Veith FJ, et al. Current status of management of type II endoleaks after endovascular repair of abdominal aortic aneurysms. Ann Vasc Surg. 2003;17:335-44.
2. Piazza M, Frigatti P, Scivere P, et al. Role of aneurysm sac embolization during endovascular aneurysm repair in the prevention of type II endoleak-related complications. J Vasc Surg. 2013; 57:934-941.
3. Owens CD, Yeghiazarians Y. Handbook of Endovascular Peripheral Interventions. New York: Springer; 2012.
4. Sacrac TP, Gibbons C, Vargas L, et al. Long-term follow up for type II endoleak embolization reveals the need for close surveillance. J Vasc Surg. 2012;55:33-40.
5. Aziz A, Menias CO, Sanchez LA, et al. Outcomes of percutaneous endovascular intervention for type II endoleak with aneurysm expansion. J Vasc Surg. 2012;55:233-1267.
6. American Society of Anesthesiologists. (2011). ASA physical status classification system. Available from http://www.asahq.org/Home/For-Members/Clinical-Information/ASA-Physical-Status-Classification-System. [Accessed March 11, 2013].
7. Karch LA, Henretta JP, Hodgson KM, et al. Algorithm for the diagnosis and treatment of endoleaks. Am J Surg. 1999; 178:225-31.
8. Uflacker R. Atlas of Vascular Anatomy an Angiographic Approach, 2nd edition. Philadelphia, PA: Lippincott Williams & Wilkins; 2007.
9. Owens CD, Yeghiazarians Y. Handbook of Endovascular Peripheral Interventions. New York: Springer; 2012.
10. Chaer RA, Gushchin A, Rhee R, et al. Duplex ultrasound as the sole long-term surveillance method post-endovascular aneurysm repair: a safe alternative for stable aneurysms. J Vasc Surg. 2009;49:845-9.
11. Schmieder GC, Stout CL, Stokes GK, et al. Endoleak after endovascular aneurysm repair; duplex ultrasound imaging is better than computed tomography at determining the need for intervention. J Vasc Surg. 2009;50:1012-7.

QUIZ

Question 1. You have just completed an arteriogram via right brachial artery access. In the recovery room, the patient complains of right hand weakness and numbness. Patient has palpable hematoma under access site. You obtain Doppler signal at radial and ulnar locations of wrist. What is the most appropriate next step?

a. Start anticoagulation for embolic event

b. Reassure patient as this is a common occurrence after brachial artery access and should resolve spontaneously

c. Recommend open exploration of access site to release hematoma of brachial sheath

d. Radiographic imaging with CT or MRI to evaluate for stroke

Question 2. After successful coil embolization of type II endoleak source of an AAA previously repaired with endograft, you recommend:

a. No follow-up imaging necessary

b. CT scan in 1 month

c. Ultrasound in 1 month

d. Both B and C at 1 month

e. Either B or C at 1 month

Question 3. Endoleak is identified immediately after placement of an endograft for an infrarenal AAA in a patient with diabetes, hypertension, and chronic kidney disease (CKD) stage 2. At 1-month follow-up, there is no change in aneurysm sac. By CT scan at 6 months, the aneurysm sac has increased by 1 cm. What is the most appropriate next step?

a. Schedule the patient for arteriogram, no preprocedure laboratories needed

b. Obtain baseline creatinine and schedule for arteriogram

c. Schedule for open operation because CKD Stage 2 is a contraindication for arteriogram

d. Obtain follow up CT scan at 1 year

Question 4. A patient underwent endovascular aortic repair with an endograft for a 5.5 cm abdominal aortic aneurysm. On completion, angiogram type Ia endoleak is identified.

What is the next step?

a. CT scan in 1 month
b. Duplex/CT prior to discharge
c. Balloon, then possible aortic extension if needed
d. Convert to open repair

Question 5. A tear in the endograft is defined as a:

a. Type I endoleak
b. Type II endoleak
c. Type III endoleak
d. Type IV endoleak

Femoral Anastomotic Aneurysms

Mitchell R Weaver, Alexander D Shepard

1 PREOPERATIVE

1.1 Indications

Asymptomatic aneurysms:
- $\geq$ 2.0–2.5 cm in diameter
- Containing a significant amount of mural thrombus

Symptomatic aneurysms:
- Local compression (venous or nerve related symptoms)
- Rupture/hemorrhage
- Infection
- Limb ischemia resulting from thrombosis or distal thromboembolism[1] (Figs. 48.1A and B)

1.2 Evidence

Complications are uncommon in femoral anastomotic aneurysms less than 2 cm; however, larger aneurysms are associated with local complications and limb ischemia.[1–3]

1.3 Materials Needed

- Table-fixed retractor system: Used for adequate exposure of operative field (Fig. 48.2A).
- Balloon occlusion catheters (#3, 4, and 5 Fr): helpful for intraluminal vascular control when standard exposure is difficult or hazardous (Fig. 48.2B).
- *Graft*: for use as arterial conduit for in-situ reconstruction. Caliber of selected conduit depends on size of inflow graft limb and outflow native artery to be reconstructed. In most circumstances it is appropriate to choose a graft intermediate in size between the larger inflow graft and the smaller outflow artery (Fig. 48.2C).
- Autotransfusion capabilities should be considered in cases of large, rapidly expanding or ruptured anastomotic aneurysms in which vascular control may be difficult to obtain (Fig. 48.2D).

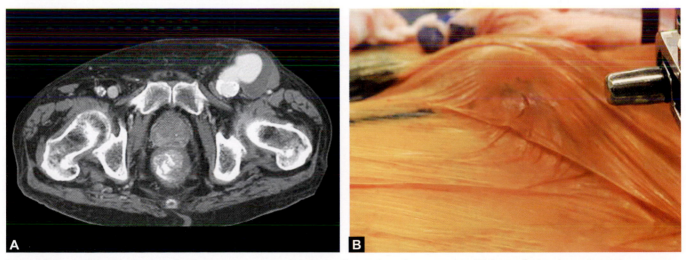

Figs. 48.1A and B: (A) CT scan demonstrating a large left femoral anastomotic aneurysm. (B) Large femoral anastomotic aneurysm presenting as large pulsatile groin mass.

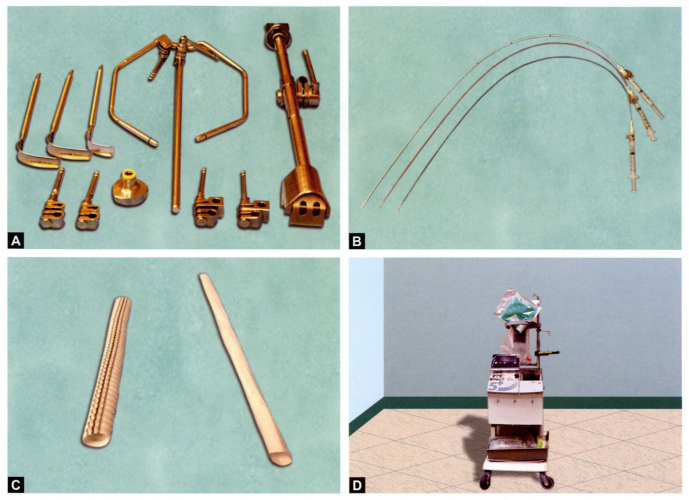

Figs. 48.2A to D: (A) Table-fixed retractor system. (B) Balloon occlusion catheter with stop-cock and syringe. (C) Prosthetic graft. (D) Autotransfusion system.

1.4 Preoperative Planning and Risk Assessment

Planning:
- CT angiography of abdomen, pelvis, and lower extremities is the preferred imaging modality; MRI is acceptable in patients with chronic kidney disease.
- Documentation of limb perfusion status should be performed by measuring Doppler-derived ankle-brachial indices (ABIs) of both lower extremities.

Risk assessment:
- ACC/AHA 2007 Guidelines on Perioperative Cardiovascular Evaluation and Care for Noncardiac Surgery[4]

1.5 Decision-Making Algorithm

- *See* Flowchart 48.1.

1.6 Pearls and Pitfalls

Pearls:
- Image all other arterial-graft anastomotic sites to rule out synchronous aneurysms.
- The finding of perianastomotic fluid and/or lack of graft incorporation are signs of a possible infectious process.
- Due to the redo nature of these operations dense scar tissue is often encountered and is best managed with sharp scalpel (#15 blade) dissection, rather than scissors.
- Exposure in a densely scarred operative field is frequently aided by initial identification and dissection of the proximal superficial femoral artery which is usually associated with relatively less scar. Once this vessel has been identified, dissection can proceed more proximally.

Pitfalls:
- When exposing densely scarred arteries, avoid entry into the plane between the adventitia and media. When

Flowchart 48.1: Decision-making algorithm.

```
          ┌─────────────────────────────────────────────────────────────┐
          │ Patient with history of femoral arterial anastomosis and      │
          │                   pulsatile groin mass                        │
          └─────────────────────────────────────────────────────────────┘
                 Active uncontrolled hemorrhage?
                      Yes    │    No
              ┌───────────────┐       ┌──────────────────────┐
              │   Urgent       │       │  Imaging (duplex      │
              │  operation     │       │  ultrasound/CT        │
              └───────────────┘       │  angiogram)           │
                                       └──────────────────────┘
```

Findings:
- < 2.0–2.5 cm
- Absent or minimal intra-luminal thrombus
- No evidence of infection
- And/or poor operative risk

→ **Observation with serial imaging**

Findings:
- Symptomatic (thrombosis, source of distal thromboemboli, or symptoms from local compression such as venous insufficiency, DVT, or femoral neuropraxia)
- > 2–2.5 cm and/or rapid expansion
- Significant intraluminal thrombus
- Evidence of infection

→ **Operative repair**

inadvertently entered, this plane often appears as an "easier" natural dissection plane. Without the support of the adventitia the resulting "exarterectomized" arterial wall is too weak to hold stitches.

- Carefully look for arterial branches coming off the distal common femoral artery and proximal most deep femoral artery, such as the medial and lateral femoral circumflex arteries. Inadvertent injury or failure to control prior to opening aneurysm can lead to troublesome bleeding and often significant blood loss.
- Avoid injury to the adjacent nerve and especially the vein.

1.7 Surgical Anatomy

- *See* Figure 48.3.

1.8 Positioning

- *See* Figure 48.4.

1.9 Anesthesia

General or regional (epidural). Avoid spinal anesthesia alone due to the potential for surgical problems, which could unexpectedly extend operative time.

2 PERIOPERATIVE

2.1 Incision

An incision can usually be made through the prior scar. Because of the complicated nature of these procedures

(i.e. redo dissection, extensive exposure, frequent prior proximal aortic surgery), these patients are at increased risk for lymphatic complications.[5] Great care should be taken to ligating any structures that appear to contain lymphatic channels. Division of overlying tissues with the cautery alone is to be avoided. Exposure using an oblique suprainguinal should be considered for proximal control of inflow artery or graft with large aneurysms (Fig. 48.5).

2.2 Steps

Attempt at control of the inflow and outflow vessels should be made before entering the aneurysm. Due to the dense scar tissue often encountered with anastomotic femoral aneurysms complete vascular control before entering the aneurysm is not always possible and in such cases balloon occlusion catheters may be useful (Fig. 48.6).

Interposition of a new prosthetic graft between old graft and host artery is the most reliable repair in most cases. The aneurysm is excised and the inflow and outflow vessels are debrided back to normal arterial wall. Anastomotic sutures should be place in normal healthy artery with good bites, creating a tension-free anastomosis. Various reconstruction options can be used. When both the superficial femoral artery and deep femoral artery are patent, every effort should be made to maintain flow to both (Figs. 48.7A to C). When the superficial femoral is

Superficial dissections

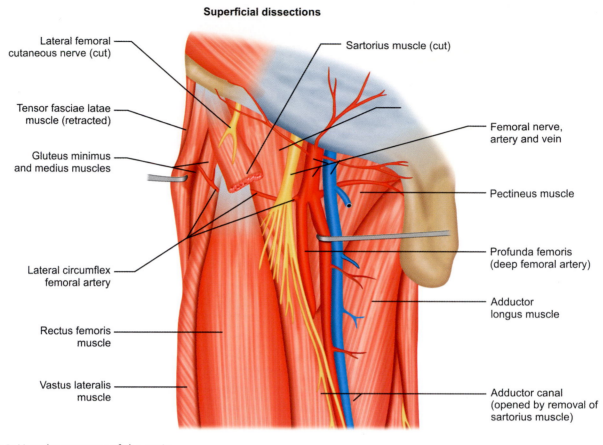

Lateral femoral cutaneous nerve (cut)

Sartorius muscle (cut)

Tensor fasciae latae muscle (retracted)

Gluteus minimus and medius muscles

Femoral nerve, artery and vein

Pectineus muscle

Profunda femoris (deep femoral artery)

Lateral circumflex femoral artery

Adductor longus muscle

Rectus femoris muscle

Vastus lateralis muscle

Adductor canal (opened by removal of sartorius muscle)

Fig. 48.3: Vascular anatomy of the groin.

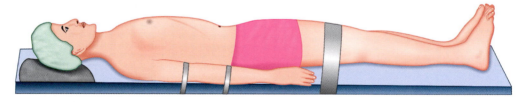

Fig. 48.4: Position patient supine on operating table.

occluded or highly diseased, reconstruction of only the deep femoral artery is necessary (Figs. 48.7D and E). Sometimes there is significant retrograde flow back up the common femoral artery-external iliac artery (e.g. to a patent isolated ipsilateral hypogastric artery) which makes preservation of an intact common femoral artery important. In this situation we recommend reconstruction of the common femoral artery by placement of an interposition prosthetic graft from the proximal common femoral artery to the distal common femoral or proximal deep femoral artery to which the graft is sewn (with or without a second interposition graft) (Fig. 48.7F).

2.3 Closure

After meticulous hemostasis is achieved, a tension-free closure of the overlying soft tissues in three layers is usually performed. In cases in which a large residual cavity is present, a more complex closure with a muscle flap may be considered to ensure adequate soft tissue coverage over the graft (Fig. 49.8).

2.4 Endovascular Alternatives

Endovascular repair of femoral anastomotic aneurysms as definitive therapy or as a bridge to open operation may

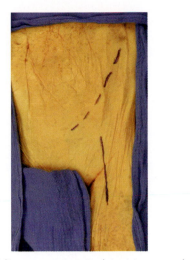

Fig. 48.5: An oblique suprainguinal incision may be used for exposure for proximal control of inflow artery or graft.

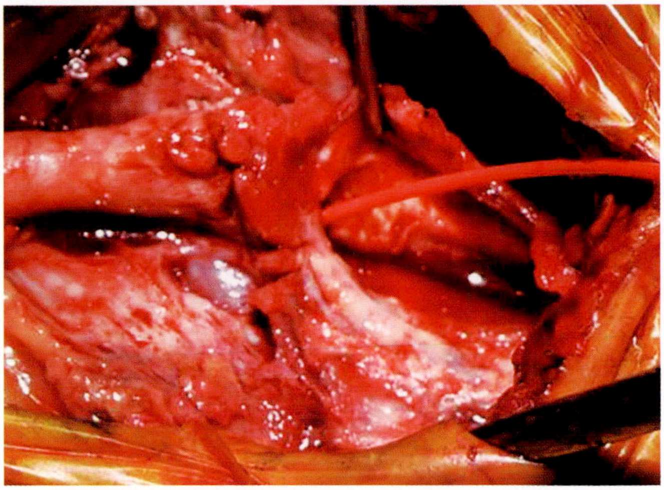

Fig. 48.6: Intraoperative image of balloon control of deep femoral artery.

be considered in patients believed to be at too high a risk for an open repair from an anatomic or physiologic standpoint.[6,7] This technique involves placing a covered stent graft from the original graft into the outflow artery (Figs. 49.9A to C). Placement of a stent graft across the hip flexion zone, however, is generally not felt to be durable and there is little to no long-term data regarding the success of this approach. To date we have never found it necessary to employ this approach.

Endovascular technical considerations:

- *Access planning*: After aortobifemoral grafting, the angle of the graft bifurcation may be too acute and the limbs too stiff to allow for tracking of a covered graft, using a retrograde approach from the contralateral common femoral artery "up and over" the bifurcation. In this setting a transbrachial access may be the only feasible approach, with the left brachial artery approach being preferred to that of the right brachial artery. An open exposure rather than a percutaneous approach to the artery is our preference due to the larger size of the sheaths required for the stent grafts.
- Must ensure that there is not significant size mismatch between the inflow graft and out flow artery that will not allow for appropriate stent graft sizing.
- If both the superficial femoral artery and profunda femoris arteries are patent there is often not an adequate distal landing zone in the distal common femoral artery to allow for stent graft attachment. In this circumstance, one of the two outflow arteries (either the deep femoral or the superficial femoral artery) must be sacrificed with coil embolization and coverage.

3 POSTOPERATIVE

3.1 Complications

- Perioperative hemorrhage
- Wound complications
  - Lymphatic
  - Infection
- Graft infection
- Graft occlusion
- Major limb amputation
- Recurrent femoral anastomotic aneurysm[1,3,4,8,9]

3.2 Outcome

- Overall good outcomes for repair of femoral anastomotic aneurysms are reported with mortality <5%. However, there are other reports of significantly higher morbidity and mortality associated with emergent repairs.
- Recurrent femoral anastomotic aneurysms are report in 6–19% of treated patients.[1,3,4,8,9]

3.3 Follow-up

Wound check in 2 weeks with follow-up ABI to document maintenance of limb perfusion:

- Yearly follow-up with physical examination and ABIs[10]
- Selective imaging (Duplex, CTA) to examine other sites for anastomotic aneurysms, or operative site for recurrent aneurysm.

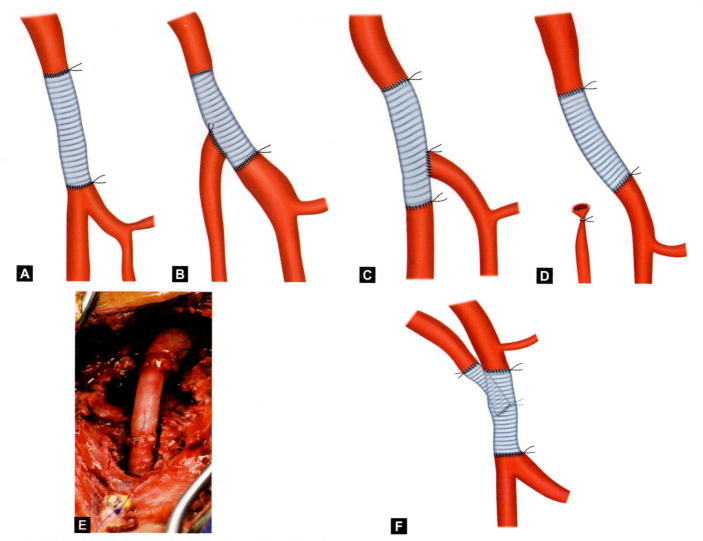

Figs. 48.7A to F: (A) Interposition graft from old graft to distal common femoral artery. (B) Interposition graft from old graft to superficial femoral artery (end to end) with end of deep femoral artery to side of graft reconstruction. (C) Interposition graft from old graft to deep femoral artery (end to end) with end of superficial femoral artery to side of graft reconstruction. (D) Cartoon representation and (E) intraoperative image of interposition graft from old graft to deep femoral artery with ligation of diseased superficial femoral artery. (F) Reconstruction demonstrating preservation of retrograde flow to iliac arterial system.

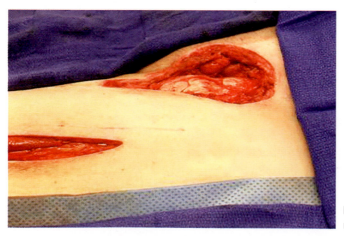

Fig. 48.8: Intraoperative image demonstrating rectus femoris muscle flap for soft tissue coverage over graft.

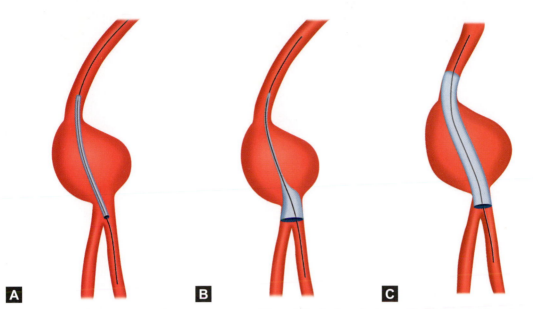

Figs. 48.9A to C: Stent graft (A) positioned across aneurysm (B) partially deployed stent graft (C) fully deployed stent graft excluding aneurysm.

REFERENCES

1. Shepard AS, Jacobson GM. Anastomotic aneurysms. In: Towne JB, Hollier LH, 2nd (Eds). Complications in Vascular Surgery. New York: Marcel Dekker; 2004.
2. Ylönen K, Biancari F, Leo E, et al. Predictors of development of anastomotic femoral pseudoaneurysms after aortobifemoral reconstruction for abdominal aortic aneurysm. Am J Surg. 2004;187(1):83-7.
3. Skourtis G, Bountouris I, Papacharalambous G, et al. Anastomotic pseudoaneurysms: our experience with 49 cases. Ann Vasc Surg. 2006;20(5):582-9.
4. Fleisher LA, Beckman JA, Brown KA, et al. ACC/AHA 2007 guidelines on perioperative cardiovascular evaluation and care for noncardiac surgery: a report of the American College of Cardiology/American Heart Association Task Force on Practice Guidelines (Writing committee to revise the 2002 guidelines on perioperative cardiovascular evaluation for noncardiac surgery). J Am Coll Cardiol. 2007;50:e159-241.
5. Tyndall SH, Shepard AD, Wilczewski JM, et al. Groin lymphatic complications after arterial reconstruction. J Vasc Surg. 1994;19(5):858-64.
6. Derom A, Nout E. Treatment of femoral pseudoaneurysms with endograft in high-risk patients. Eur J Vasc Endovasc Surg. 2005;30(6):644-7.
7. Klonaris C, Katsargyris A, Vasileiou I, et al. Hybrid repair of ruptured infected anastomotic femoral pseudoaneurysms: emergent stent-graft implantation and secondary surgical debridement. J Vasc Surg. 2009;49(4):938-45.
8. Marković DM, Davidović LB, Kostić DM, et al. False anastomotic aneurysms. Vascular. 2007;15(3):141-8.
9. Ernst CB, Elliott JP, Ryan CJ, et al. Recurrent femoral anastomotic aneurysms: A 30-year experience. Ann Surg. 1988;208(4):401-9.
10. Norgren L, Hiatt WR, Dormandy JA, et al. TASC II Working Group. Inter-society consensus for the management of peripheral arterial disease (TASC II). J Vasc Surg. 2007; 45(Suppl S):S5-67.

SECTION

6

Venous

Inferior Vena Cava Filter

Neil Moudgill

1 PREOPERATIVE

1.1 Indications

- Thromboembolism with an absolute contraindication to anticoagulation
- Thromboembolism while receiving anticoagulation
- *Relative indication*:
  - Proximal thromboembolism with poor cardiopulmonary reserve
  - Venous thromboembolism in an individual with a high risk of bleeding
  - Massive pulmonary embolism and a perceived inability to tolerate further embolization
- *Contraindications*:
  - Ability to receive anticoagulation

1.2 Evidence

- *A clinical trial of vena caval filters in the prevention of pulmonary embolism in patients with proximal deep vein thrombosis*[1,2]:
  - Prospective Randomized trial that assigned 400 patients randomly to receive standard anticoagulation therapy versus inferior vena cava (IVC) filter and anticoagulation.
  - After 12 days of randomization the IVC filter group experienced significantly less recurrent thromboembolism (1% vs 5%).
  - At 2-year and 8-year follow-up, there was no significant difference in symptomatic pulmonary embolism or survival.
  - At 2-year and 8-year follow-up, the IVC filter group was significantly more likely to experience recurrent deep venous thrombosis.
- *High utilization rate of vena cava filters in deep vein thrombosis*:

- Prospective registry that enrolled 5,451 patients from 183 study sites
- 781 patients reviewed
- Fourteen percent (781) of the total population underwent IVC filter placement

1.3 Materials Needed

- Fluoroscopy table and C-arm, or Intravascular ultrasound
- Contrast material if performing with fluoroscopy
- Inferior vena cava filter kit
- Micropuncture access kit
- Medium stiffness .035 guidewire

1.4 Preoperative Risk Assessment

Low risk:
- No comorbidities, stable patient, no prior venous interventions
- Femoral or jugular access available

Intermediate risk:
- Compromised hemodynamics requiring noninvasive support
- Obesity (difficulty with fluoroscopic guidance)
- Renal insufficiency

High risk:
- Unstable patient
- Extensive venous thromboembolism
- Femoral and jugular access unavailable

1.5 Preoperative Checklist

Sign in:
- Correct patient.
- Review updated history since pre-operative evaluation.
- Mark surgical site.

- Evaluate groins and abdomen for abnormalities (infection, rash, injury, etc.).
- Assess lower extremity pulses and document baseline for future reference.
- Examine lower extremities.
- Review preoperative laboratory studies prior to entering operating room.

Time out:
- Verify correct patient.
- Verify correct position.
- Verify antibiotic administration.
- Verify pertinent patient comorbidities (cardiac, pulmonary, renal, etc.).
- Review patient allergies and ensure no materials to be used will elicit allergic response.
- Review critical procedural details with team members in operating room.
- Ensure necessary equipment is functional and appropriate staff available.
- Ensure endograft is available and present in the operating room.

Sign out:
- Review essential case details, any deviations from initial plan.
- Ask anesthesia for summary of care rendered from their standpoint.
- Discuss plan for immediate postoperative care specifics and patient's proposed location prior to transfer from operating room.

1.6 Decision-Making Algorithm

- *See* Flowchart 49.1.

1.7 Pearls and Pitfalls

Pearls:
- The left renal vein is typically the lower of the two renal veins.
- The left renal vein is most commonly visualized at the level of the L1–L2 vertebral body.
- If the cava appears large, measurement with a marking catheter is useful to ensure that the selected device is appropriate for deployment.
- An iliac venogram should be performed to visualize reflux into the contralateral iliac venous system.

Pitfalls:
- Inadequate marking of the lowest renal vein may result in misdeployment of the filter.
- Nonvisualization of reflux into the contralateral iliac system can result in inadequate caval interruption as a result of caval duplication.
- Angled deployment of the caval filter will result in difficult during future retrieval.
- Suprarenal deployment should be corrected if an infrarenal location is available.
- An undersized filter may embolize into the cardiac circulation if deployed.

1.8 Surgical Anatomy

- *See* Figure 49.1.

1.9 Positioning

- *See* Figure 49.2.

1.10 Anesthesia

- Local anesthesia with monitored anesthesia care is appropriate for most caval interruption procedures.

Flowchart 49.1: Decision-making algorithm.

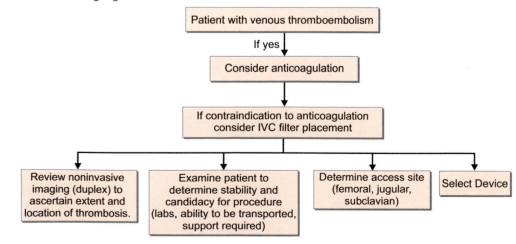

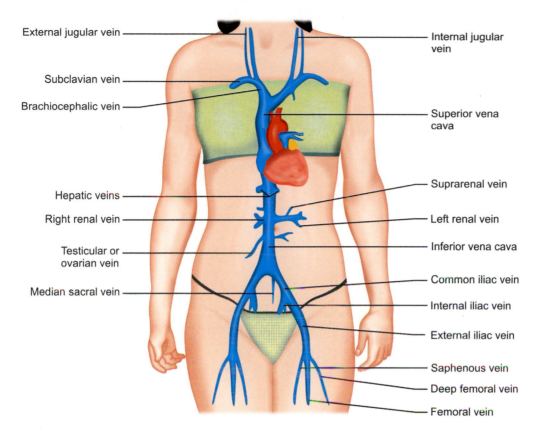

External jugular vein

Subclavian vein

Brachiocephalic vein

Hepatic veins

Right renal vein

Testicular or
ovarian vein

Median sacral vein

Internal jugular
vein

Superior vena
cava

Suprarenal vein

Left renal vein

Inferior vena cava

Common iliac vein

Internal iliac vein

External iliac vein

Saphenous vein

Deep femoral vein

Femoral vein

Fig. 49.1: Surgical anatomy.

- Any acute changes in hemodynamic or pulmonary status should be addressed aggressively and conveyed to the surgical team. This may be a result of pulmonary venous thromboembolism.
- If the patient is therapeutically anticoagulated during the procedure, any complaints of back pain from the patient should be relayed to the surgical team. This may be a result of caval rupture or injury.
- Direct pressure will be held for several minutes at the completion of the procedure.

2 PERIOPERATIVE

2.1 Incision

- *See* Figure 49.3.

2.2 Procedure

- An iliac venogram and cavogram are performed after sheath access is obtained. The renal veins are identified and marked prior to sheath advancement.
- The filter is deployed in the infrarenal vena cava.

2.3 Closure

- *See* Figure 49.4.

3 POSTOPERATIVE

3.1 Complications

Most common complications:
- Access site hematoma
- Malaligned IVC filter

Least common complications:
- Caval rupture or injury
- Filter embolization

3.2 Outcomes

Expected outcomes:
- Caval interruption with continued caval flow
- Infrarenal deployment
- Successful prevention of pulmonary embolus

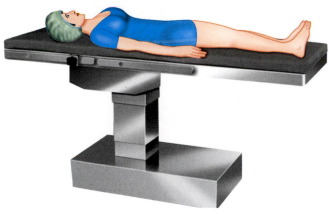

Fig. 49.2: Positioning. The patient is positioned supine with foot of bed positioned at patient's feet.

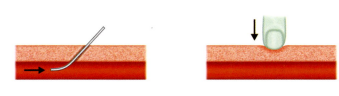

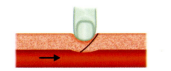

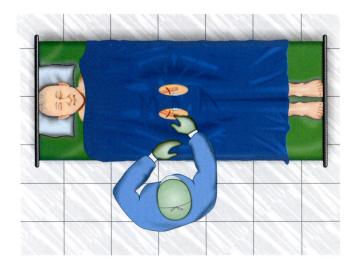

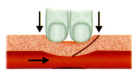

Fig. 49.4: Manual pressure is held over the femoral vein after sheath removal.

Fig. 49.3: The femoral vein is punctured and access is obtained via standard Seldinger technique.

Femoral artery

Crease of groin
(Inguinal ligament)

Femoral vein

3.3 Follow-Up

- If the filter is intended to be placed in a temporary fashion, clear follow-up instructions regarding the timing of retrieval should be provided for the patient.
- Expected filter removal in 3–6 months.

3.4 E-mail an Expert

- *E-mail address*: nmoudgil@health.usf.edu

3.5 Web Resources/References

- Rutherford's Vascular Surgery, 7th edition.
- eMedicine: IVC filter placement.
- http://emedicine.medscape.com/article/1377859-overview#a01

REFERENCES

1. Decousus H, Leizorovicz A, Parent F, et al. A clinical trial of vena caval filters in the prevention of pulmonary embolism in patients with proximal deep-vein thrombosis. Prévention du Risque d'Embolie Pulmonaire par Interruption Cave Study Group. N Engl J Med. 1998;12;338(7):409-15.
2. Jaff MR, Goldhaber SZ, Tapson VF. High utilization rate of vena cava filters in deep vein thrombosis. Thromb Haemost. 2005;93(6):1117-19.

QUIZ

Question 1. An IVC filter is indicated in which patient?

a. A 23-year-old male with intracranial hemorrhage and right lower extremity DVT
b. A 56-year-old patient with chronic DVT currently on warfarin therapy
c. A 2-year-old male with DVT
d. A 47-year-old woman with leg swelling and negative venous duplex for DVT

Question 2. When placing an IVC filter, what anatomic structure(s) are most likely to correlate with the position of the renal veins?

a. The transverse colon
b. The T1 vertebral body
c. The L5 vertebral body
d. The L2 vertebral body

Question 3. Reflux of contrast into the contralateral iliac system is helpful to exclude what anatomic variation?

a. Left sided cava
b. Caval duplication
c. Aberrant Iliac vein
d. Incomplete cava

ANSWERS: 1. a   2. d   3. b

Lower Extremity Venous Thrombolysis, Angioplasty and Stenting

CHAPTER 50

Bruce Zwiebel, Scott Perrin

1 PREPROCEDURAL EVALUATION

1.1 Indications/Contraindications

Indications:
- *Emergent*:
  - Phlegmasia cerulea dolens
  - Inferior vena cava thrombosis with or without extension into the renal veins
- *Nonemergent*:
  - Symptomatic lower extremity edema caused by iliofemoral deep venous thrombosis (DVT) ± femoral popliteal DVT.

- *Contraindications*:
  - Active bleeding
  - Thombocytopenia (platelet count <50 K)
  - Recent gastrointestinal bleeding (<3 months)
  - Recent ischemic stroke (<6 months)
  - CNS lesion predisposed to bleeding (tumor, aneurysm, arteriovenous malformation)
  - Recent ophthalmologic surgery (<3 months)
  - End stage liver disease
  - Renal insufficiency, glomerular filtration rate (GFR) <30
  - Septic thrombophlebitis
  - Advanced chronologic age of >75–80 years
  - Pregnancy

1.2 Evidence

Use of catheter-directed thrombolysis:
- Catheter-directed thrombolysis (CDT) via infusion of thrombolytics was shown to completely dissolve acute thrombus in 80% of patients in a 473-patient prospective multicenter registry and in a pooled analysis of 19 observational studies involving over 1,000 patients[1,2] (Level B, class IIa).

- CDT resulted in fewer occurrences of post-thrombotic syndrome and improved quality of life at 16-month interval follow-up[3] (Level B, class IIb).
- CDT resulted in more complete symptom resolution at 5 years compared with anticoagulation alone[4] (Level B, class IIb).
- CDT resulted in a higher rate of normal venous function and less valvular reflux at 6 months in a small population of patients with proximal DVT5 (Level B, class IIb).[5]

Use of venous stents in the iliac veins and inferior vena cava (IVC):
- Primary patency rates of stents placed along the iliofemoral segment for all causes range from 50% to 85%. Secondary patency rates are reported in the 90–100%.[6]
- The initial technical success rate for treatment of IVC occlusion with stent placement is 88% with primary stent patency of 80% and secondary patency of 87%.[7]

1.3 Materials Needed

- General angiography tray
- Micropuncture kit
- Ultrasound machine
- 7-Fr vascular hemostatic sheaths (5–10 cm in length)
- 0.035 Glidewire(s), exchange length
- 5-Fr 100-cm hockey stick catheter
- Mechanical thrombectomy systems (Angiojet or Trellis thrombectomy devices) with associated catheters (Fig. 50.1)
- Recombinant tissue plasminogen activator (tPA, alteplase)
- Infusion catheter (± ultrasound assisted e.g. EKOS), 40–50 cm working length with associated infusion pump and machine (Fig. 50.2)

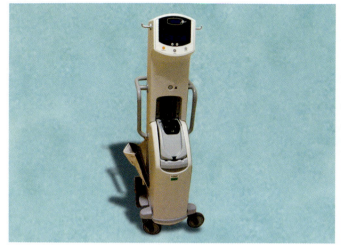

Fig. 50.1: Angiojet machine for use with Angiojet thrombectomy catheters. The machine has two different settings: mechanical thrombectomy and power pulse spray.

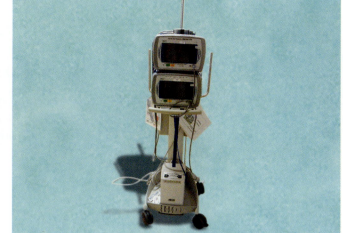

Fig. 50.2: EKOS machine for use with EKOS ultrasound-assisted thrombolysis infusion catheters that are available in various working lengths. Typically working lengths of 40–50 cm are used for treatment of the iliofemoral and femoral popliteal segments from popliteal access.

- Assortment of self-expanding stents in the range of 8–24 mm diameter and 60–120 mm length
- Assortment of angioplasty balloons in the range of 8–24 mm diameter and 40–80 mm length.

1.4 Preprocedural Planning and Risk Assessment

Preprocedural planning:
- Laboratory testing including basic metabolic panel, PT, PTT, INR, and platelet level
- Ultrasound Doppler evaluation of the affected limb(s)
- CT or MR venography of the abdomen and pelvis to evaluate for iliac or caval extension (time of flight MR venography without contrast can be performed if there is renal insufficiency and patient is able to follow commands)
- CT pulmonary angiography can be used to evaluate for pulmonary embolus if patient has a history of PE or has signs/symptoms on PE
- Obtain patient consent for procedure. Suggested wording for the procedure consent form is as follows:
  - "Lower extremity venography with possible thrombolysis, venoplasty, stent placement, possible IVC filter, possible central venous access."

Risk factors for complications and/or procedural complexity:
- Age
- Chronic DVT

- Acute and/or chronic pulmonary embolus
- Renal insufficiency
- Morbid obesity
- Compromised venous access sites (internal jugular vein or popliteal veins)
- Inability to lay prone
- Prior IVC filter placement or venous stent placement
- History of underlying thrombotic disorder
- History of underlying anatomic lesion predisposing to thrombosis
  - May–Thurner syndrome (Cockett's syndrome)
  - Postradiation change
  - Retroperitoneal fibrosis
  - Intrapelvic or retroperitoneal tumor compression

1.5 Preoperative Checklist

Sign in:
- Patient identification and consent
- Correct patient positioning (prone for popliteal access)
- Laboratory parameters within acceptable range
- Foley catheter in place
- Central venous access or two large bore IV sites.

Time out:
- All needed equipment is available
- tPA is ready and mixed in preparation for possible overnight infusion at 0.5–1 mg/h as well as for use in the thrombectomy catheter device and/or bolus doses in aliquots of 4–6 mg.

Sign out:

- Check for infusion catheter functionality and appropriate infusion rates (see intraprocedural section for suggested infusion rates).
- Intensive care unit (ICU) admission with hemorrhage precautions if patient is having overnight infusion with tPA.
- Clear liquid diet with nothing by mouth (NPO) at midnight for recheck venogram in the morning.
- If single-session catheter-directed thrombectomy is performed then patient should be placed on heparin weight-based protocol with transition to long-term (6-month) coumadin or low-molecular-weight heparin.
- All patients should have compression stockings as well as sequential compression devices.

1.6 Decision-Making Algorithm

- *See* Flowchart 50.1.

1.7 Pearls and Pitfalls

Pearls:

- Variant anatomy of the popliteal vein in its relationship to the popliteal artery should be considered. Careful sonographic interrogation of the popliteal fossa as well as

the surrounding superficial venous system may provide additional information as to the presence of collateral formation and alternative access sites.

- Difficulty with popliteal access could be indicative of chronic popliteal DVT with recanalization and collateral formation.
- Determining salvageable segments of vein based on the angiographic appearance of acute versus chronic DVT is crucial in deciding how effective thrombolysis is going to be. Recognizing and catheterizing the correct deep venous (Figs. 50.3A and B and 50.4A and B) segments and avoiding any collateral vessels are essential for effective thrombolysis.
- Place the appropriate length of infusion catheters in order to provide adequate thrombolysis of the more acute appearing clot while avoiding unnecessary infusion of tPA into the systemic circulation.
- Initial placement of 7-Fr sheaths as well as use of exchange length wires will make planned interventions easier with less exchanges. Largest angioplasty balloons (in the size range of 8–14 mm diameter) will go through a 7-Fr sheath.
- If there is a significant amount of acute appearing thrombus on initial venography, consider initial catheterdirected thrombectomy and power pulse spray for tPA bolus delivery for debulking of thrombus before placement of infusion catheters.
- Currently, the maximum available stent size for caval and iliac venous stents is 24 mm diameter.

Flowchart. 50.1: Decision-making algorithm for patients with lower extremity edema.

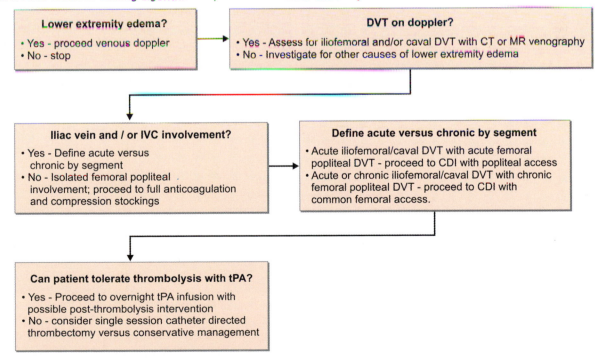

- The ultimate goal of stent placement for the iliac veins and cava is to restore "in-line" flow and long-term patency is highly dependent on adequate inflow from the femoral popliteal segment as well as adequate outflow into the IVC back to the right atrium.

Pitfalls:

- Morbid obesity with superimposed lower extremity edema can make popliteal venous access difficult or impossible. Consider using a curved array probe instead of a linear

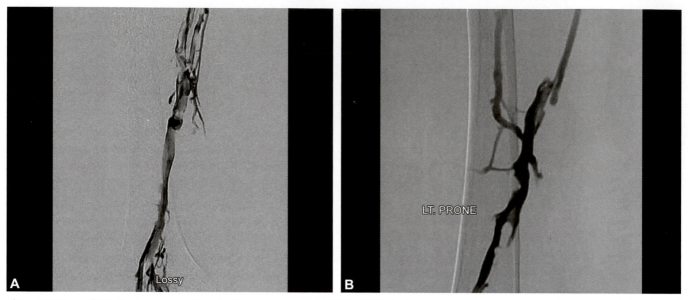

Figs. 50.3A and B: Acute versus chronic femoral popliteal DVT. (A) Left lower extremity venogram via contrast injection of the popliteal vein demonstrates primarily acute DVT which appears as central luminal filling defects that expand the vessel diameter. There is also mild collateral filling as well. (B) Left lower extremity venogram via contrast injection of the popliteal vein demonstrates primarily chronic DVT which manifests as smaller diameter vessels suggesting recanalization with accompanying collateral formation.

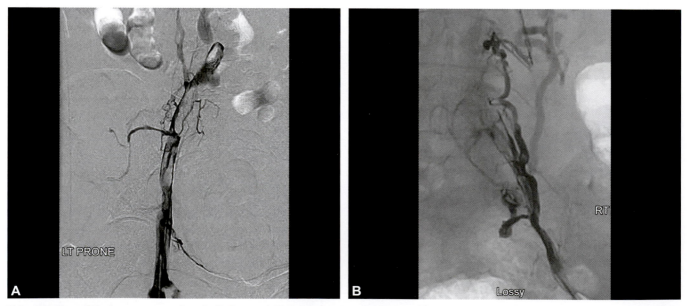

Figs. 50.4A and B: Acute versus chronic iliofemoral DVT. (A) Contrast injection of the left common femoral vein demonstrates acute appearing thrombus within the left external iliac and common iliac veins with no in line flow to the IVC. (B) Contrast injection of the right common femoral vein in a different patient demonstrates extensive collateral formation with likely chronic occlusion of the right common iliac vein.

probe to increase the insonation depth in order to visualize the popliteal vein more effectively.

- Care should be taken to avoid through and through puncture of the popliteal vein into the popliteal artery especially if tPA is considered for overnight infusion as puncture of the artery can lead to higher risk of hemorrhagic complications.
- Rapid post-thrombolysis evaluation with venography is essential as once the tPA infusion is stopped there is possibility for rethrombosis secondary to stagnant flow. The decision window for additional intervention such as the need for additional infusion time versus venoplasty and/or stent placement is therefore narrow.

1.8 Pertinent Anatomy

- *See* Figure 50.5.

1.9 Patient Positioning

- For planned interventions involving the femoral popliteal and iliofemoral segments, the preferred access site is the popliteal vein.
- If the patient cannot tolerate the prone position because of pain then consider the use of general anesthesia.
- If there is chronic femoral popliteal DVT by history, it may be necessary to access the common femoral vein(s) with the patient in the supine position.

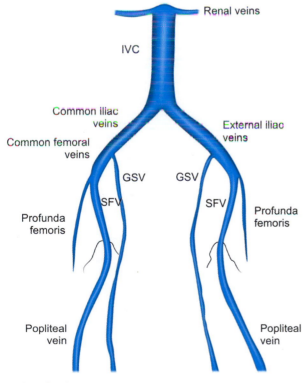

Fig. 50.5: Pertinent anatomy.

- If there is caval thrombosis, either evidenced by pre-procedural ultrasound or CT/MR examination, then consider the internal jugular vein as an alternative access site although this is less preferred because of patient comfort and possible bleeding/hematoma which could compromise the airway.

1.10 Anesthesia

- At least 8 hours of NPO status is required. Monitored conscious sedation with IV fentanyl and versed with continuous vital sign monitoring is preferred during the procedure. Alternatively general anesthesia can be employed if the patient cannot tolerate prone positioning under conscious sedation.

2 PERIOPERATIVE

2.1 Venous Access

- A 7–9 MHz linear array ultrasound transducer is used to interrogate the popliteal fossa. The popliteal vein can be readily identified by its more superficial position on top of the popliteal artery which is the deeper of the two major vessels in the popliteal fossa. Depending on the presence or absence of thrombus, the popliteal vein may or may not be compressible but will certainly not be pulsatile, a feature which can readily be used to distinguish it from the underlying artery. Use of both color flow as well as spectral Doppler waveform with augmentation can be helpful.
- Once the 21-gauge micropuncture needle tip is confirmed in the lumen of the popliteal vein, a small amount of contrast can be injected and/or the micropuncture 0.018 wire can be advanced under fluoroscopy for additional confirmation.
- Placement of a 5–10 cm 7-Fr sheath is preferable for stable access because it will accept most of the larger profile balloons that may be required for intervention in the cava and/or iliac vasculature after initial thrombolysis.

2.2 Venography

- Hand injection of the access sheath side arm is preferred for imaging the deep venous system. Injection of approximately 10–15 mL is usually sufficient to allow for visualization of the femoral popliteal segment. Manual augmentation and/or slight Trendelenburg positioning can aid in the flow of contrast centrally. Additionally, a 5-Fr hockey stick catheter can be advanced into the common femoral vein for imaging of the iliofemoral segment as well as the IVC. The entire venous outflow from the access site to the right atrium should be imaged before any intervention is planned. Decision should then be made whether to proceed to overnight infusion versus catheter-directed thrombectomy with or without overnight tPA infusion.

2.3 Catheter-Directed Thrombectomy

- If there is a significant amount of acute thrombus and/ or the patient cannot tolerate overnight tPA infusion, catheter-directed thrombectomy can be performed with either the Trellis system or Angiojet system. Stable wire access is obtained through the affected venous segments into the suprarenal IVC. If using the Angiojet system, the Angiojet catheter is set to "power pulse spray" mode and approximately 10–15 mg of tPA in a total volume of 250 mL of normal saline is pulse sprayed into the clot, while the catheter is advanced in back and forth along the affected segments over the wire at approximately 1 cm/s. Once the tPA dose is instilled along the affected segments, a dwell time of 20–30 minutes is then observed to allow for adequate time for tPA-induced clot destabilization. After this dwell time, the Angiojet catheter is then set to aspiration mode and the Angiojet is then advanced again over the affected segments in a back and forth motion at 1 cm/s for clot aspiration (Figs. 50.6A and B). Care should be taken to monitor the total thrombectomy volume that should be kept under 250–300 mL in patients with normal renal function and <150 mL in patients with compromised renal function as high thrombectomy volumes can cause significant renal tubular dysfunction from hemoglobinuria.

2.4 Infusion-Based Catheter Thrombolysis

- Infusion based thrombolysis is preferred over single-session thrombectomy because there is overall better clot clearance. An infusion time of at least 8 hours is needed to allow for clearance of acute thrombus. A dose of 0.5–1 mg/h is utilized based on the patient's overall risk of bleeding, the extent of thrombosis as well as the time until the patient can return to the interventional radiology suite. The side arm port of the access sheath is infused with 400 units/h of heparin. There is little evidence on the use of monitoring fibrinogen levels during catheter-directed tPA thrombolysis but the patient must be monitored closely in an ICU setting with hemorrhage precautions. An indwelling Foley catheter allows for hourly assessment of urine output.

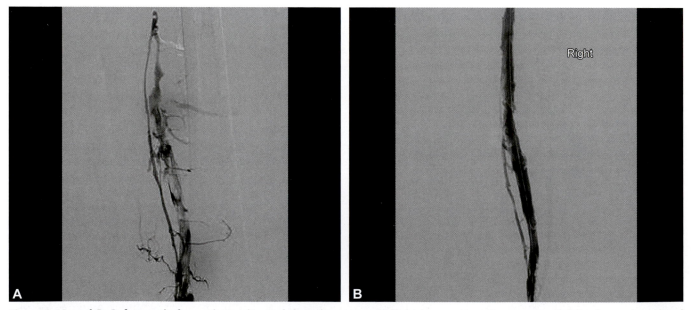

Figs. 50.6A and B: Before and after catheter-directed thrombectomy. (A) Right lower extremity venogram of the femoral popliteal segment demonstrates extensive, acute appearing DVT. (B) Repeat right lower extremity venogram in the same patient after treatment with 10 mg of tPA delivered via Angiojet thrombectomy catheter in power pulse spray mode with subsequent catheter-directed thrombectomy.

Patients are placed on a clear liquid diet after catheter placement and made NPO at midnight in anticipation for recheck venogram scheduled for the next day typically although if the initial infusion catheter placement is performed in the morning then the recheck venogram with intervention can be performed in the afternoon on the same day.

2.5 Postthrombolysis Assessment

- This portion of the procedure is critical to long-term success and begins with initial repeat venography to assess the degree of residual acute thrombus (if any) as well as the degree of chronic changes and/or underlying/offending stenosis, and most importantly the overall hemodynamics after clot dissolution (Figs. 50.7A and B).
- Rapid post-thrombolysis evaluation is essential as once the tPA infusion is stopped, there is possibility for rethrombosis. Deciding to proceed with additional thrombolytic infusion time versus performing venoplasty and/or stenting needs to be made quickly.

2.6 Iliac and Caval Angioplasty and Stenting

- In order to re-establish in-line flow across the iliac and caval segments affected by chronic DVT and/or

extrinsic compression, it is important to choose the appropriate diameter and length of the stent needed so as to maximize luminal diameter and minimize number of stents placed.
- For chronic iliac DVT and/or extrinsic compression, primary angioplasty has an extremely low success rate but angioplasty prior to stent placement is helpful for not only pushing chronic thrombus against the vein wall but also helpful in determining the appropriate luminal size needed for stent selection (Figs. 50.8A and B and 50.9A and B.
- *Sizing considerations*: As a rule of thumb, the infrarenal IVC will usually accept the largest available stent which is a 24-mm stent. The common iliac veins usually accept 12–14 mm diameter stents and the external iliac veins usually accept 8–10 mm stent diameters.

2.7 Hemostasis

- Following intervention after thrombolysis, the wires, catheters, and sheaths are removed and manual compression is held at the access sites for approximately 10–15 minutes with additional placement of pressure dressings to prevent further access site bleeding. All patients should be left on full anticoagulation with heparin weight-based protocol and/or started immediately on Coumadin versus low-molecular-weight

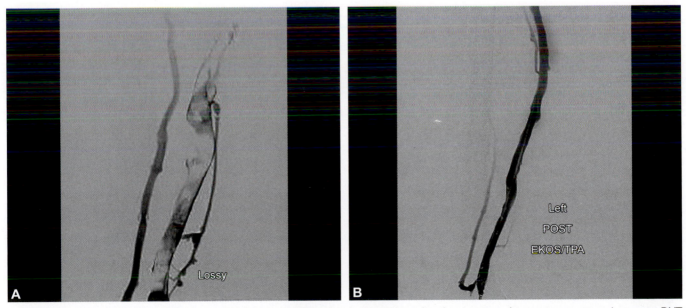

Figs. 50.7A and B: Before and after overnight thrombolysis. (A) Left femoral popliteal venogram demonstrates extensive acute DVT in the popliteal and superficial femoral veins with collateral venous filling. (B) Repeat venogram of the same patient after overnight thrombolysis demonstrates complete resolution of acute DVT with normal filling of the left popliteal and superficial femoral veins.

heparin injections. Also all patients should be placed in thigh high compression stockings with sequential compression devices. Ambulation should be encouraged approximately 12 hours after termination of the procedure.

3. POSTPROCEDURAL CONSIDERATIONS

3.1 Complications[1]

- Venous access site bleeding (8–11%)

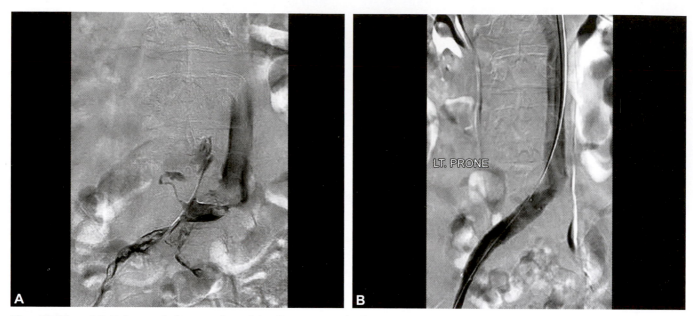

Figs. 50.8A and B: Before and after stenting of the iliac veins and inferior vena cava. (A) Left common iliac venogram demonstrates long segment narrowing of the left iliac system with associated thrombus at the iliocaval junction. (B) Repeat left iliac venogram in the same patient after overnight thrombolysis and subsequent placement of a 14-mm Luminexx stent in the left common iliac vein restores in-line flow to the IVC.

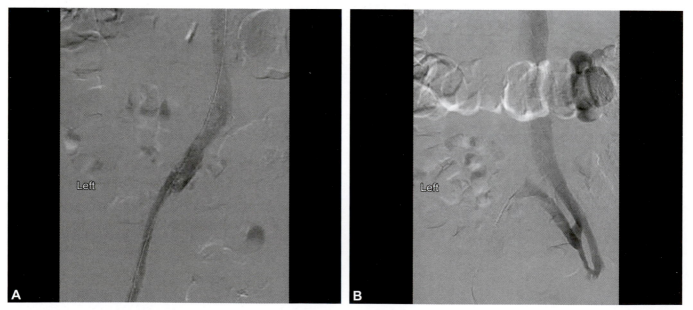

Figs. 50.9A and B: May–Thurner syndrome, Pre and Post Stenting. (A) Injection of the left common iliac vein after overnight thrombolysis demonstrates classic extrinsic compression defect at the left iliocaval junction caused by the crossing right common iliac artery. (B) A 14-mm Luminexx stent was placed across the site of extrinsic compression to restore in-line flow to the IVC.

- Intracranial bleeding (0.4%)
- Symptomatic pulmonary embolus (1.3%)
- Fatal pulmonary embolus (0.2%)

3.2 Expected Outcomes

- Decreased lower extremity swelling and decreased chance of post-thrombotic syndrome[3-5]
- Iliac and caval stents have relatively good patency rates at 1 year >70%.[6,7]

3.3 Follow-Up

- At least 24 hours of observation is recommended following lower extremity thrombolysis to ensure adequate postprocedural hemostasis as well as adequate anticoagulation with coumadin versus low-molecular-weight heparin and lack of rethrombosis.
- Coumadin or low-molecular-weight heparin for 3–6 months at minimum is recommended.
- A follow-up lower extremity venous Doppler after completion of anticoagulation is helpful to re-establish baseline appearance of the lower extremity venous structures to serve as a comparison for future examinations if symptoms reoccur.
- All patients who receive iliac stents should be maintained on lifelong coumadin if possible with INR in the range of 2–3.

3.4 E-mail an Expert

- *E-mail address*: bzwieb@tampabay.rr.com

REFERENCES

1. Mewissen MW, Seabrook GR, Meissner MH, et al. Catheter-directed thrombolysis for lower extremity deep venous thrombosis: report of a national multicenter registry. Radiology. 1999;211(1):39-49.
2. Vedantham S, Thorpe PE, Cardella JF, et al. Quality improvement guidelines for the treatment of lower extremity deep vein thrombosis with use of endovascular thrombus removal. J Vasc. Int Radiol. 2006;17(3):435-47; quiz 48.
3. Comerota AJ, Throm RC, Mathias SD, et al. Catheter-directed thrombolysis for iliofemoral deep venous thrombosis improves health-related quality of life. J Vasc Surg. 2000;32(1):130-7.
4. AbuRahma AF, Perkins SE, Wulu JT, et al. Iliofemoral deep vein thrombosis: conventional therapy versus lysis and percutaneous transluminal angioplasty and stenting. Ann Surg. 2001;233(6):752-60.
5. Elsharawy M, Elzayat E. Early results of thrombolysis vs anticoagulation in iliofemoral venous thrombosis. A randomised clinical trial. Eur J Vasc Endovasc Surg. 2002; 24(3):209-14.
6. Nazarian GK, Bjarnason H, Dietz CA Jr, et al. Iliofemoral venous stenoses: effectiveness of treatment with metallic endovascular stents. Radiology. 1996;200(1):193-9.
7. Razavi MK, Hansch EC, Kee ST, et al. Chronically occluded inferior venae cavae: endovascular treatment. Radiology. 2000;214(1):133-8.

QUIZ

Question 1: A 66-year-old female presents with lower extremity swelling worsening over the past 3 weeks that is limiting her daily activities. An ultrasound shows extensive bilateral lower extremity DVT. The patient has no contraindication to full anticoagulation. On admission, the patient has a creatinine of 2.3 that is above her baseline creatinine of 0.9. Which of the following pre procedural tests would most affect subsequent management of this patient?
a. Conventional venography of the lower extremities
b. CT pulmonary angiogram
c. CT venography of the pelvis
d. Doppler evaluation of the kidneys.

Question 2: A 55-year-old male with glioblastoma multiforme with prior craniotomy for tumor resection approximately 4 months ago presents with acute bilateral lower extremity swelling found to be secondary to extensive lower extremity DVT. Patient has an overall poor performance status. What is the best therapeutic option for this patient?

a. Catheter-based overnight thrombolysis with infusion of tPA
b. Full anticoagulation with Lovenox or Coumadin
c. Single-session catheter-directed thrombectomy with power pulse Angiojet
d. Conservative management with compression stockings and sequential compression devices.

Question 3: A 68-year-old male patient has lower extremity edema and shortness of breath. The patient has a history of coronary artery disease and subsequent congestive heart failure. A bilateral lower extremity venous ultrasound reveals nonocclusive thrombus in both the right and left popliteal veins. Which of the following would be the most appropriate management?
a. CT pulmonary angiogram
b. Conventional lower extremity venogram with possible thrombolysis

c. Full anticoagulation with coumadin or low molecular weight heparin

d. Both choices A and C.

Question 4: A 46-year-old female with symptomatic ilio-femoral DVT diagnosed with CT venography is brought to the interventional radiology department for overnight infusion thrombolysis. After obtaining popliteal vein access under ultrasound guidance, left lower extremity venography is performed and reveals the following: findings of chronic femoropopliteal DVT:

What is the next step?

a. Attempt wire cannulation so as to gain access into the iliofemoral segment so that the infusion catheter can be placed

b. Abandon the popliteal access and obtain access at the common femoral vein

c. Abandon the popliteal access and obtain access at the right internal jugular vein

d. Placed stents along the visualized thigh vein so as to restore luminal patency.

Question 5: After placement of the infusion catheter for planned overnight thrombolysis and subsequent secure-ment of the infusion catheter and access site with sterile dressing, there is an error message at the IV infusion pump stating that the infusion catheter is occluded and the thrombolytic cannot be infused. What is the next step?

a. Attempt to inject the infusion catheter with a 1-mL syringe of normal saline

b. Remove the infusion catheter over a wire and insert a new infusion catheter

c. Examine the length of the infusion catheter for possible kinks

d. None of the above.

Surgical and Pharmacomechanical Venous Thrombectomy

Sharon Kiang, David Rigberg

1 PREOPERATIVE

1.1 Indications

- Extensive/severe deep vein thrombosis (DVT) resulting in phlegmasia cerulean dolens
- Patients with DVT refractory to anticoagulation
- Patients with progressive DVT despite aggressive medical therapy
- Patients with DVT associated with May–Thurner syndrome

1.2 Evidence/Background

- Acute iliofemoral occlusion is defined as complete or partial thrombosis of the any part of the iliac vein and/or the common femoral vein with or without associated femoropopliteal DVT, in which symptoms have been present for 14 days or less or for which imaging indicates that venous thrombosis has occurred within the past 14 days or less.[1]
- There are three objectives in the treatment of iliofemoral occlusion: (1) prevent propagation of DVT and subsequent pulmonary embolism (PE), (2) provide symptomatic relief for the patient, and (3) prevent the development of post-thrombotic syndrome (PTS).
- Etiology for acute iliofemoral occlusion may be secondary to de novo DVT, stenosis from previous DVT, iatrogenic injury to the iliac, and femoral veins from previous procedures or from external compression (May–Thurner syndrome, tumors).
- Treatment options include systemic anticoagulation, angioplasty, catheter-directed thrombolysis, thrombo-mechanical lysis, stenting, open vein reconstruction, or a combination of these modalities.
- Forty-four percent of patients with untreated iliofemoral DVT will have venous claudication and 49% to 60% with develop PTS within 2 years.[2–4]

1.3 Materials Needed

Wires:
- 0.035 stiff angled Glidewire (Terumo Interventional Systems, Inc., Somersent, NJ)
- 0.035 Bentson wire (Cook Medical, Bloomington, IN)

Catheters:
- 5-Fr short Pinnacle introducer sheath (Terumo, Somerset, NJ)
- 5-Fr Pigtail catheter (Cook Medical, Bloomington, IN)

Thrombolysis devices:
- Angiojet (Possis Medical, Minneapolis, MN)
- Trellis (Bacchus Vascular, Santa Clara, CA)
- EKOS (EKOS Corp, Bothell, WA)

Lytics:
- Tissue plasminogen activator (TPA; Alteplase, Genentech, San Francisco, CA)

1.4 Preoperative Risk Assessment

Planning:
- *Imaging*:
  - Imaging is important in the diagnosis of iliofemoral occlusion as clinical examination can be inconsistent due to the variation of presenting symptoms. At present, the modalities available include duplex ultrasonography, venography, CT venography (CTV), and MR venography (MRV) imaging. Imaging can confirm the diagnosis, distinguish the etiology of occlusion, and the extent of iliofemoral vein occlusion.
- *Duplex ultrasonography*:
  - In the hands of an experienced operator, duplex US with manual compression can be extremely sensitive and specific in infrainguinal DVT although its utility may be limited in the visualization of the

iliac veins due to overlying bowel gas, obesity, and noncompressibility of the region.

- Criteria for the diagnosis of acute venous occlusion by Doppler ultrasound include failure of vein to collapse on direct compression, visualization of thrombus within the normally echo-free lumen, and absent or abnormal venous pulsation on Doppler scanning.[1]

- One main advantage of duplex US is its non-invasiveness and accessibility in the outpatient setting. In addition, it is much more cost-effective compared to the other modalities. Other advantages of duplex include not only its ability to identify thrombus, but it ability to identify hematomas, aneurysms, lymphedema, thrombophlebitis, and abscesses. This makes duplex US a useful initial screening tool and should be obtained as the initial imaging evaluation in a patient with iliofemoral DVT.

- *CT venography*:
  - The CTV is one of the most frequently ordered diagnostic tests when evaluating patients in the in-hospital setting. Advantages of this modality is that it is technician independent, causes the patient no pain since it does not requires soft tissue contact with an ultrasound probe and can be obtained at most hospitals at any time.
  - The modern spiral CTV has a sensitivity of 100% and a specificity of 96% and in one study was found to detect previously unsuspected venous thrombosis at a prevalence of 1.1%.[2,3]

- A CTV is also useful in that it can possibly differentiate new from old thrombus, visualize completely occluded veins and can help delineate soft tissue abnormalities that could be causing extrinsic compression of the iliac vein (Fig. 51.1).

- The applicability of CTV can be limited given its use of iodinated contrast and radiation. Patients with renal failure may not be able to undergo this study, as it may exacerbate their kidney renal failure while radiation is contraindicated in pregnancy and children. Additionally, CTV is an expensive test, making it unsuitable as a first line study. CT venography should be obtained if the duplex ultrasound is nondiagnostic or if there are soft tissue aberrations that merit further visualization.

- *MR venography*:
  - Like CTV, MRV can visualize intraluminal thrombus and can delineate whether the thrombus is new versus old. It has a sensitivity of 100% and specificity of 95%.[4] Likewise, MR is valuable in visualizing the surrounding soft tissue and can detect surrounding soft tissue finding such as lymph nodes, soft tissue sarcomas, venous aneurysms, and venous malformations that may be contributing to iliofemoral DVTs (Fig. 51.2).
  - However, unlike CTV, MRV can be utilized during pregnancy and is deemed as a safer modality in patients with renal failure.
  - Contraindications for this modality include patients with pace makers or other ferromagnetic clips and patients with claustrophobia may not be able to

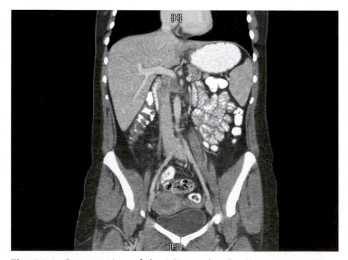

Fig. 51.1: Compression of the LCI vein by the RCI artery in May–Thurner syndrome.

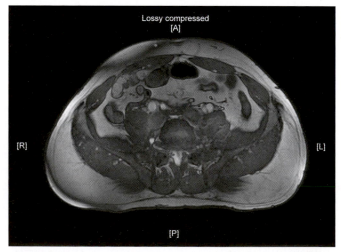

Fig. 51.2: MRV of bilateral common iliac vein (CIV) occluded with thrombus. (MRV: MR venography).

undergo the examination, as it requires a prolonged time in a small enclosed space. MR venography is also an extremely expensive test that requires dedicated MR machines personnel. This sometimes makes the MRV a difficult test to obtain and may be even unavailable in some smaller hospitals. MRV is recommended if the duplex US is nondiagnostic and if there are contraindications to obtaining a CTV. If there are concerns of soft tissue abnormalities in the region of the iliac vein or if there is concern of a venous vascular malformation, MRV should be obtained.

• *Contrast venogram*:
  – Despite the options for noninvasive imaging, contrast venogram remains the gold standard for the evaluation of iliofemoral vein. It has a sensitivity of 100% and it allows direct visualization of the iliofemoral vein to the IVC when it is accessed in a retrograde fashion from the CFV (Fig. 51.3).
  – The findings typical of iliofemoral thrombosis include abrupt vessel cutoff in the case of total occlusion or a visualization of a filling defect with contrast flowing on either side of the filling defect known as "tram-tracking" (Fig. 51.4).
  – One major determinant of how successful this modality is in evaluation iliofemoral thrombosis is that it is highly operator dependent. It has been reported that contrast venogram is nondiagnostic in 18% of the cases due to misinterpretations, artifacts, superimposition of the vessels.[5] Thus, an experienced operator, usually a vascular surgeon, is necessary to obtain the necessary fluoroscopic fields to visualize the thrombus.

  – The major drawbacks of this modality are that it is invasive and some patients have adverse reactions to the contrast that is required for this study. In addition, nephrotoxicity and phlebitis have been reported. Furthermore, this modality requires fluoroscopy, which is contraindicated in pregnancy, children, and patients who cannot tolerate prolonged fluoroscopy time. The summation of these drawbacks makes contrast venogram inappropriate as the initial diagnostic tool.

• *Intravascular ultrasound*:
  – Intravascular ultrasound (IVUS) is an endovascular imaging modality that utilizes an ultrasound probe at the end of a catheter to visualize luminal area during angiography (Volcano Corp., San Diego, CA).
  – Intravascular ultrasound can visualize the vessel lumen by assessing the circumferential area, the craniocaudal diameter and the anterior–posterior diameter. Therefore, it is much more sensitive and specific to detecting external compression of the iliac vein secondary to May–Thurner syndrome or from malignancy (Fig. 51.5).[5-9]

Risk assessment:

• *Low risk*:
  – Focal DVT
  – No evidence of PTS, prior intervention, or stents
  – Young age, no renal dysfunction, no cardiopulmonary compromise, no history of bleeding diathesis

• *Intermediate risk*:
  – Contrast allergy
  – Recurrent DVT

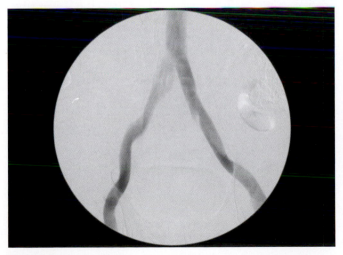

Fig. 51.3: Normal diagnostic venogram.

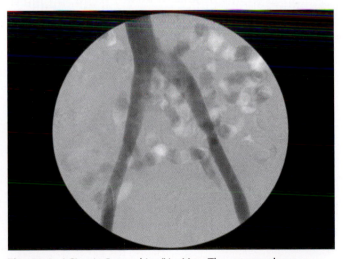

Fig. 51.4: LCI vein "pancaking" in May–Thurner syndrome.

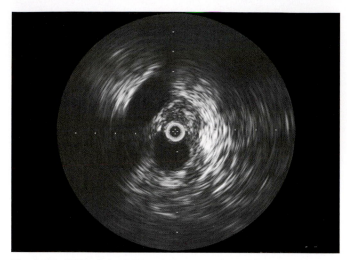

Fig. 51.5: IVUS of the RCIA crossing over the LCIV in May–Thurner syndrome. (RCIA: Right common iliac artery; LCIV: Left common iliac vein).

- DVT secondary to May-Thurner syndrome or evidence of external compression
• *High risk*:
  - Age older than 65
  - High cardiopulmonary risk [Congestive heart failure (CHF), Chronic obstructive pulmonary disease (COPD)]
  - History of PE or PE refractory to anticoagulation
  - DVT with evidence of PTS
  - Chronic renal insufficiency

1.5 Preoperative Checklist

• All patients should have a basic metabolic panel to evaluate for creatinine and a coagulation profile checked.
• All patients should be treated with Lovenox preoperatively. If there is anticipation for stent placement, patients should be placed on Plavix preoperatively as well.

Sign in:
• Patient identity, procedure, and reason for procedure are reviewed.
• Prior to taking the patient back to the operating room, their treatment leg should be marked and examined for the extent of edema as a baseline examination prior to intervention. Any evidence of ulcers or tissue loss needs to be documented.
• If access is planned for multiple sites (i.e. bilateral femoral veins versus politeal and/or internal jugular

approach), those sites should be marked as well. At this time, positioning of the patient (supine or prone) should be reviewed.
• Anesthesia approach: MAC versus general anesthesia reviewed.
• Review of allergies and last dose of anticoagulants (Lovenox, Coumadin, Plavix , ASA).

Time out:
• Introduction of all team members.
• Verbal confirmation of all sites to be accessed.
• Review of all critical equipment: wires, catheters, pharmacomechanical devices (Angiojet EKOS, Trellis etc.), availability of TPA.
• Preoperative imaging reviewed.

Sign out:
• Completion venogram reviewed.
• Correct procedure recorded.
• List of all medication received and last documented ACT level.
• Review that patient will remain immobile for 1 hour postoperatively with gentle pressure over the access site for 1 hour.
• Review of postoperative anticoagulation required in PACU and at time of discharge.

1.6 Pearls and Pitfalls

Pearls:
• Review appropriate imaging prior to procedure to review the veins that are patent and are eligible for cannulation.
• Always visualize and compress the vein under ultrasound visualization to confirm patency and to make sure there is not DVT at the site of entry.
• Always obtain an initial venogram to evaluate for the venous outflow since the outflow can be via a collateral and not to the vena cava.
• During the procedure, obtain venograms in both the AP and LAO positions to fully visualize luminal narrowing from all directions.
• Utilizing IVUS can identify residual luminal narrowing from thrombus, in addition to venography.

Pitfalls:
• When accessing the vein, avoid injuring the artery since that may lead to hematoma formation.
• Watch out for venous collaterals and avoid injuring these collaterals since this can lead to venous injury. Accidentally accessing these collaterals may mislead the surgeon into thinking it is the true venous lumen.
• Do not force wires or catheters if there is resistance as this can cause caval injury.

- Pharmacomechanical lysis of the deep venous system can often cause discomfort to the patient. The anesthesia should be notified as this portion of the procedure is beginning so they are prepared to sedate the patient for comfort.

1.7 Positioning

- Patients can be placed supine or prone depending on the site necessary for access.
- The patient should be placed supine on the operating table with their arms secured at the side of their body if the groin or the neck will be used for venous access.
- The patient should be placed prone if the popliteal vein will be used for venous access.

1.8 Anesthesia

- Most venous thrombectomy cases can be performed under MAC sedation. MAC sedation can be used as long as the patient can comfortably remain immobile for the duration of the case.
- Pharmacomechanical lysis of the venous system can be uncomfortable for the patient. When the surgeon is preparing to start this portion of the case, the anesthesia team should be prepared to administer additional medication.

2 PERIOPERATIVE

2.1 Percutaneous Puncture of the Femoral Vein

Duplex identification of the femoral vein:
- The ipsilateral femoral vein is identified using duplex ultrasound (Fig. 51.6).
- An arterial needle is then used to puncture the femoral vein. Under fluoroscopy, a Bentson or stiff glidewire is then inserted through the arterial needle into the femoral vein, through the iliac vein into the vena cava. The arterial needle is then withdrawn over wire from the patient and passed off the field.
- A 5-Fr short introducer sheath is then placed over wire into the femoral vein for access.
- If the contralateral femoral vein needs to accessed, the above steps can be used to obtain access.

2.2 Diagnostic Venography

- The initial diagnostic venography is performed to confirm sheath placement, visualization of the iliofemoral junction and the visualization of the vena cava.

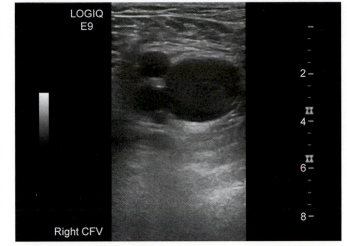

Fig. 51.6: Ultrasound image of the CFV, SFA, and profunda. (CFV: Common femoral vein; SFA: Superficial femoral artery).

- Contrast agent is injected through the side port of the 5-Fr sheath under fluoroscopy. If there is bilateral femoral access, then simultaneous injection through both 5-Fr sheaths can be performed to visualize the bilateral iliofemoral region simultaneously.
- The initial venogram should be of adequate quality to identify either the iliofemoral stenosis, DVT or concomitant collateral veins (Figs. 51.7 and 51.8). If these cannot be adequately identified or there is insufficient visualization of the venous system in general, repeat injection with a larger quantity of contrast may be repeated.
- Once the venous system is visualized, a 5-Fr marker pigtail catheter may be placed over the Bentson wire. This can allow measurement of the length of the iliofemoral region (from the bifurcation of the vena cava to the femoral head) as a preliminary estimate of the length of stents that may be required.

2.3 Intravascular Ultrasound

- If the initial venogram is not diagnostic of the iliofemoral stenosis, IVUS can be used as a diagnostic and confirmatory modality to visualize the area of normal and abnormal vein caliber. As previously mentioned, the IVUS is a catheter based tool with an ultrasound at the tip of the catheter for intraluminal measurement of diameter.
- The IVUS probe and catheter is passed over the Bentson wire into the vena cava. With the IVUS device initiated, a slow withdrawal from the vena cava, pass

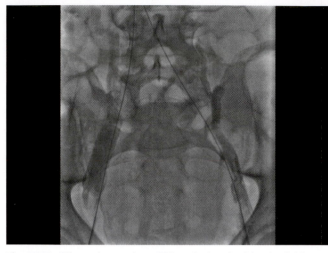

Fig. 51.7: Bilateral complete CIV occlusion (guidewires). Venous outflow of the lower extremities is via collaterals (lateral to the glidewires).

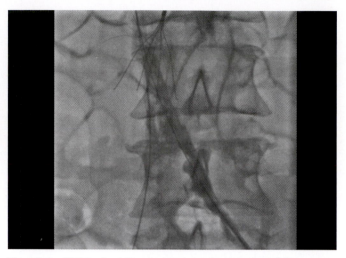

Fig. 51.8: DVT in the LCI vein. Note the irregularity of the venous contour and the luminary filling defect due to thrombus.

the bifurcation into the iliofemoral region. During this passage, it is important to note the distal and proximal parts of the vein that are of normal caliber as these two sites will serve as the proximal and distal landing zones for the stent (Fig. 51.9).

2.4 Angiojet (Possis Medical, Minneapolis, MN)

- If the initial diagnostic venogram and IVUS demonstrated an iliofemoral DVT, pharmacomechanical lysis is recommended prior to placement of an iliofemoral stent.
- With the Bentson wire in the iliocaval venous system, the DVX catheter is passed over the Bentson wire into the vena cava. The Angiojet is primed with TPA per manufacturer's protocol and power pulse mode initially utilized with 6–8 mg of TPA per segment treated.
- The Angiojet can then be reactivated in regular thrombectomy mode after a 15-minute dwell time.
- A completion venogram should be performed to visualized resolution of the DVT.

2.5 Stenting of the Iliofemoral

- If the venography and IVUS studies identify an iliofemoral venous stenosis after treatment of the DVT, a stent can be placed.
- Diameter of stent required will be based primarily on the measurements obtained by IVUS while the length

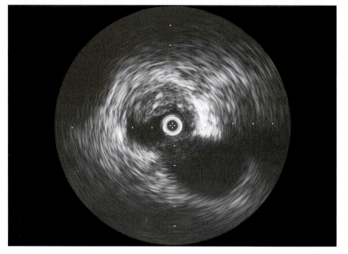

Fig. 51.9: IVUS image of bifurcation of the vena cava. Thrombus present in the RCIV.

of the stent will primarily be based by the length as measured by the pigtail catheter.
- The length of the stent should span the distance from the distal normal caliber vein to the proximal normal caliber vein (Fig. 51.10).
- Two types of stents are used primarily for the iliofemoral region: the self-expending nitinol stent (Protégé, eV3, Plymouth, MN) and the stainless steel stent (Wallstent, Boston Scientific, Watertown, MA). The decision to use either stent is based on the venographic and IVUS findings. Self-expanding stents may be used for veins without significant scarring and contraction, while

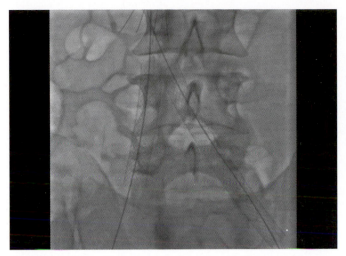

Fig. 51.10: Bilateral iliac stents for chronic CIV occlusion after serial lysis.

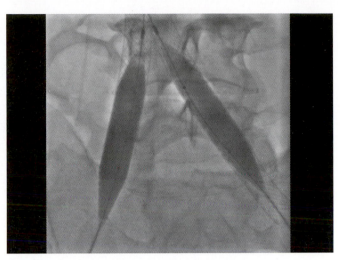

Fig. 51.11: Balloon angioplasty of bilateral CIV.

the stainless steel stents are used for veins with evidence of scarring.
- Once the stent has been appropriately deployed, postdilation of the stents with appropriate balloons are necessary to ensure full expansion of the stent and to prevent migration (Fig. 51.11).

2.6 Completion Venography

- A completion venography should be performed after the iliofemoral stent placement to visualize the expansion of the iliofemoral stenosis and the resolution of associated venous collaterals (Fig. 51.12).
- If there are persistent venous collaterals, it may that the stent is incompletely expanded. Repeat balloon dilatation may be necessary.

2.7 Closure

- The femoral vein short sheath can be pulled and manual pressure held over the venous puncture site.
- Patients will need to remain supine for at least 1 hour.
- Operative management of iliofemoral DVT
- *Exposure of the iliofemoral vein*:
  - A longitudinal inguinal incision is made with complete dissection of the common femoral vein, femoral vein, saphenofemoral junction, and the profunda femoris vein.
- *Infrainguinal femoral thrombectomy*:
  - Usually perform a longitudinal venotomy starting at the level of the saphenofemoral junction.

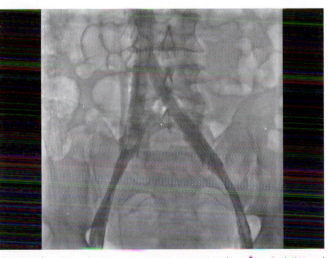

Fig. 51.12: Completion venogram: patent in-line flow in bilateral CIV after angioplasty and stent placement. Note that the previous collateral veins are now diminished.

- Local thrombectomy is performed at the venotomy site. Evaluate and exsanguinate the leg with an esmark and milk clot from below.
- For persistent clot, particularly at the knee, the posterior tibial vein is used as an access site. Steps are usually needed to deal with passing a balloon against the valves:
  - A No. 3 Fogarty balloon catheter is passed from below and brought out at the common femoral vein.
  - A small piece of silastic tubing is used to pull a No. 3 or 4 Fogarty down to the PT vein. Each balloon is inserted into a side of the tubing, and

these are gently inflated to hold the catheters in place as the lower catheter is used to pull the upper catheter down.

- The Fogarty balloon is then passed from below to top until all thrombus is extracted. The catheter is "dragged" back down for repeated passes as described above.
  - Following the infrainguinal balloon-catheter thrombectomy, the infrainguinal venous sheath is then accessed and flushed using copious amounts of heparinized saline.
  - The infrainguinal venous system is then filled with rTPA (4 to 5 mg in 200-cc saline). This is then allowed to dwell for the remainder of the procedure.
  - If the infrainguinal venous thrombectomy fails due to chronic thrombus in the femoral vein, the vein is then ligated below the profunda, and direct thrombectomy is then performed on the profunda vein.
- *Iliac thrombectomy*:
  - A No. 8 or 10 thrombectomy catheter is passed part way into the iliac vein several times to extract as much thrombus as possible before advancement of the catheter into the vena cava.
  - The iliocaval thrombectomy is then performed with fluoroscopic guidance. Positive end-expiratory pressure should be applied to reduce the risk of pulmonary embolus.
  - Completion venography is performed at the end to ensure the quality of flow and that all bulky thrombus has been removed.
- *Arterial venous fistula: This is not always performed, but can assist in the patency of the thrombectomized venous segments*:
  - The venotomy is closed with running monofilament suture or patched if needed secondary to narrowing.
  - The previously ligated proximal saphenous vein is then exposed. The segment of vein is then anastomosed to the side of the superficial femoral artery (anastomosis 3.5–4 mm in diameter).
  - A cuff of PTFE is then wrapped around the saphenous AVF and a 4-0 permanent monofilament suture is looped around the PTFE and clipped. This is buried subcutaneously, and can be used for ligation of the AVF in the future.
  - Common femoral vein pressures should be measured with the AVF open and obstructed. If the pressures increase with AVF flow, then the iliac vein needs should be examined for residual thrombus/obstruction.

- *Closure*:
  - Meticulous control of bleeding and lymphatics is required.
  - A closed suction drain is placed in the wound.
  - The wound is then closed with multilayered running absorbable suture.

3 POSTOPERATIVE

- The patient needs to be anticoagulated on heparin or Lovenox postoperatively. This can be transitioned to Coumadin.
- External pneumatic compression garments should be applied to both legs when the patient is not ambulating. Elastic compression stockings (30–40 mm Hg ankle gradient) are used in all patients to reduce post-thrombotic sequelae.

3.1 Complications

Most common complications:
- Minor bleeding
- Recurrent DVT (Fig. 51.13)
- Ipsilateral edema
- Phlegmasia cerulean dolens
- Delayed wound healing
- Wound hematoma
- Wound infection

Least common complications:
- Rupture of vein during procedure
- Pulmonary embolism

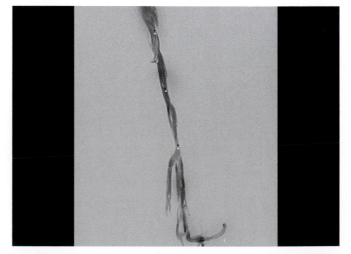

Fig. 51.13: Example of a stenosed vein due to chronic DVT in post-thrombotic syndrome.

- Stroke
- PTS
- Arterial injury

3.2 Outcomes

Endovascular pharmacomechanical thrombectomy:
- Pharmacomechanical venous thrombectomy has a success rate of 70% to 100%.
- Reduces the incidence of PTS.
- Long-term venous patency is reported at 84% in 5 years.
- Valvular competence is preserved at 80% in 5 years and 56% in 10 years.

Surgical thombectomy:
- Surgical thrombectomy may provide long-term iliac venous patency with rates approximately 80% when combined with the creation of an arteriovenous fistula.
- At 5 years, 37% patients were symptom free and 36% had valvular competence.
- PTS was absent or mild in 69% of three level thromboses, 75% of iliofemoral thromboses, and 82% of isolated iliac vein thromboses.

3.3 Follow-Up

- Follow up venous duplex to evaluate for recurrent DVT and venous patency.
- Compliance with anticoagulation (Lovenox transitioning to Coumadin).
- Minimalization of extremity swelling by being compliant with compression stocking and leg elevation.

3.4 E-mail an Expert

- *E-mail address:* drigberg@mednet.ucla.edu

REFERENCES

1. Vedantham S, Grassi CJ, Ferral H, et al. Reporting standards for endovascular treatment of lower extremity deep vein thrombosis. J Vasc Interv Radiol. 2005;17:417-34.
2. Prandoni P, Lensing AW, Prins MH, et al. Below-knee elastic compression stockings to prevent the post-thrombotic syndrome. Ann Intern Med. 2004;141:249-56.
3. Brandjes DP, Buller HR, Heijboer H, et al. Randomized trial of effect of compression stockings in patients with symptomatic proximal-vein thrombosis. Lancet. 1997; 349:759-62.
4. Delis KT, Bountouroglou D, Mansfield AO. Venous claudication in iliofemoral thrombosis: long-term effects on venous hemodynamics, clinical status, and quality of life. Ann Surg. 2004;239:118-26.
5. Kearon C, Ginsberg JS, Hirsh J. The role of venous ultrasonography in the diagnosis of suspected deep venous thrombosis and pulmonary embolism. Ann Intern Med. 1998;129:1044-9.
6. Weinmann EE, Salzman EW. Deep-vein thrombosis. N Engl J Med. 1994;15:1630-41.
7. Zontsich T, Turetschek K, Baldt M. CT-phlebography. A new method for the diagnosis of venous thrombosis of the upper and lower extremities. Radiology. 1998;38:586-90.
8. Burke B, Sostman HD, Carroll BA, et al. The diagnostic approach to deep venous thrombosis. Which technique? Clin Chest Med. 1995;16:253-68.
9. Allie DE, Hebert CJ, Lirtzman MD, et al. Novel simultaneous combination chemical thrombolysis/rheolytic thrombectomy therapy for acute limb ischemia: the power pulse spray technique. Catheter Cardiovasc Interv. 2004; 63:512-22.

QUIZ

Question 1: Current indications for either open or thrombomechanical venous thrombectomy include which of the following:
a. Phlegmasia cerulea alba in a patient with a recent cerebral bleed
b. Isolated soleal vein DVT
c. Phlegmasia cerulea dolens in a patient 4 days postoperative from a thoracotomy
d. 40-year-old woman with May–Thurner syndrome and intermittent leg swelling

Question 2: Access of a tibial vein for open venous thrombectomy is best attained via the:
a. Posterior tibial vein at the ankle
b. Dorsalis pedis vein
c. Anterior tibial vein laterally
d. Posterior tibial vein at the calf level

Question 3: Regarding stents in the iliac veins:
a. Self-expanding stents should not be used because of poor radial force.
b. Balloon expandable stents should not be used because of the risk of arterial compromise.
c. Either stent may be appropriate depending on clinical factors.
d. Unlike in arteries, postdeployment dilatation of venous stents is contraindicated.

Question 4: The gold standard for venous imaging ilio-femoral DVT is:

a. CT venography because it has 100% sensitivity and 96% specificity and can be used in children and pregnant women.

b. Duplex ultrasonography because it is not dependent on the operator and can visualize lesions above the inguinal ligament.

c. Contrast venogram because it allows direct visualization of the iliofemoral vein to the IVC when accessed in a retrograde fashion.

d. MR venography because it is easily obtainable and can be utilized in patients with pacemakers.

Question 5: The initial diagnostic venogram demonstrates a large filling defect in the common iliac vein without in-line contrast flow to the vena cava. Your next step should be:

a. Force a wire through to the filling defect because all thrombus is soft and can be traversed with any wire.

b. Start pharmacomechanical lysis with Angiojet.

c. Repeat contrast venogram in a LAO position to obtain different view point.

d. Abort the procedure as the lesion is completely occlusive and schedule the patient for exploratory laparotomy.

Question 6: Postoperative care and follow-up for patients after a pharmacomechanical thrombectomy include all the following EXCEPT:

a. Use antiplatelet therapy alone

b. Anticoagulation with Lovenox and/or Coumadin

c. Use of external pneumatic compression garments or compression stockings to reduce swelling

d. Obtain an outpatient duplex to evaluate for venous patency

Question 7: Initial assessment of patients being evaluated for venous thrombectomy should investigate the following:

a. Prior history of DVT and/or PE

b. Use of medications including warfarin, heparin, ASA, or Plavix

c. Order a metabolic panel and coagulation laboratories

d. All of the above

ANSWERS:

1. c   2. d   3. b   4. c   5. c   6. a   7. d

Endovenous Therapy for Varicose Veins, RFA, and Laser

Jean Marie Ruddy, Ravi K Veeraswamy

1 PREOPERATIVE

1.1 Indications

- CEAP classes 2 to 6 (Clinical severity, Etiology, Anatomy, Pathophysiology)
  - 2: simple varicose veins only
  - 3: ankle edema of venous origin
  - 4: skin pigmentation
  - 5: healed venous ulcers
  - 6: open venous ulcers
- Greater saphenous vein (GSV) valvular incompetence by duplex
  - Retrograde flow > 0.5 seconds after calf compression
- Endovenous therapy of varicose veins is contraindicated in patients with concurrent deep venous thrombosis (DVT) or absence of other venous outflow.

1.2 Evidence

- When compared to surgical saphenous vein stripping and stab phlebectomy, radio frequency ablation (RFA) and laser ablation are equally effective in obliterating reflux in the treated vein and have similar recurrence rates. Between these two energy modalities, neither demonstrated superiority.
- With either endovenous ablation procedure, wound infection risk is decreased by 70% compared to conventional surgical techniques, pain scores are significantly reduced, and return to normal activities occurs at least 2 days sooner than with surgical stripping.[1–4]

1.3 Materials Needed

- Ultrasound
- 14-gauge vascular access needle
- Guidewire

- Tumescent anesthesia solution
  - 1 L lactated Ringer's solution
  - 500 mg 1% lidocaine
  - 1 mg epinephrine
  - 12.5 mEq sodium bicarbonate
- Treatment catheter [Figs. 52.1A (RFA) or B (laser probe)]
- ACE bandage or compression stockings

1.4 Preoperative Risk Assessment

Endovenous varicose vein therapy may be safely performed on patients who can:

- Tolerate local anesthetic
- Lay flat for a sustained period of time
- Wear compression hose in the postoperative period

1.5 Perioperative Checklist

Sign in:
- Mark side of planned procedure
- Confirm informed consent

Time out:
- Patient identity
- Correct side
- Correct procedure
- Patient allergies

Sign out:
- Debrief regarding equipment problems
- Home instruction packet for patient

1.6 Decision-Making Checklist

- *Patient presents with Clinical severity, Etiology, Anatomy, Pathophysiology (CEAP) class 2–6 lower extremity superficial venous insufficiency*:
  - Conservative management with compression and leg elevation

- Wound care as needed for ulceration
- Antibiotics for acute infections
- Patient perception of continued discomfort and lifestyle limitations
- Nonhealing ulcers with documented reflux or perforator vein underlying the ulcer
  - Proceed with endovenous varicose vein therapy

1.7 Pearls and Pitfalls

Pearls:
- Use of tumescent anesthetic to minimize the risk of thermal injury
- Initiate venous ablation 2–3 cm proximal to saphenofemoral junction to avoid deep extension of superficial thrombosis

Pitfalls:
- Patient compliance with postintervention compression
- Operator knowledge of specific technology and ablation system

1.8 Surgical Anatomy

- *See* Figures 52.2A and B.

1.9 Positioning

- *See* Figure 52.3.

1.10 Anesthesia

- Continuous pulse oximetry, heart rate monitoring, and blood pressure monitoring
- Oral anxiolytic 1 hour prior to procedure, potential intravenous redose depending on patient comfort

- Local anesthetic at venous access site
- Tumescent anesthetic injected along GSV treatment zone

2 PERIOPERATIVE

2.1 Incision

- *See* Figures 52.4A and B.

2.2 Steps

- *See* Figures 52.5A to E.

2.3 Closure

- *See* Figure 52.6.

3 POSTOPERATIVE

3.1 Complications

Common complications:
- DVT
- Endovenous heat-induced thrombosis (EHIT)
- Phlebitis
- Saphenous nerve injury
- Epidermal thermal injury
- Hyperpigmentation[5]

3.2 Outcomes

Expected outcomes:
- With current technology, RFA and laser ablation are nearly 100% effective in accomplishing venous obliteration at the time of the index procedure.

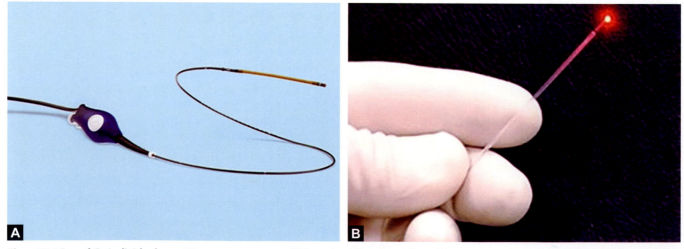

Figs. 52.1A and B: Individual practitioners may use an RFA probe (A) or laser fiber (B).

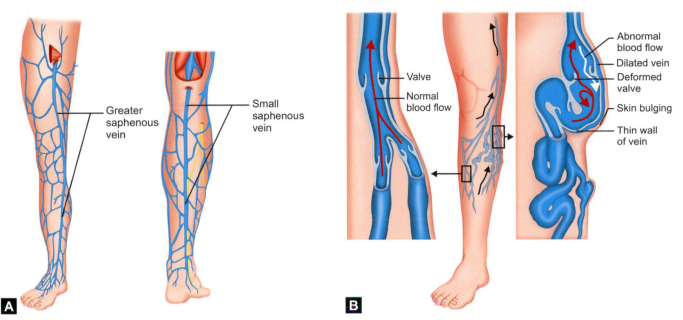

Figs. 52.2A and B: (A) The greater saphenous vein runs superficially along the medial aspect of the leg from the medial malleolus to the groin where it goes deeper to join the femoral vein. The small saphenous vein is in the subcutaneous adipose tissue of the posterior lower leg and goes deep to join the popliteal vein. (B) When vein valves become incompetent, the reversed, stagnant flow causes dilation and remodeling of superficial veins to form thin-walled varicosities that bulge through the skin.

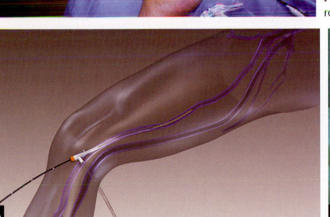

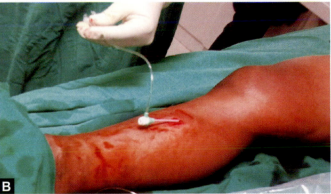

Fig. 52.3: The patient should be positioned with the leg externally rotated and prepped from the toes to groin.

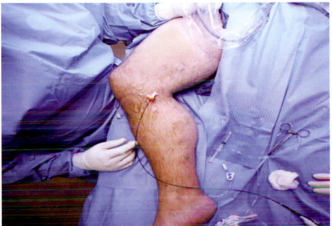

Figs. 52.4A and B: The saphenous vein may be percutaneously accessed at (A) or below (B) the knee with subsequent insertion of a short sheath and the treatment probe.

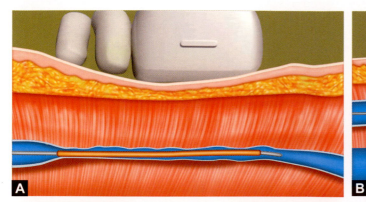

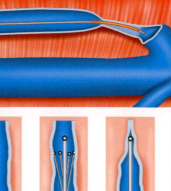

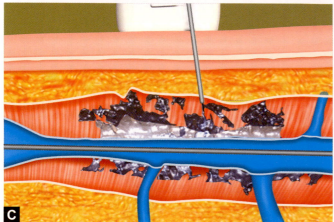

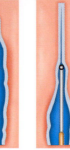

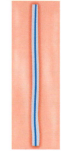

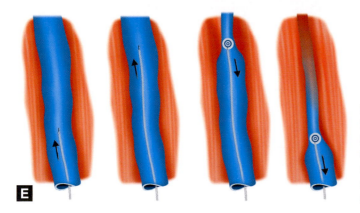

Catheter inserted in refluxing vein	Catheter positioned, electrodes deployed	RF energy heats and contracts vein wall	Catheter slowly withdrawn, closing vein	Denuded vein is physically narrowed

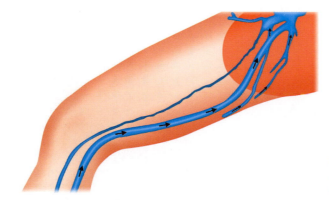

Figs. 52.5A to E: After percutaneous venous access, the probe is advanced under ultrasound guidance (A) until situated approximately 2 cm from the saphenofemoral junction (B). (C) Tumescent anesthesia is then injected along the length of the greater saphenous vein treatment area. (D) The RFA probe is then slowly retracted at 0.5–1 cm/s. (E) The laser probe is then slowly retracted at a speed dictated by the laser intensity.

Fig. 52.6: At procedure completion, the greater saphenous vein is sclerosed and lacks flow. Pressure is held after sheath removal for hemostasis.

- When evaluated 2–3 years postprocedure, as many as 15% of patients treated with endovenous ablation may have recurrent varicosities, a value which is not significantly different than the 20% observed after surgical vein stripping.
- At long-term follow-up, the Venous Clinical Severity Score (VCSS) and quality-of-life survey measurements are no different between endovenous ablation and surgical therapy, emphasizing that the advantage of these minimally invasive techniques is demonstrated in the immediate postprocedure period with lower pain scores, fewer complications, and faster return to activity.[6,7]

3.3 Follow-Up

- Duplex ultrasound at one week to look for DVT
- Duplex ultrasound at 1 month
- Clinic visits as needed for recurrence

3.4 E-mail an Expert

- *E-mail address*: rveeras@emory.edu and j.m.ruddy@emory.edu

3.5 Web Resources/References

- http://www.nwgavein.com/Varicose-Veins
- http://www.venacure-evlt.com/Laser-Vein
- http://www.radiologyinfo.org/en/info.cfm?pg=varicoseabl
- http://www.cooltouch.com/ctev.aspx
- http://www.angiodynamics.com/products/venacure-evlt

REFERENCES

1. Siribumrungwong B, Noorit P, Wilasrusmee C, et al. Systematic review and meta-analysis of randomised controlled trials comparing endovenous ablation and surgical intervention in patients with varicose veins. Eur J Vasc Endovasc Surg. 2012;44:214-23.
2. Almeida JI, Kaufman J, Gockeritz O, et al. Radiofrequency endovenous Closure FAST versus laser ablation for the treatment of great saphenous reflux: a multicenter, single blinded, randomized study (RECOVERY study). J Vasc Interv Radiol. 2009;20:752e9.
3. García-Madrid C, Pastor Manrique JO, Gómez-Blasco F, et al. Update on endovenous radio-frequency closure ablation of varicose veins. Ann Vasc Surg. 2012;26:281-91.
4. Lohr J, Kulwicki A. Radiofrequency ablation: evolution of a treatment. Semin Vasc Surg. 2010;23:90-100.
5. Harlander-Locke M, Jimenez JC, Lawrence PF, et al. Management of endovenous heat-induced thrombus using a classification system and treatment algorithm following segmental thermal ablation of the small saphenous vein. J Vasc Surg. 2013;58(2):427-32.
6. Lurie F, Creton D, Eklof B, et al. Prospective randomised study of endovenous radiofrequency obliteration (closure) versus ligation and vein stripping (EVOLVeS): two-year follow-up. Eur J Vasc Endovasc Surg. 2005;29:67-73.
7. Perälä J, Rauto T, Biancari F, et al. Radiofrequency endovenous obliteration versus stripping of the long saphenous vein in the management of primary varicose veins: 3-year outcome of a randomized study. Ann Vasc Surg. 2005;19:669-72.

QUIZ

Question 1. Endovenous therapy of varicose veins is contraindicated in patient with:
a. Venous ulcers
b. Lifestyle limiting varicose veins
c. Deep venous thrombosis
d. Arterial insufficiency

Question 2. Utilization of tumescent anesthesia decreases the risk of:
a. Superficial thrombophlebitis
b. Wound infection
c. Procedure failure
d. Thermal injury

Question 3. Following endovenous ablation, complications include all of the following except:
a. Pneumonia
b. DVT
c. Superficial thrombophlebitis
d. Saphenous nerve injury

Question 4. What percentage of patients have successful venous obliteration at the conclusion of their primary endovenous ablation procedure?
a. 50%
b. 30%
c. 75%
d. 100%

Question 5. The primary imaging modality utilized in follow-up for venous ablation procedures is:
a. Computed tomography
b. Duplex ultrasound
c. Magnetic resonance venography
d. X-rays

ANSWERS: 1. c 2. d 3. a 4. d 5. e

53

Deep Femoral Vein Harvest for Arterial Reconstruction

Michael M McNally, Adam W Beck

1 PREOPERATIVE

1.1 Indications

- Autogenous aortoiliac/femoral reconstruction
- Autogenous arteriovenous fistula creation
- Central venous bypass

1.2 Evidence

- There are no randomized control trials or systematic reviews on deep femoral vein harvest. Multiple institutional experiences for various uses of deep femoral vein can be cited from the literature. Listed below are important selected articles regarding first descriptions, including technique, of deep femoral vein use for various indications.[1-4]

1.3 Materials Needed

- *See* Figures 53.1A and B.

1.4 Preoperative Risk Assessment

Low risk:
- Thin patient with no venous insufficiency

Intermediate risk:
- Obese patient
- History of deep vein thrombosis (DVT) or chronic venous insufficiency
- History of phlebitis.

High risk:
- *Cardiac*: unstable angina, myocardial infarction (MI) within 6 months, decompensated congestive heart failure (CHF), significant arrhythmia, critical aortic stenosis
- *Pulmonary*: severe chronic obstructive pulmonary disease (COPD), FEV1 <60%, $Pa\text{CO}_2$ >45 mm Hg

- *Renal*: ESRD on dialysis
- Morbid obesity, body mass index (BMI) $\geq$ 30

1.5 Preoperative Checklist

Sign in:
- Patient identification confirmation
- Patient identifies site of operation and planned procedure
- Patient allergies

Time out:
- Surgeon and anesthesiologist confirm patient name and planned procedure
- Anticipated surgery critical events
- Antibiotics
- Imaging

Sign out:
- Instrument, sponge, and needle count
- Key concerns for patient recovery discussed by anesthesia, nursing, and surgeon.

1.6 Decision-Making Algorithm

See Flowchart 53.1.

Preoperative lower extremity duplex ultrasonography:
- *Assessment*:
  - Vein size (>5 mm)
  - Vein patency
- *Contraindications*:
  - Vein scarring and recanalization after prior thrombosis
  - Vein duplication (if individual duplicated veins are <5 mm)
  - Congenital vein hypoplasia

1.7 Pearls and Pitfalls

Pearls:
- During vein harvest, preserve the major branches of the superficial femoral and popliteal arteries that serve as important collateral arterial pathways.

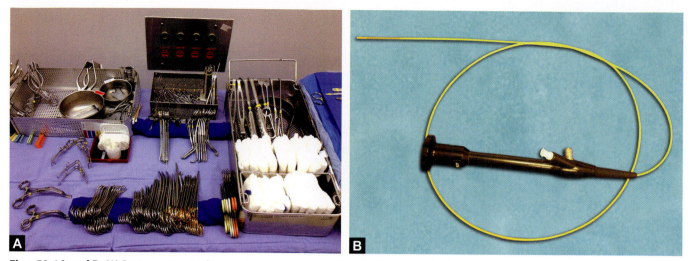

Figs. 53.1A and B: (A) Basic open vascular tray. Vascular tray should include scalpel, Bovie cautery, Metzenbaum scissors, 2-0 silk suture ligature, 3-0 silk, 4-0 Monocryl suture, 5-0 and 6-0 Prolene suture. (B) Femoral vein is typically everted for complete valve excision, but angioscopy can be used to confirm complete valve lysis if the surgeon elects not to evert the vein when lysing the valves.

Flowchart 53.1: Decision-making algorithm.

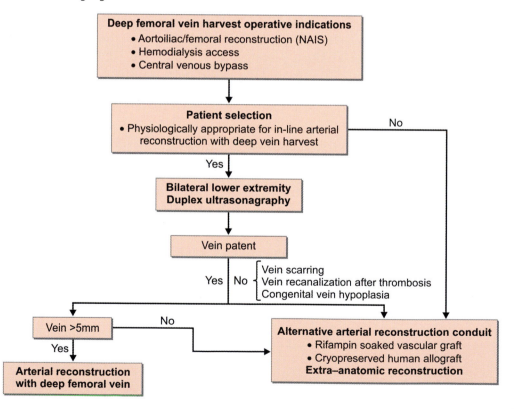

- Identify and preserve the saphenous nerve, which runs parallel to the femoral vein in the mid-thigh.
- Secure ligation (i.e. double ligation or [preferred] suture ligation of large branches) is crucial to prevent hemorrhage.

- Oversew the femoral vein remnant at the common femoral vein such that there is no stump, but also preserve unimpeded venous outflow from the profunda femoris vein.

- Evert the vein (usually on the inner cannula of a pool sucker) and completely excise the vein valves to prevent postoperative stenosis. Alternatively, retrograde passage of a valvulotome with angioscopy can be performed for valve lysis. Valve excision allows for a nonreversed (transposed) configuration that allows an anastomosis of the larger diameter proximal vein to a larger vessel (i.e. terminal aorta or central vein).

Pitfall:

- Previous ipsilateral saphenous vein harvest is not an absolute contraindication to femoral vein harvest, but increases the risk of compartment syndrome and need for fasciotomy.

1.8 Surgical Anatomy

- *See* Figures 53.2A and B.

1.9 Positioning

- *See* Figure 53.3.

1.10 Anesthesia

- General anesthesia

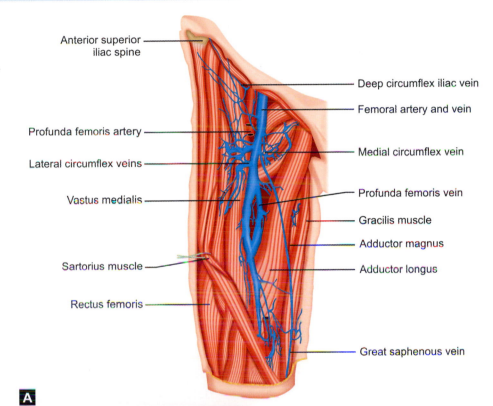

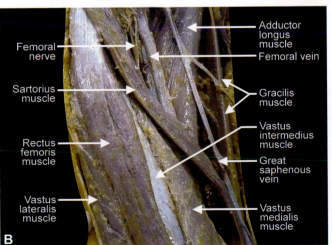

Figs. 53.2A and B: (A) Femoral vein anatomy. The femoral vein lies medial to the femoral artery and courses beneath the sartorius muscle (retracted medially). The great saphenous vein originates from the proximal femoral vein and runs medially in the thigh. The anterior superior iliac spine and insertion of the sartorius muscle at the knee level serve as landmarks for exposing the femoral vein. An incision along this line will prevent creation of a flap while removing the femoral vein. (B) Femoral vein anatomy (cadaver). Only the proximal one third of the femoral vein is exposed without dissection and medial retraction of the sartorius muscle.

2 PERIOPERATIVE

2.1 Incision

- *See* Figure 53.4.

2.2 Steps

- *See* Figures 53.5A to C.

2.3 Closure

- *See* Figure 53.6.

3 POSTOPERATIVE

3.1 Complications

Most common complications:
- Venous hypertension
- Compartment syndrome (more common when saphenous vein previously harvested)
- Hematoma
- Wound infection

Least common complications:
- Venous thromboembolism
- Saphenous neuralgia

3.2 Outcomes

Expected outcomes:
- *Venous morbidity*:
  - *Short term*:
    - Increase in leg circumference with mild edema
    - 11% patients of 61 study patients with reflux in popliteal or tibial veins at 37-month follow-up. Less than one third had edema without skin changes (C3). No patients with major chronic venous changes (C4–C6).[5]
  - *Long term*:
    - *Case-control study 16 patients with 70-month follow-up*: 85% without significant venous insufficiency, 15% major chronic venous morbidity (C3–C6).[6]

3.3 Follow-Up

- Operative dressings and ACE wrap taken down postoperative day 1.
- Continue ACE wrap for compression therapy to alleviate symptomatic lower extremity edema.
- Once mobile, provide thigh high mild to moderate compression hose, depending on symptoms.
- Surgical follow-up visit in 2 weeks to inspect surgical sites.

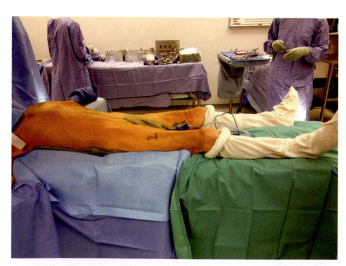

Fig. 53.3: Supine position. Place patient in the supine position with arms alongside torso or abducted on arm boards and the lower extremities prepped circumferentially to the toes. The torso is prepped as appropriate for any suprainguinal arterial reconstruction. The leg can be supine during the initial dissection, but can be externally rotated with knee flexed at 30° to facilitate exposure of the more distal popliteal vein near the knee.

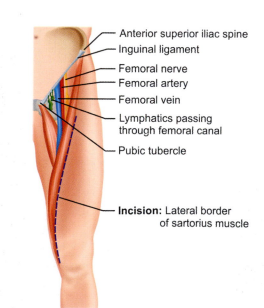

Fig. 53.4: Incision. Landmarks of the anterior superior iliac spine and the medial knee identify the lateral border of the sartorius muscle, highlighted here by the dotted blue line. The lateral incision is required in order to avoid removing the segmental blood supply to the sartorius muscle, and to prevent creation of a thin flap.

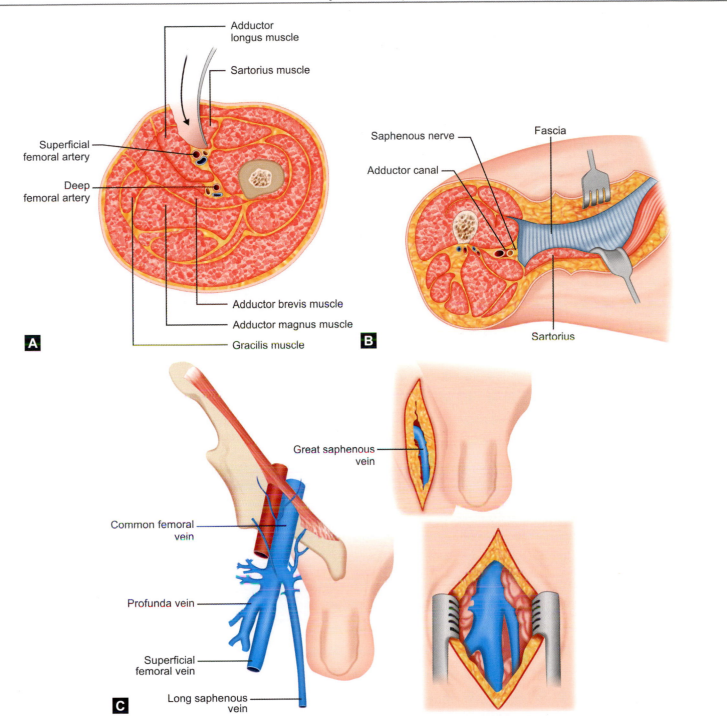

Figs. 53.5A to C: (A) Approach and dissection plane to expose the femoral vein in the right leg. Dissection is carried down between the sartorius muscle and adductor longus muscle. (B) Exposure of the femoral vein and adductor canal. The incision and dissection is carried through the fascia lata. The sartorius muscle is retracted medially to expose the roof of the adductor canal. After the fascia is divided, sharp dissection is used to separate the femoral artery and vein throughout their course in the thigh. Secure ligation of multiple large braches of the femoral vein is crucial to avoid bleeding complications when the vein is placed in the arterial circulation and pressurized. Additionally, the saphenous nerve should be identified and preserved to prevent saphenous neuralgia. (C) Proximal femoral vein transection. The proximal femoral vein should be mobilized and clamped at the level of the confluence with the common femoral vein. The femoral vein should be transected and oversewn flush with the profunda femoris vein in order to prevent a stump that could serve as a potential nidus for deep venous thrombosis and pulmonary embolus. The distal femoral vein can be mobilized to the length appropriate for the arterial reconstruction, and can include harvest of the proximal above the knee popliteal vein. At this point, perform vein eversion with complete valve excision.

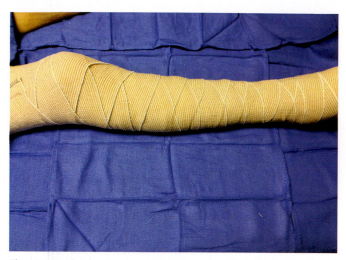

Fig. 53.6: Thigh closure and ACE wrap. The fascia is closed over closed suction drains (2 when the entire femoral vein is harvested) with a running 2-0 Vicryl suture. A deep dermal closure is completed with interrupted 3-0 Vicryl sutures. The skin is closed with 4-0 Monocryl suture and Dermabond. The lower extremity is ACE wrapped from toes to proximal thigh.

3.4 E-mail an Expert

- *E-mail address*: adam.beck@surgery.ufl.edu

SUGGESTED READINGS

Smith ST, Clagett GP. Femoral vein harvest for vascular reconstructions: pitfalls and tips for success. Semin Vasc Surg. 2008;21(1):35-40.

Valentine RJ, Wind GG. Vessels of the thigh (Chapter 16). In: Anatomic Exposures in Vascular Surgery, 2nd edition. Philadelphia: Lippincott Williams & Wilkins; 2003.

REFERENCES

1. Clagett GP, Bowers BL, Lopez-Viego MA, et al. Creation of a neoaortoiliac system from lower extremity deep and superficial veins. Ann Surg. 1993;218:239-49.
2. Clagett GP. Replacement of infected aortic prostheses with lower extremity deep veins. In: Yao JST, Pearce WH (Eds). Arterial Surgery: Management of Challenging Problems. Stamford, CT: Appleton & Lange; 1996. pp. 257-64.
3. Huber TS, Ozaki CK, Flynn TC, et al. Use of superficial femoral vein for hemodialysis arteriovenous access. J Vasc Surg. 2000;31:1038-41.
4. Hagino RT, Bengtson TD, Fosdick DA, et al. Venous reconstructions using the superficial femoral-popliteal vein. J Vasc Surg. 1997;26:829-37.
5. Timaran CH, et al. Late incidence of chronic venous insufficiency after deep vein harvest. J Vasc Surg. 2007 Sep; 46(3): 520-5; discussion 525.
6. Modrall JG, Sadjadi J, Ali AT, et al. Deep vein harvest: predicting need for fasciotomy. J Vasc Surg. 2004;39:387-94.

QUIZ

Question 1. Which one of the following is a contraindication to deep vein harvest?
a. 44-year-old female with history atrial fibrillation on anticoagulation
b. 65-year-old male with a history of bilateral lower extremity iliac, femoral, and popliteal vein DVTs from an MVC 15 years ago
c. 52-year-old male in need of NAIS for aortic reconstruction preoperative duplex ultrasound showing 6-mm femoral vein
d. 58-year-old male with history of obesity (BMI 32), COPD, chronic kidney disease (GFR 25) with preoperative duplex ultrasound showing femoral vein 5.5 mm

Question 2. Which one of the following is NOT true?
a. It is important to oversew flush the junction of the femoral vein with the common femoral vein to allow unimpeded venous outflow from the profunda femoris vein.
b. Using a valvulotome with angioscopy or alternatively eversion of the vein graft with direct vein excision are two methods to prevent rare incidences of vein graft stenosis from retained valves
c. An incision medial to the sartorius muscle allows exposure to the deep femoral vein
d. The segmental blood supply to sartorius muscle enters on the inferior-medial muscle edge

Question 3. Which one of the following is not a common complication of deep femoral vein harvest?
a. Surgical site wound infection
b. Mild lower extremity edema without skin changes
c. Hyperpigmentation of lower extremity with active venous ulcer
d. Lower extremity compartment syndrome

ANSWERS:

1. a   2. d   3. c   4. a

Central Venous Port Placement

Alexis Powell

1 PREOPERATIVE

1.1 Indications

- Long-term intermittent venous access needs in patient with poor overall venous status
- Chemotherapy
- Frequent transfusions or blood draws
- Plasmapheresis
- Total parenteral nutrition (TPN)

1.2 Contraindications

- Systemic infection
- Severe, uncorrectable coagulopathy
- Inability to cannulate target vein (thrombosed, stenotic, completely occluded).

1.3 Evidence

- Port devices are associated with a lower risk of complications (specifically infection and thrombosis) without an increase in overall cost compared to peripherally inserted central venous catheters (PICC lines).[1-2]

1.4 Materials Needed

- General surgery all-purpose kit (needle driver, hemostat, scissors, forceps, scalpel)
- Nonabsorbable suture for port securement
- Bovie cautery
- Concentrated heparinized saline flush (1,000 U/mL)
- Commercially available mediport placement kit containing access needle, guidewire, dilator, subcutaneous tunneling device, catheter, and access port device (Fig. 54.1)
- Fluoroscopy equipment (optional) (Fig. 54.2)
- Portable ultrasound (optional) (Fig. 54.3)

1.5 Preoperative Risk Assessment

Low risk:
- In general, this is a very low risk procedure.

High risk:
- Patients with severe cardiopulmonary disease preventing ability to lie in Trendelenburg position.

1.6 Preoperative Checklist

Preoperative orders: NPO after midnight, hibiclens shower, IV hydration if needed:
- *Intraoperatively*: Timeout (correct patient, position, procedure), preoperative antibiotic dose (Ancef 1 g IV), proper skin preparation (alcohol/Betadine based prep, Ioban dressing)

1.7 Pearls and Pitfalls

Pearls:
- Use of ultrasound guidance promotes easy vein access and lessens chance of injury to nearby structures (i.e. arterial cannulation).
- Always advance the dilator under live fluoroscopy.
- Maintain control over wire at all times (never let go of the guide wire).
- Ideally, catheter tip should lie at atrial–caval junction or just below it.
- Check final catheter position under fluoroscopy to ensure no catheter kinks (typically at the junction of clavicle and first rib).

Pitfalls:
- Preoperative evaluation with physical exam and ultrasound will avoid intra-operative complications with thrombosed veins.
- Trim catheter to patient-specific length (avoid too long, too short tip placement).
- Make sure port is easily palpable under skin for easy access.

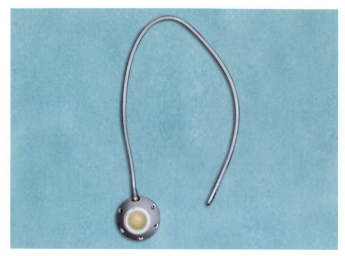

Fig. 54.1: Port catheter kit.

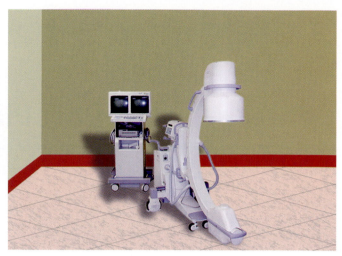

Fig. 54.2: Fluoroscopy equipment.

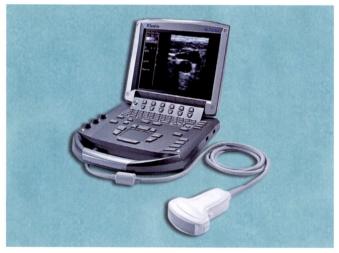

Fig. 54.3: Portable ultrasound.

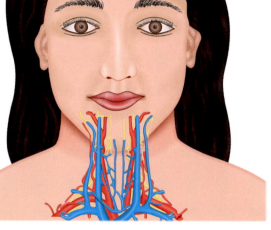

Fig. 54.4: Venous anatomy of the neck and infraclavicular region.

- Ensure port is secured to pectoralis major fascia to avoid post placement migration/flipping of port.

1.8 Surgical Anatomy

- *See* Figure 54.4.

1.9 Positioning

- *See* Figure 54.5.

1.10 Anesthesia

- Local anesthesia (Lidocaine/Marcaine) ± MAC anesthesia (monitored anesthesia care)

2 PERIOPERATIVE

2.1 Internal Jugular Vein Placement

- Place patient in 15° Trendelenburg position, surgically prep out neck and chest (superior: angle of mandible, inferiorly: nipple, medially: sternal notch, laterally, shoulder).
- Identify the sternocleidomastoid (SCM) triangle landmarks (two heads of SCM, clavicle).
- Anesthetize skin (neck and subcutaneous pocket area 1–2 cm below clavicle).
- Use handheld ultrasound to identify internal jugular (IJ), and access with 18-gauge introducer needle under ultrasound guidance (Fig. 54.6).

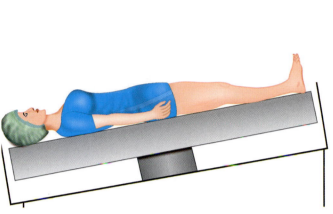

Fig. 54.5: Patient should be placed supine, in slight Trendelenburg, with neck turned toward the contralateral side.

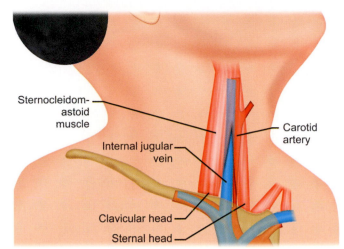

Fig. 54.6: Vein access.

Sternocleidom-
astoid
muscle

Carotid
artery

Internal jugular
vein

Clavicular head

Sternal head

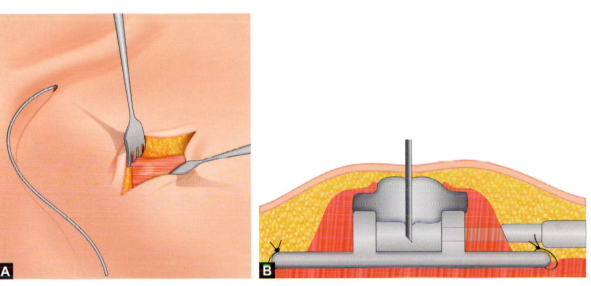

Figs. 54.7A and B: Create a subcutaneous "pocket" for port.

- Pass the guidewire and remove needle. Check wire position [superior vena cava (SVC)] with fluoroscopy.
- Nick the skin at wire entry site with No. 11 blade (Figs. 54.7A and B).
- Incise skin 1–2 cm below clavicle approximately 4–6 cm in length.
- Use electrocautery to dissect to level of pectorals major fascia and create subcutaneous pocket with combination of blunt dissection and cautery.
- Place port in pocket and secure in place with nonabsorbable suture (3-0 Prolene) (Figs. 54.8A and B).
- Utilize port dilator to create subcutaneous tunnel between pocket and guidewire site.

- Bring catheter through subcutaneous tunnel and trim to patient length. This can be done by marking the atrial–caval junction under fluoroscopy with a hemostat and appropriate trimming of catheter.
- Advance the vessel dilator and sheath introducer together over the wire (using gentle rotational motion) under live fluoroscopy, leaving 1–2 cm of sheath exposed.
- Release the locking mechanism if present, and remove the vessel dilator and wire, leaving the sheath in place. Put thumb over exposed opening of sheath to minimize blood loss and prevent air embolism.
- Insert catheter into the sheath and advance to full length (Fig. 54.9).

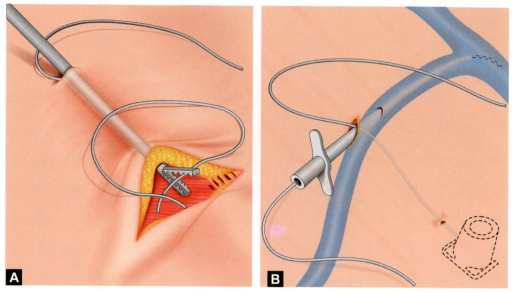

Figs. 54.8A and B: Port placement.

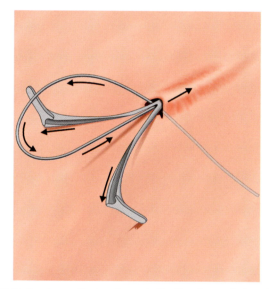

Fig. 54.9: Passing catheter through the "peel-away" sheath.

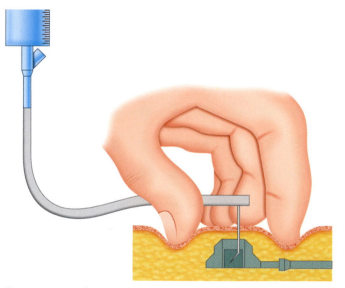

Fig. 54.10: Verify easy access of port with Huber needle (draws back blood, flushes easily) and "lock" port with concentrated heparin solution (1,000 U/mL).

- Grasp the peel-away sheath handles and pull outward and upward, with care to hold catheter in place during sheath removal.
- Verify catheter tip position using fluoroscopy.
- After appropriate hemostasis, irrigate port pocket and close in multiple layers. Puncture skin can be closed with single monofilament suture or glue (Figs. 54.10 and 54.11).
- Check postprocedure chest X-ray to ensure lung inflation (Fig. 54.12).

- Access the subclavian vein with 18-gauge introducer needle aiming toward the sternal notch at the junction of the medial and middle third of the clavicle.
- Pass the guidewire and remove needle. Check wire position SVC with fluoroscopy.
- Follow the steps for placement of IJ mediport.

Note that mediport placement kits vary in port-catheter connection site, one may prefer to trim catheter to appropriate length and attach to port site post placement (Figs. 54.13A and B).

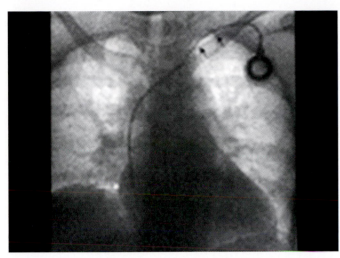

Fig. 54.11: Spot fluoroscopy to verify tip position, and ensure no kinking of catheter.

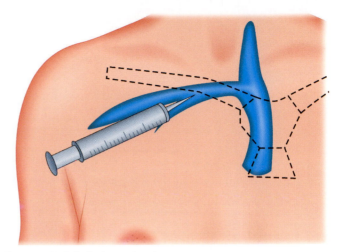

Fig. 54.12: Subclavian vein placement.

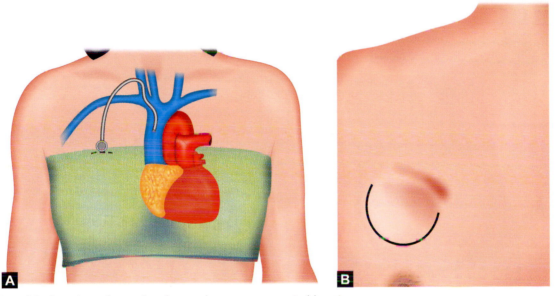

Figs. 54.13A and B: Overview of completed port placement anatomical location.

3 POSTOPERATIVE

3.1 Complications

Most common complications:
- Infection (port pocket or catheter related systemic infection)
- Pneumothorax
- Arterial injury (puncture, cannulation)
- Venous thrombosis

Least common complications:
- Venous air embolus
- Port migration
- Cardiac arrhythmias
- Cardiac perforation with cardiac tamponade

3.2 Outcomes

- Patient may have postoperative tenderness at area of port pocket immediately postprocedure.
- Incision should heal within 10–14 days of procedure.
- Port may be accessed immediately with proper technique.

3.3 Follow-Up

- Immediate postprocedure upright chest X-ray to evaluate catheter tip position and lung inflation.
- Port may be accessed immediately.
- Heparin flush (100 unit/mL) after each use or monthly during periods of inactivity.
- Difficulty with access should prompt chest X-ray to evaluate position, venogram if occlusion or malpositioned port is suspected.
- Follow up with surgeon for port removal once no longer in use or patient wishes removal of port.

3.4 E-mail an Expert

- *E-mail address*: apowell@health.usf.edu

REFERENCES

1. Groeger JS, Lucase AB, Thaler HT, et al. Infectious morbidity associated with long-term use of venous access devices in patients with cancer. Ann Intern Med. 1993;119:1168-74.
2. Patel GS, Jain K, Kumar R, et al. Comparison of peripherally inserted central venous catheters (PICC) versus subcutaneously implanted port-chamber catheters by complications and cost for patients receiving chemotherapy for non-haematological malignancies. Department of Medical Oncology, Flinders Centre for Innovation in Cancer, Flinders Medical Centre/Flinders University, Bedford Park, SA, 5042, Australia. Epub. Support Care Center, September 2013.
3. Wheeless CR, Roenneburg ML. Subclavian Port-A-Cath. Atlas of Pelvic Surgery, online edition. (2013). Access from www.atlasofpelvicsurgery.com/10MalignantDisease/2SubclavianPort-A-Cath/cha10sec2.html. [Accessed August 28, 2014].

QUIZ

Question 1. Postprocedure chest X-ray is useful for determining:
a. Catheter tip position
b. Presence of pneumothorax
c. Absence of catheter kinking
d. All of the above

Question 2. Proper catheter tip location for mediport placement is at:
a. Junction of SVC and right atrium
b. Junction of IJ and subclavian vein
c. Right ventricle
d. Inferior vena cava (IVC)

Question 3. Ultrasound evaluation and periprocedural use can be used:
a. To avoid accidental arterial cannulation
b. To determine vein patency and absence of thrombus
c. To facilitate first-stick venous cannulation
d. All of the above

ANSWERS:
1. d   2. a   3. d

Index

Note: Page number followed by *f* and *fc* indicates figures and flowcharts, respectively.